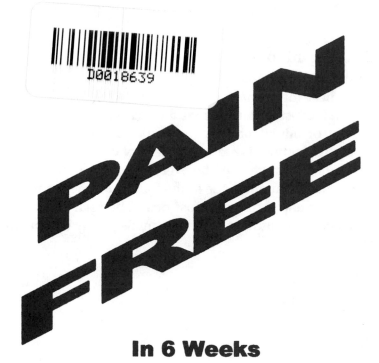

# PAIN FREE

## In 6 Weeks

**How to find the causes and cures for your pain, regardless of its label, including chronic back pain, chronic knee pain, arthritis, fibromyalgia, damaged discs, sciatica, tendonitis, bursitis, and neuralgia. Also included are cystitis, prostatitis, colitis, lupus, endometriosis, Raynaud's, Gulf War Syndrome, angina, and even end-stage cancer.**

## SHERRY A. ROGERS, M.D.

### 2001

**Sand Key Company Inc.**
**PO Box 40101**
**Sarasota, FL 34242**
**www.prestigepublishing.com**

*Pain Free* In 6 Weeks

Sherry A. Rogers, M.D.

Copyright © 2001

All rights reserved, including the right to reproduce this book or portions thereof in any form whatsoever.

Sand Key Company, Inc.
PO Box 40101
Sarasota, FL 34242

1-800-846-6687
www.prestigepublishing.com

Library of Congress Card Catalog Number:

ISBN: 1-887202-03-X
Printed in the United States of America

## Dedication

I am constantly surrounded by God's miracles, and His unfathomable ways. But by far His greatest gift to me has always been my precious Luscious, who grows more luscious every day! As the enormously talented Barbra Streisand says in her album, *A Love Like Ours* (1999 Sony Music Entertainment Inc., Columbia Records, NY),

"Just one lifetime won't be enough time for us, we need more for all this love."

# Foreword

Prisoner of pain, queen of drugs. Just when I had exhausted every specialist, every medication and thought there was no way out, I discovered a whole world of control that is within the grasp of everyone.

Pain is pervasive. Just look at the drug and grocery store shelves lined with painkillers. It would be an unusual bathroom cabinet or gym bag that did not contain a few drugs for pain as well.

And pain knows no boundaries, attacking every system. Do you have chronic back pain, knee or shoulder pain, or the total body pain of fibromyalgia? Or is it the devastating migratory pain of rheumatoid arthritis or the nagging pain of osteoarthritis, degenerative arthritis or that of an old injury? Have you been told you have to learn to live with it or that you are getting older? Funny, the other joints are just as old, yet they don't hurt.

The pain of migraine, angina, tic doloreux, TMJ, colitis, endometriosis, PMS, Gulf War Syndrome, diabetic neuropathy, cystitis or prostatitis all share one thing: there is no recognized cure. But buck up, for there is nothing further from the truth. In fact you can even learn how to turn off the morphine-resistant pain of metastatic, end-stage cancer within hours.

If you want complete control over pain so that you never have to suffer again, read on.

# Introduction

## The Pain Epidemic

There is no question – we are people in pain! Over fifty million Americans suffer from some form of connective tissue (bone, cartilaginous joints, discs, muscle, tendon or ligament) disease.

The labels given to these "incurable" pain syndromes include osteoarthritis, rheumatoid arthritis, fibromyalgia, and chronic degenerating back discs. Not limited to these, there is gout, ankylosing spondylitis, psoriatic arthritis, lupus arthritis, polymyalgia rheumatica, Sjogren's syndrome, carpal tunnel syndrome, Crohn's arthritis, and much more.

The rheumatic or painful joint and other connective tissue diseases (muscle, tendon, ligament, fascia) are rarely cured, but merely "managed" with countless drugs. Many of these drugs, methotrexate as an example, can go on to cause cancer. Over 65 billion dollars is spent each year for no cure, merely management complete with not only high cost, but many side effects and ineffective pain relief.

The ironic twist is that total wellness is available to the vast majority of these suffers. And most of the treatments are non-prescription, non-toxic, and available to everyone. So let's see what pain cures apply to you.

# Table of Contents

i

# Chapter 1

## What is Your Pain Trying to Tell You?

### Plain and Simple, Drugs Destroy

When you have pain, do you "Reach for Aleve"? This and its over-the-counter cousins like Motrin (ibuprofen), Advil, Naproxyn, Orudis and prescription drugs like Indocin, Tolectin, Lodine, Feldene, Clinoril, Anaprox, Toradol, Nalfon, Voltaren, Celebrex, and Vioxx fall into a category of drugs called NSAIDs (non-steroidal anti-inflammatory drugs) with some of the most dangerous side effects known.

Since side effects of drugs constitute the 3rd cause of death in the U.S., it should come as no surprise that over 6000 people die from NSAIDs a year. Why don't you hear about it? Because the symptoms slowly come on over the years, masquerading as labels like congestive heart failure, kidney disease with fluid retention, suicidal depression, or idiopathic liver disease. The ones who don't die have the misery of cataracts, ulcers, macular degeneration, hearing loss, ringing of the ears, memory loss, headaches, heartburn, fibromyalgia, chronic fatigue, and much more.

For example, one out of four people get ulcers or other intestinal problems from NSAIDs, but are labeled irritable bowel or heartburn and treated with additional drugs which produce further side effects. No wonder statistics show that once you start taking a gut drug you increase your chances of cancer 43 times! For once you start with a drug, you are propelled into the vortex of more drugs either for the side effects of the first or the progression of underlying causes that were ignored in the first place.

1

But worse is that these **pain-relievers actually cause bone deterioration,** ironic because they are taken for relief of bone pain. That's right, they actually cause the condition for which they are being taken to get much worse, often requiring surgery. No wonder we have been hurled into an epidemic of hip and knee replacements!  And if that were not enough reason to find the real cause of pain, common pain relievers cause the leaky gut syndrome.  The leaky gut can then go on to cause food and chemical allergies, vitamin and mineral deficiencies that accelerate aging, and auto-immune diseases where the body destroys its own tissues.  These include labels like rheumatoid arthritis, lupus arthritis, multiple sclerosis, amyotrophic lateral sclerosis (Lou Gehrig's Disease), thyroiditis, colitis, and more.  These nastiest of conditions destroy tissues much like a cancer.

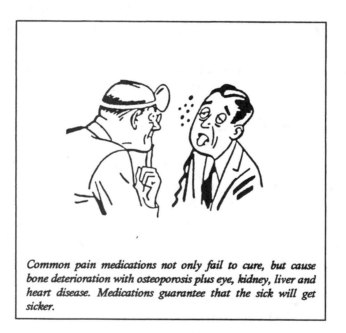

*Common pain medications not only fail to cure, but cause bone deterioration with osteoporosis plus eye, kidney, liver and heart disease. Medications guarantee that the sick will get sicker.*

NSAIDs not only increase your risk of being hospitalized by 4-fold, but are implicated in contributing to at least one in five cases of heart failure, for which one treatment is now cutting out part of the heart!   But that pales when you consider the side effects of steroids used to mask pain.  For they can cause death of the tiny femoral artery in the neck of the long thigh bone (femur), requiring attempts to artificially replace the ball and socket bone (with a poor at best prognosis).

And methotrexate, a drug commonly used for arthritis and other recalcitrant pain conditions, as a form of chemotherapy, can actually cause cancer later on down the road.  No wonder the prestigious *Journal of the American Medical Association* teaches us that prescription drugs kill well over 100,000 people each year in hospitals alone.  And this does not count those who die at home, in accidents, with non-prescription drugs or whose deaths were not recognized as being connected to drugs and their myriad insidious side effects.

Drugs are designed to merely shut down a chemical pathway that is malfunctioning.  For example, the malfunction of the cell membrane's inflammatory chemistry triggers a prescription of anti-inflammatory drugs, but this allows the underlying condition to accelerate and worsen: **the sick get sicker, quicker.** Better to find the true underlying cause and fix what is broken and get on with the joy of life.  That is what this book is about.

### Princess of Pain and Queen of Drugs

For a couple of decades, I had enough pain and drugs to qualify me for the Pain Hall of Fame. After years of relentless suffering, you can imagine my surprise in discovering that the pain was totally within my control all along.  It was just that none of the top-of-the-line physician specialists I consulted had the slightest glimmer of understanding for the mechanisms involved with my pain. Nor did the thousands of dollars of medical texts I own or physician courses I attended even hint at the true causes, much less the acutal cures for pain that I am going to show you how to master for yourself.

And had it not been for a combination of fortuitous God-directed events superimposed on an unrelenting need to be out of pain, this physician too, would still be among the ranks of physicians who will never know how to give each individual personal power over his pain. But once I found that I could not only control but cure my pain, and realized in fact that anyone could, I knew my next mission was to spread the word to fellow sufferers.

It all began as the classic story with ruptured lumbar discs in my 20's when I lifted the heavy end of a boat away from me. What a way to remind me of the simple physiologic fact that I am not as strong holding something three feet away from me as I am holding it close to me. At the moment I lifted the heavy bow away from me, its weight viciously yanked me forward, crushing my L5-S1 disc with lightning pain. I ended up in the emergency room that night, for the first time in my career as a patient instead of as the doctor, and with Demerol for the first time in my life. I recovered uneventfully and didn't think much of it for the next 10 years.

Increasingly I had more back pain, but as a physician I had an endless supply of various drugs that were always around to relieve it and keep me going. I was also "breaking" in a new horse and trying to learn how to jump. But I was the only thing that got broken, being thrown off numerous times. I recall one day in particular when my horse startled and I felt that unmistakable lightening bolt down my spine again.

As the years rolled by, I had repeated back injuries with increasingly more back pain. But I was so busy and looked forward so much to riding the horses on weekends that I couldn't let the pain get in my way. So I merely drugged myself with whatever I had: aspirin, Darvon® (propoxyphene), codeine, muscle relaxants and every brand of prescription non-steroidal anti-inflammatory drug (NSAID's) that was made.

During those days, I was also busy collecting large flat field stones from the pastures and corn fields to make a 500 foot long stone wall to edge my perennial garden. This didn't help my back either, but I was driven to complete this dream project. I wasn't going to let any old back pain hold me down. After all, I was only in my 30's, far too young to be limited by physical problems and I was an invincible physician to boot. When I took up tennis that really stretched me to my limit. And when I water-skied backward, the serious falls would leave me in pain for days. The solution was inevitable: more drugs.

As if I didn't have enough damage, a few more bucks off the horse crushed more backbones and their discs. I would have to slither out of bed on my stomach like a beached whale in the morning, and get up an hour early to work the stiffness out. Eventually even that was worthless and often I had to be carried crying in pain to the bathroom. I would be bed-ridden for days on end unable to eat or move and racked with pain regardless of what I did and what I took. There was no combination of drugs or position in a bed full of pillows that could offer relief from the pain.

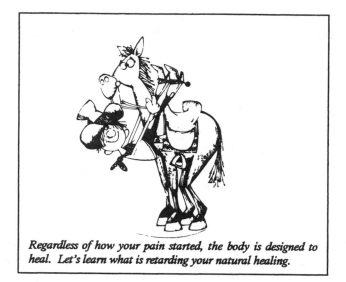

*Regardless of how your pain started, the body is designed to heal. Let's learn what is retarding your natural healing.*

By the time I went to one of my orthopedic friends to evaluate my ruptured disc, he laughed and said, "You don't even have a disc anymore. You have brutalized it for so long you have ground it up and spit it out, and now you are working on degenerating a couple of other ones above it."

I had the classic lumbo-sacral deteriorated disc with degeneration of the vertebral bodies (backbones). Arthritic spurs that were beginning to form on the vertebral bodies periodically jabbed my muscles making me rigid with muscle spasms. And the intermittently bulging discs pressed on my sciatic nerve sending pain down the back of my left leg, creating classic sciatica.

Following the wisdom of my orthopedic specialists, pretty soon I had tried every prescription brace and corset made. I even hung like a monkey from bars at the medical school while doctors and medical students deftly enclosed my torso in plaster. When it dried, they sawed it off and sent it away to have a custom-made brace that I was strapped into every day via 6 one inch leather straps. I used this brace (called a Raney Jacket) to allow me to do a little gardening, water skiing and horseback riding. For without activity after just using my mouth and brain all week in the office, I would have gone stark raving mad. It was horribly uncomfortable and squeezed me so much in order to produce some stabilization of the lumbo-sacral area that it gave me a hiatus hernia, varicose veins and hemorrhoids. Some days I swear I was bug-eyed from it! But it enabled activity, and that made it worth the price.

The pain continually worsened as I tried harder to ignore it and mask it with drugs, DMSO, and a TENS unit (battery operated electrical stimulator); I eventually got to a stage where I thought my life was over. Here I was only in my 30's and I couldn't even bend over to pick up a glove, I couldn't go grocery shopping because I could not bend enough to pick out the items from the shelves and carrying the grocery bags was torture. I couldn't empty a wastebasket at home. I couldn't have any fun. All I could do was see patients and painfully sit to read, study, and write.

I would walk around the farm on weekends in tears nostalgically looking at all the projects I had planned on doing: creating little gardens here, and little terraces there, and winding rock walls in other spots. I thought my life was over. By now I had seen the best orthopedic surgeons at my medical school. They offered a fusion of my back with a piece of my hip and a lifetime of drugs. Neither I nor any of my specialists ever dreamed that the power to completely get rid of all that life-sapping pain was totally within my control. And to this day they do not. But it is that control I now excitedly give to you.

## Types of Pain

There are actually many types of pain other than degenerative discs with or without sciatica. Arthritis in the back can be caused by trauma or old injury, but other forms of arthritic pain include deteriorating or degenerating bones and discs from osteoporosis and osteoarthritis, or the inflammatory destruction from lupus arthritis, rheumatoid arthritis, and even psoriatic arthritis that accompanies severe skin and nail psoriasis.

But you don't have to have any form of arthritis in order to be wracked with pain, for *inflammation and toxicity* in tissues from a myriad of causes can rival the worst arthritis pain. Tendonitis, bursitis, myositis, fibrositis, muscle spasms, dermatomyositis, or the catchall term fibromyalgia are the labels medicine uses for these types of pain. Later on I'll explore the different organs like the brain, heart, face, gut, bladder, and prostate which also can be the targets for nasty pain syndromes. And I won't overlook the indescribable pain of metastatic cancer as the ultimate type.

## The Reason for Pain

Did you every wonder why we have pain? It is to warn and protect us. It serves to keep us from touching the fire that would burn off our hands. We get pain and swelling from a sprained ankle as a warning not to use it while it is healing, and the swelling serves as a mini cast to hold things in place. Pain is designed to facilitate healing by keeping us from using the area. But healing is a limited process. It should not be chronic. Why should we suffer with pain for the rest of our lives because of one injury? The answer is we should not.

There is no teleological or protective mechanism or reason for having chronic suffering after one particular injury. Therefore, it is up to us to find out why the body is still having pain and what it is trying to tell us.

## Pain Means Inflammation:
## Inflammation Means Reaction to or
## Rejection of Something

If there is continual pain in an area that signifies there is an irritation, an inflammatory response. What is the body reacting to that forces it to continually release chemical mediators from cells, sending signals to bring in inflammatory repair cells and allergic cells? What offender or invader is the body chemistry trying to reject or gobble up?

Wherever there is pain, there must also be inflammation, with varying degrees of swelling, redness, or tenderness. It is through inflammation that the body defends and heals itself. It uses enzymes to penetrate and dissolve debris from injured or infected tissues, and white cells to gobble it up and cart it away. It is these extra cells that in the process of trying to clean up and protect us, also put out chemicals or mediators that produce the chemistry of pain. Whatever it is that we are reacting to, the reaction will persist as long as the body has not conquered the stimulus or trigger. Real healing, as with cuts and fractures, occurs over a finite period of time. We get over it. It has an end, as opposed to chronic inflammation that perpetuates the chemical messages of pain.

Never lose sight of the fact that only when there is a persistent trigger (that the body is reacting to and cannot conquer) does it continue to produce inflammation and pain. My goal is to help you discover what the cause is and get rid of pain once and for all.  Inflammation and resultant **pain should never be chronic**.  And when you choose to cover up or mask pain with medications, it allows you to ignore finding the true underlying causes.  The chronic inflammation inevitably progresses to much more serious damage and tissue destruction, while the drugs used cause their own damage as well as create new diseases.

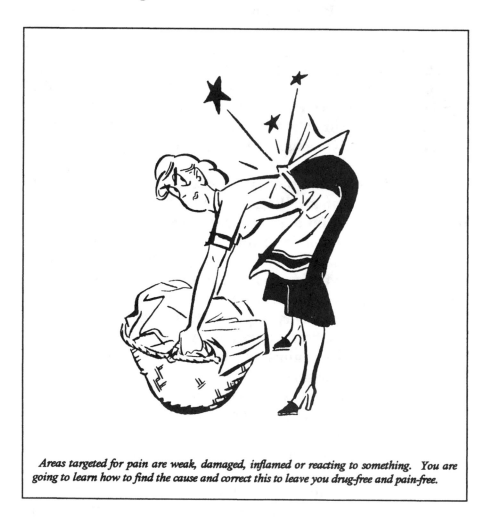

*Areas targeted for pain are weak, damaged, inflamed or reacting to something.  You are going to learn how to find the cause and correct this to leave you drug-free and pain-free.*

## If Everything Heals, Why Should Pain be Chronic?

When you cut your finger, it doesn't bleed and stay open forever unless there is something else wrong. If there is a non-healing infection from a sliver in a diabetic, the persistence of inflammation alerts us to remove the sliver and regulate the diabetes before healing can be completed. When you break your wrist, you don't have pain forever. So why should a back or any other source of chronic pain be an exception? Every chronic condition has an underlying cause that can be remedied. It is these causes you are going to learn to identify and correct.

A target organ can be any organ in your body, any area, any tiny little spot or a whole side. It merely is the place that disease or inflammatory reaction settles into in a particular person. For example, with too much tennis, one person may have a sore back, another a sore knee, another "tennis elbow". And they could all have the same cause or totally different ones.

When someone develops food allergies, vitamin or mineral deficiencies, or chemical sensitivities, these too, can then turn on the chemistry of inflammation. It is also common for this reactive inflammation to target a place of previous damage or injury, like the old back injury. Areas of previous damage are particularly vulnerable for becoming target organs for inflammatory reactions due to allergies. For these areas may be weaker, due to years of uncorrected mineral deficiencies, for example, or having a poorer blood and lymphatic supply from the previous injury. But more on that later.

Fortunately, we now have the tools with which to identify the triggers to our damaged target organs that keep them

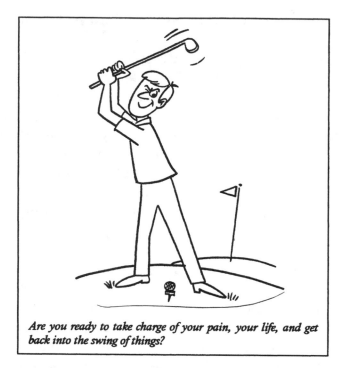

*Are you ready to take charge of your pain, your life, and get back into the swing of things?*

chronically inflamed and in pain. We can identify the triggers, turn off the inflammation by fixing the problem, and once and for all, *stop the vicious cycle of pain*. Are you ready to learn how to become **pain-free at last**?

### Message in a Nutshell

Never give up hope of curing your pain. Just because medical specialists may have told you "There is nothing that can be done" or that "You have to learn to live with it", nothing could be further from the truth. You haven't even begun to learn how to uncover all the possible remedial causes.

# Chapter 2

## The Nightshade Nemesis

### The Hidden Answer to Crippling Pain

What would cause me to be pain-free for weeks on end, enjoying two hours of singles tennis a day, only to suddenly get slammed? The mystery of why I went from great to bed-ridden in severe pain for weeks on end was finally solved.

Despite pills and braces, my attacks of pain began getting more and more unpredictable and steadily more incapacitating. They were especially bad every time I went to a Caribbean island in the British West Indies where I have spent the last 20 Christmases to visit friends. Most often within 48 hours of arriving, I would be mysteriously bedridden with back pain, unable to move and in extreme agony. Anticipating the trip for months on end, I looked forward to so many island activities in a setting where I am totally relaxed. Yet the irony was that sometimes within hours of arriving, I was mysteriously flat out in bed unable to move sometimes for days. I had to be carried to the bathroom in severe pain.

My husband and I would wrack our brains for the possible causes, for it was much too consistent to be a mere fluke. All sorts of questions played through our heads: was this pain from carrying the luggage, was it the stress that I endured while getting ready to leave, was it the grinding of my lumbo-sacral bones from walking on the sandy beach, or from snorkeling with over-sized fins? We never could figure it out until numerous repetitive episodes finally drove the point home. I was a victim of the **nightshade nemesis**.

Years ago a wonderful horticulturist, Dr. Norman Childers, Ph.D., while teaching at Rutgers University in New Jersey, had a special interest in studying the Solonaceae family of plants, often called the "deadly nightshades". Because animals would be found crippled and sometimes dead after they had grazed in pastures containing these plants, he became an avid student of the mechanism of this mysterious crippling toxicity caused by one botanical family. The world owes him a tremendous debt of gratitude. I had to restrain myself from literally kissing his feet when I first met him at my home, for his diligent and humble discovery saved not only my sanity, but the lives of thousands of others.

### "Too Easy to Believe"

Dr. Childers discovered and proved with his own money in research studies that over 74%-90% of the people who ache and hurt, regardless of their diagnostic label or type or arthritis, have a sensitivity to nightshades. It didn't matter if they had arthritis of old age or degenerated back discs with sciatica, heel spurs, a "bad shoulder", bum knees, or lupus or rheumatoid arthritis. It didn't matter if they had fibromyalgia or tendonitis or joint or muscle pain that was undiagnosable. The label given to their type of pain was of no consequence.

For once the person had a diet free of nightshades for 3 months, over three-fourths of them were totally out of pain. I have proven this over and over again with myself and with hundreds of my patients who are also indebted to Dr. Childers. And age is just as irrelevant as the type of pain. The children who have been brought to my office wracked in pain from rheumatoid arthritis would bring tears to the eyes of the most stoic. They had consulted the best

14

rheumatologists at the medical centers and had the best drugs that money could buy. Then they were turned out to pasture as incurable, sentenced to a lifetime of destructive drugs.

Yet these victims of juvenile rheumatoid arthritis are now totally free of pain and deformity as long as they adhere, as I must also, to the nightshade-free diet. They now enjoy dancing and soccer and all the fun activities of normal childhood. Their parents actually cried tears of gratitude when the daily frustration of seeing their children in agony ended.

Another example, a young tall real estate agent, comes to mind who had to stop playing basketball because of incapacitating knee pain. But stopping the nightshades was all he really had to do in order to be pain-free and able to resume the sport. People in their 80's and 90's relieved of decades of arthritis or pain, regardless of their individual medical labels are amazed that they have never heard of this veritable cure that is within the grasp of every person. Yet rarely does a doctor know about it, much less recommend it. And every time I first mention it to anyone, they invariably reply that it is just "too hard to believe" that the solution could be so simple, so easy.

My scenario progressed to a point where once I got slammed with the pain, I was locked in it for two incapacitating weeks, followed by 2-3 more weeks of manageable (drugged but walking) pain. After a few more weeks of lesser pain, the pain would mysteriously leave, just as quickly as it had come. I would wake up one morning and it would be totally gone. I was later to learn that this is when the antigen-antibody complexes drop off the target organ. I must admit, that before I knew what the cause was, and that it would dramatically come to an end in less than three months, it was very difficult to not throw myself at the mercy of medicine. Pain has a way of wearing you down to a point where you'll beg a surgeon to operate.

So let's show you how to do a nightshade-free diet. For the odds are in your favor that you, too, are a victim of the nightshade nemesis.

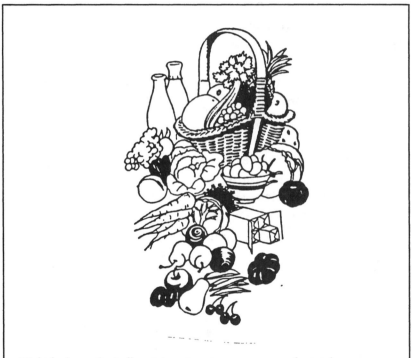

*Nightshades are basically potatoes, tomatoes, peppers, eggplant, tobacco, cayenne, chili, paprika. There is still plenty to eat.*

# Foods That Cripple

**Nightshades include potatoes, tomatoes, peppers, eggplant, tobacco, and spices.** Before you jump to the conclusion that this is pretty simple, take a look at the hidden sources for these cripplers in our food:

## Potato

In the potato category, the number one vegetable in the U.S., obvious sources are baked potatoes, mashed potatoes, French fries, scalloped potatoes, pierogies, and foods that contain potato products. For one place that can really foul up your detective work and keep you in pain is by unknowingly ingesting soups, biscuits and breads that are made with potato water, or processed foods (some yogurts and frozen seafoods) that contain potato starch, **modified food starch,** modified vegetable protein (or MVP), **modified vegetable starch,** or **hydrolyzed vegetable protein.**

Potato starch is also in gluten-free baking powders. Potato starch is often used as a binder in artificial seafoods as well, like mock crab (that is really seasoned whitefish). And don't overlook sausages, meatballs, motzah, blintzes, and other Passover foods, gravies, potato chips, stews and stuffing. And do not forget vodka! This is merely fermented potato peelings. Sweet potato and yams are safe, as they are in a different botanical family. Also do not have fish and other fried foods that have been cooked in the same oil they make French fries in. The same precaution goes for lobster boiled in the same water as salt potatoes.

Potato starch is also a common filler in prescription and non-prescription medications. Your doctor or pharmacist can call the company to learn whether it is currently in your brands.

However, this is no guarantee that the source will not change in the future. Also some vitamins and other supplements contain nightshade antigens, especially some brands of lycopenes (tomato) and lipoic acid (potato).

## Tomato
Tomatoes are obviously found in ketchup, spaghetti sauce and pizza. In vogue now, sun-dried tomatoes are added to many dishes. Many different condiment sauces like A-1 Steak Sauce, Worcestershire Sauce, and even brown sauces invariably contain tomato or other nightshades. But do not overlook baked beans, bolognas, barbecue sauces, meat loaf, gravies, and salad dressings like Thousand Island. There are also tomato relatives that are uncommon but sometimes cultivated in home gardens like tomatillo and ground cherry. Obviously, tomato juice and a bloody Mary would be out.

## Peppers
Peppers include red, green, yellow, orange, jalapeno, chili, and pimento. Those microscopic red flecks in your pasta that you cannot see during a candle light dinner are crushed ground red pepper that can leave me bedridden for days and in severe pain for 2-3 months. Green pepper is nearly invisible as tiny shavings in cabbage salad and cooked into many dishes. Stuffed olives in deviled eggs contain pimentos, another nightshade pepper.
**Note:** Black peppercorns are not in the same botanical family and they are safe to have.

## Spices
Spices of the nightshade family include cayenne, chili, curry, ground red pepper, crushed red pepper, and paprika. Cayenne and crushed red pepper can provide a wonderfully paralyzing accompaniment to garlic dishes like olive oils used

for dipping Italian bread.  Paprika is often hidden on nuts and sprinkled over grilled fish and even on raw fish at the mongers.

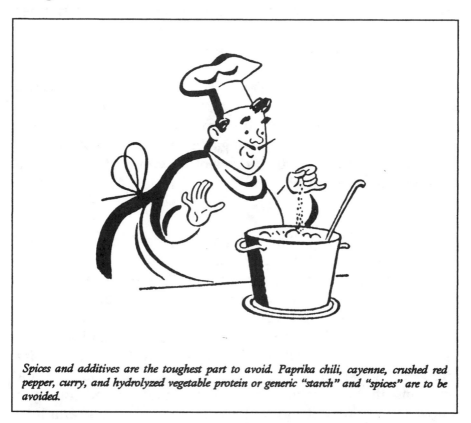

*Spices and additives are the toughest part to avoid. Paprika chili, cayenne, crushed red pepper, curry, and hydrolyzed vegetable protein or generic "starch" and "spices" are to be avoided.*

Even the spine of the lemon wedge is dipped in red paprika! Seasoning mixes like Shake and Bake® type coatings, snack crackers and cocktail crackers, mayonnaise, Hollandaise sauce, relishes, and seasoned salts contain hidden nightshades, depending upon individual recipes and the creativity of the chef.  Nearly all processed foods and commercial salad dressings contain nightshade spices.  And in case you are into surprise salads containing edible flower blossoms, be sure to pass up the **petunias**.

Curry contains a number of spices. The formula for curry usually includes several nightshades in secret amounts and combinations: **cayenne, paprika, chili, ground red pepper** as well as safe non-nightshade spices of fenugreek, coriander, cumin, turmeric, celery seed, mace, ginger, pepper (black or white), salt, cloves, allspice, caraway, and garlic.

So you can readily see that you curry fans can easily create your own unique blends by carefully eliminating the nightshades and balancing the remaining ingredients to your taste. For example, ample fresh garlic more than makes up for the lack of cayenne. With all those other wonderful spices, the nightshades will not be missed. And if you find pure curry leaf, that is fine.

Any ingredient list that includes "spices" or unspecified "natural flavorings" usually contains one or more of the nightshade spices namely cayenne, chili, paprika, ground red pepper, or curry. Therefore, it is **mandatory to avoid "spices" when they are unspecified.** Avoid sauces, especially Thai, barbecue, Cajun, Mexican, Southern, and Jamaican dishes as well as tobasco sauce and Worcestershire. Prepared mustards usually contain paprika also. Avoid anything that comes your way that is pink or red until you know exactly why it has that color. Paprika, for example, is used more liberally than salt in some restaurants, on garlic breads and as a dusting on the main dish prior to presentation.

**Eggplant**
Eggplant (aubergine) is also a nightshade, but is rarely disguised, being prepared as eggplant Parmesan, eggplant lasagna, or stuffed eggplant.

## Tobacco

Tobacco is probably the most addicting and therefore toughest nightshade family member for people in pain to quit. Each puff on a cigar or cigarette is like an intravenous injection of nightshades. Sometimes it takes years of smoking before the chronic pain sets in. Many prisoners of pain will never stop hurting until they stop smoking and then it takes 2-8 months to detoxify this from the body.

The nightshades are particularly difficult to avoid if you do not remember the following:

- Tomato is commonly hidden in brown meat sauces and gravies.
- Potato is hidden as potato water or modified food starch in many breads, biscuits, seafood and meat mixtures and soups; and vodka is distilled from fermented potato.
- Eggplant
- Peppers, red, green, orange, yellow, and hot. These are hidden in many foods such as salads and pastas, clams casino, oysters Rockefeller and deli meats. As more people eat processed foods and get lower in zinc and other important nutrients their ability to taste food dwindles and so restaurants make foods more exciting with these spicy flavors.
- Cayenne is hidden in the word "spices" in many soups, seafood dishes, especially crab cakes, conch fritters, and chili con carne.
- Paprika is hidden in most salad dressings under the guise of "spices", in all sorts of condiments, in sandwich spreads, mayonnaise and mustard, deli meats, and added liberally to grilled fish and roasted nuts. It is probably the most difficult nightshade to avoid.
- Tobacco, one of the toughest addictions.

If the nightshade-free diet does not clear you within 3 months, you may have other hidden food sensitivities. To identify them, do the rare food or diagnostic diet in the *E.I. Syndrome, Revised*. For example, citrus fruits, red meats or wheat products are culprits for a hefty proportion of people whose arthritis is triggered by nightshades. Basically, for the diagnostic diet, you list all the foods you eat frequently or at least every two weeks. Then eliminate them. This may reduce you to brown rice and steamed vegetables. Once you are pain-free, introduce every third day an old favorite. It generally will tell you within 2 days if it is a culprit.

If the diagnostic diet doesn't clear you in 1 month, you should do the macrobiotic diet in *The Cure is in the Kitchen*. First read *You Are What You Ate* which is the primer for the strict phase macrobiotic diet with which many people have cleared absolutely everything they ever had including end-stage cancers that had already failed chemotherapy, surgery, and radiation. If that diet doesn't agree with you, the live food diet as described in our publications in progress should be done. A recipe book to get you started is Baker's, *The Gourmet Uncook Book* (available at this publisher 1-800-846-6687). Basically 85% of the diet is raw fruits and vegetables and soaked or sprouted grains, beans, seeds and nuts.

Because unsuspected food allergy is such a common cause of chronic inflammation and pain, you owe it to yourself to rule out a cause over which you have 100% control. Furthermore, there is no diagnostic test that can take the place of the actual food elimination trials mentioned. For one reason, foods can cause allergy by over a dozen mechanisms. But blood tests used to identify food allergies can only identify food allergy caused by one or two mechanisms. So there are many false negatives that can only be found through dietary trials.

## Nightshade Substitutes

I was devastated at the thought of never making my scrumptious scalloped potatoes again, and irked at having to leave all those French fries on a plate when my stomach was only half full. But have a double helping of coleslaw, salad or vegetable, which is healthier for you anyway. Jerusalem artichokes sautéed in garlic and oil can be a substitute for potatoes. Kohlrabi, cauliflower or turnips can be boiled and mashed with or without cheese, butter or herbs.

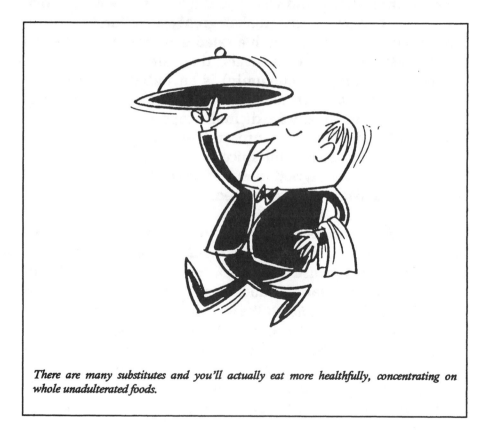

*There are many substitutes and you'll actually eat more healthfully, concentrating on whole unadulterated foods.*

For French fries make your own, which will be far healthier anyway, since they will not contain the damaging trans fatty acids that commercial ones are cooked in. Peeled **sweet** potatoes cut into French fry strips, oiled with olive oil and a little salt and **black** pepper are baked on a cookie sheet in a 350 degrees F. oven for 20 minutes. Cornstarch, arrowroot, and kudzu are all wonderful thickeners to replace potato starch and potato water.

Pastas can be just as exciting without tomatoes, it all depends upon your creativity and tastes. Oil and garlic, soy or shoyu sauce, or cheese sauces make great substitutes. Small amounts of grated beet root in a salad can impart a pretty red color and lend phytochemicals that are good for you. Turmeric (or tumeric, curcumin) is an Indian herb or spice that has healing benefits and imparts a pretty yellow color to foods. Garlic has many medicinal properties, like lowering cholesterol and blood pressure and lessening the chance of blood clots. It is a superior spice when a hot zesty flavor is called for, as are a myriad of spices that you merely need to acquaint yourself with. Experiment.

There are 3 cookbooks that contain great recipes for standards without nightshades. *Macro Mellow* for example has homemade mayonnaise and mock tomato sauce, *Nightshade-Free Cooking* has tartar sauce and barbecue sauce, and *Arthritis: A Diet to Stop It* has salad dressings and more. You'll never miss nightshades with all these ideas (all from 1-800-846-6687). And an added benefit is that by making your own salad dressings, mayonnaise and condiments, you avoid the body-damaging trans fatty acids that are in all foods containing hydrogenated vegetable or soybean oil.

## The Deadly Nightshades
## Mimic the Need for Disc Surgery

In the past when I had heard the term "Deadly Nightshades", I thought it only pertained to a species of weed that caused toxic problems in animals that were turned out to graze in pastures containing nightshades. But I have developed over the years a serious respect for the nightshade family for it almost forced me and many of my patients to undergo needless disc surgeries and/or back fusions. Others were slated for surgery of knees, hips, heels (spurs), wrists (carpal tunnel syndrome) and shoulders before they found the pain-free nightshade solution.

Fortunately, God is very persistent in his teaching of physicians who only know about drugs and surgery as answers to medical problems. My ruptured discs were only my first initiation into the world of real pain. Factor in the years of being repeatedly thrown off horses, collecting large fieldstones to make a 500-foot long stone wall, water skiing, totaling 5 cars, and numerous other repressed activities that severely beat up my back. After 3 badly damaged discs and being strapped into a plaster cast for 6 years, I became the queen of drugs. Only in my 30's, and thoroughly believing that my physical life was over, I consulted the best orthopedic surgeons and followed all of their advice. But not one knew about the **food factor in chronic back pain.**

Remember that areas of previous damage and injury, with their compromised blood supply due to scar tissue, become an easy mark or target organ for our food sensitivities. One deterrent to making the connection is that one tiny mouthful may not trigger the pain for 48 hours. By then you may have forgotten what you ate. And it is dose related. So a small amount here and there may not affect you. Then one day you are mysteriously slammed with pain for seemingly no reason, because nightshades silently accumulate in your system until you reach a high enough dose to produce pain. Then, the pain usually does not leave until 1 to 3 months later, further clouding any analysis. However, once the kernel of suspicion is planted in your brain, it becomes much easier to figure out whether nightshades are only a part of or constitute the entire cause of your pain. For avoiding them strictly for 3 months will give you a clear answer.

One lady was signed and sealed for back surgery in 2 weeks. She came to the office as a last resort to see if there was another option. When we put her on the diet, her pain was completely gone within a week. Eight years later she is still pain free and has never had that surgery.

An elderly gentleman scheduled for a hip replacement found tomatoes were the source of his pain. In spite of degenerative changes on x-ray (from the years of NSAIDs) he had no pain once he was totally off all nightshades. He learned how to rebuild the degenerating bone (see chapter 5) and remains pain-free and active. Another man had painfully incapacitating swelling of his thumb joint, another bilateral knee pain, all unimproved with drugs. The nightshade-free diet provided the solution.

I was offered disc repair, back fusion, and a plethora of medications. Never having succumbed to the surgery, I now at 57 have no back pain and play daily tennis, water ski backwards, can lift a 100-lb. sack of oats and I'm only 5'2". Give me one bite of red pepper and within 2 days I'm bed-ridden and have severe pain for 6-9 weeks.

As a doubting physician, I have probably knowingly tested the nightshades 2 dozen times with serious consequences each time. When I have potatoes, my thumb and finger joints swell up so that they look like banjos and feel like they have been hit with a sledgehammer. My large toe joints also swell, making walking painfully impossible, except in wooden clogs. But if I went to a conventional physician, I would be diagnosed as having osteoarthritis with bunions and a Motrin® deficiency. I would be told there is no known cause or cure and only chronic medicines could be recommended. There is no search for cause as it is assumed there is none.

A fellow golfer who had always complained of aching knees and neck, solved his problem after merely stopping his daily lunch of French fries and hamburgers with tomato slice and ketchup; a nightshade special.

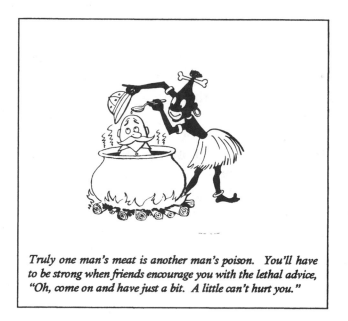

*Truly one man's meat is another man's poison. You'll have to be strong when friends encourage you with the lethal advice, "Oh, come on and have just a bit. A little can't hurt you."*

## Avoidance is the Key

Clearly, for those who want freedom from pain, start by avoiding all members of the nightshade family right this moment for three months. That means that you will need to rigorously question everything that enters your mouth. You will disgustedly find that many waiters and waitresses do not want to be bothered with your questions, regarding the ingredients of the recipes. I have repeatedly found that many have neither the knowledge to answer ingredient questions nor the inquisitiveness or courtesy to pursue the answers in the kitchen. In fact, often they do not know what vegetables have accompanied the main courses they have been serving all night! So be it. You are responsible for your health, not them.

Have a salad with no dressing or olive oil and lemon. Substitute rice (unseasoned) for potatoes, have meat without sauce, or fish specified without sauce or paprika, but baked or broiled with lemon or wine. Instead of French fries, have a double order of salad or vegetable. Unfortunately, classic recipes are frequently substituted for cheaper or more antigenic ingredients in this era. You have to know your restaurant's kitchen well before you make any leap of faith. For example, coleslaw or rice are often jazzed up with green peppers or contain surprise hot spices, as do dressings and sauces. And the ubiquitous use of mayonnaise and special sauces in sandwiches has to be substituted with butter. At home you can make your own.

28

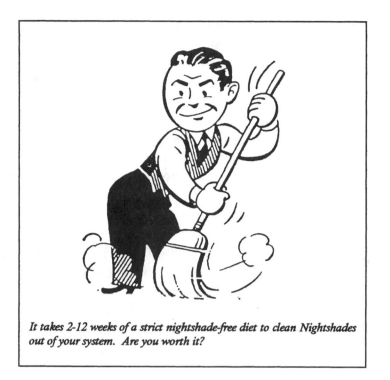

*It takes 2-12 weeks of a strict nightshade-free diet to clean Nightshades out of your system. Are you worth it?*

## You May Not Hurt Enough to do the Diet

The thing that always cracks me up is the person who bitterly complains about how pain has devastated his life, but is obviously not sick enough to do the diet. For he offers up every excuse I have heard in 30 years of medicine for why he would not be able to accomplish the diet. The bottom line is that he just does not hurt enough. For when he does, the diet is a piece of cake.

Some have other gains in maintaining their disability; it enables them to avoid certain obligations; it punishes someone with their constant martyrdom and pain; it serves as a means of manipulation or control, or it helps them get the attention and care they crave. That is fine. But when you are ready to be pain-free, try the diet.

Others say they are mostly on the diet, and only cheat a little, or only once in a while. Then they moan about how the diet is not the answer for them. Let me tell you now, so there is no mistake. You are either on the diet, or off. There is no half way. Do not kid yourself or others. Just like you are either pregnant or you are not. You are not a little bit pregnant. You either have cancer, or you do not. There is no half way. And so it is with the diet.

It is truly a challenge to cook and order without nightshades, but it is worth every effort, and becomes easier with practice. But an extra benefit is that more of your foods are made from scratch with far superior quality ingredients. In addition, avoiding hidden nightshades rules out a host of processed and unhealthful additive-laden foods in place of more whole foods.

Since one indiscretion can lead to months of agony, are you willing to take that chance? For recipe books that are nightshade-free, don't forget Childer's *Arthritis: A Diet to Stop It*, Vogel's *The Nightshade-Free Cookbook*, and *Macro Mellow* (all from 1-800-846-6687). They also make great gifts for hostesses (plus chances are someone in that household will benefit). In chapter 4 I'll show you how a nightshade allergy can appear in anyone at any time. So never let down your guard.

One of the worst emerging problems I see now, however, are with nutrients. More vitamin C powders and lipoic acid, for example, are made from potato. Likewise, lycopenes are usually from tomato. Cayenne is a common ingredient in herbal heart, arthritis, and digestive combinations. Even a company you have relied on for years can suddenly switch their source for vitamin C, for example, from beet to potato. Don't hesitate to call the company and ask the source.

It is not enough that the hidden nightshade sources come in the most innocent sounding forms as "hydrolyzed vegetable protein", "natural flavorings", "modified vegetable starch", "spices" and more. Now thanks to GM (genetically modified) foods you can scratch another food from your list — soy. Although it is not a nightshade, thanks to Monsanto's genetic engineering, they have incorporated the petunia gene into the soybean as part of the genetic machinery. Since this is a nightshade, it can cause a nightshade reaction in susceptible persons, just as the famed *New England Journal of Medicine* article showed how incorporation of Brazil nut antigen into soy caused allergic reactions, sometimes fatal, in folks allergic to Brazil nuts. They removed the Brazil nut gene, but I wouldn't hold my breath for the same to happen for the petunia gene.

Because so many of us can be stricken with pain for weeks and months due to nightshades, you may want to copy the following letter and use it for going to restaurants. It puts the waitress/waiter and chef on notice. If your symptoms are not as severe you may want to modify the letter.

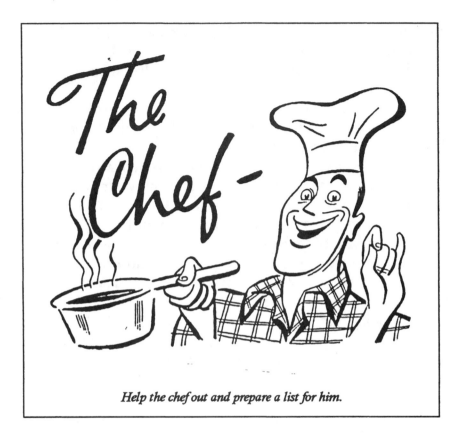
*Help the chef out and prepare a list for him.*

Dear Chef,

I have a violent allergy to one category of foods that is life threatening. This family of foods, the "deadly nightshades", includes **potatoes, tomatoes, peppers, eggplant** (aubergine), **and spices.** Unfortunately it is not that simple, for there are multiple hidden sources for these in foods:

**Potato**
In the potato category, obvious sources would be baked, mashed or scalloped potatoes, French fries, and potato chips. But violent reactions occur in me from hidden sources of potato, like **potato starch**, or **potato water** in soups, stews, breads, biscuits, donuts, stuffings, gravies, sauces. Another hidden source is processed foods, including some frozen seafoods and sausages that often contain modified food starch, potato starch, **modified vegetable protein** (sometimes only designated on the

package by MVP), or **hydrolyzed vegetable protein** (HVP). This also means that foods like fish or calamari could not be fried in oil in which French fries were cooked, likewise, lobster could not be boiled in water to which salt potatoes were cooked, and use no vodka in cooking.

## Tomato
Tomatoes, spaghetti sauce, tomato juice, Bloody Mary mix, sun-dried tomatoes and pizza. Most condiment sauces like steak sauces, Worcestershire sauce, tobasco sauce, barbecue sauces, and even brown sauces invariably contain tomato or other nightshades in the form of peppers and spices. Other sources include baked beans, bolognas and other deli meats, meat loaf, and salad dressings.

## Peppers
Peppers **include red, green, yellow, orange, jalapeno, chili,** and **pimentos** (in stuffed olives, for example).

## Spices
This is the sneakiest category of hidden nightshades, but the reactions have been near lethal in the past. Spices of the deadly nightshade family include **cayenne, chili, ground red pepper, crushed red pepper, curry, and paprika.**

Any ingredient lists, as in **salad dressings** as an example, that include "**spices**" or unspecified "**natural flavorings**", cannot be used. Only if the exact spices are specified and not in the list of nightshades can anything be used. Spreads like **mayonnaise** and condiments like **prepared mustards** usually contain **paprika** and/or potato starch. **Hollandaise sauce** usually contains a pinch of **cayenne**, but is deadly for me. Likewise, do not use paprika on broiled fish, garlic breads, on the spine of lemon wedges, or as a final garnish for the dish.

(Some of you may want to add this to your letter to better obtain the chefs attention.) **Because I can die from one hidden ingestion**, I avoid any dish that is red and ethnic dishes, especially Thai, Tex-Mex and barbecue, Cajun, Mexican, Southern, and Jamaican.

What can I eat? Lots of other vegetables, including sweet potatoes (a different botanical family) and many other spices like black pepper (again not in the same family), garlic, ginger, basil, rosemary and more. All fresh unprocessed meats, fowl and seafoods, wines and fruits are safe, providing the precautions above are taken.

33

I have spent 2 months in a hospital bed because a chef did not read the package in which frozen lobster for a soufflé came. **Potato starch** was the ingredient (on the package label) that caused the reaction.

Fortunately there are many wonderful whole foods left for me to eat. **So when in doubt, leave it out.**

Most appreciatively,

## Thank You, Dr. Norm Childers

Before I close the "Childers' chapter", I must bow down and humbly thank Dr. Norm Childers, for his tireless efforts in researching all of this and explaining it so thoroughly in his wonderful book that I heartily recommend. An advocate of a nightshade-free diet himself, he is an example of how taking control of his own health sets him apart from others his age. In 1997, he took time from his busy schedule where he still works at the University of Florida at Gainesville to drive several hours to my home in his orchid 1976 Cadillac convertible. Having not a gray hair on his head, this vigorous gentleman has a gorgeous head of thick dark wavy hair. You can imagine how astounded I was to learn that he was 86! I still consult with him 4 years later at the University where at 90 he continues his research.

Although he is not a medical doctor, I suspect he has saved more lives than any dozen medical physicians I know rolled into one. He certainly saved my life and that of hundreds of patients and thousands of readers. We are eternally grateful.

*References: see back of book for all references.*

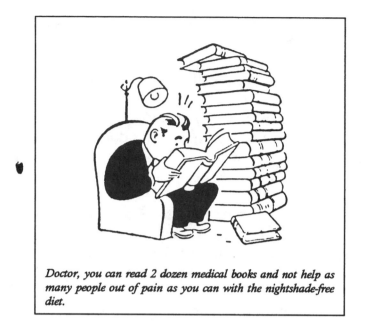

*Doctor, you can read 2 dozen medical books and not help as many people out of pain as you can with the nightshade-free diet.*

## Mechanisms and Science for Physicians

Because animals would be found crippled and sometimes dead after they had been turned out to graze in pastures containing nightshade plants, Dr. Childers became an avid student of the mechanism of the crippling toxicity caused by this botanical family. The family of **Solonaceae** is the number one category of vegetables ingested in the U.S., since potatoes are the number one most frequently ingested vegetable and tomato is number two (Krebs-Smith 1996). It contains 90 genera and over 2,000 species (D'Arcy 1985, Heiser 1987). The veterinarian literature documents the nightshade alkaloids as capable of producing arthritis, with heart, lung, circulatory, and bone damage as well as cancer and death (Spoerke 1994, West 1952, Durrell 1952).

The *alkaloids are bound to tissues and bioaccumulate,* which means the toxicity can slowly add up without producing any symptoms until it reaches a critical level, months or years later (Nigg 1996, Alonzie 1978, Claringbold 1982). By then, sensitivity is the last thing suspected, since these foods had been ingested with impunity for a lifetime. But similar is the story of a high cholesterol diet and its damage as well. Man can likewise wallow in fatty meals until the fateful day of his first (and last?) heart attack, never aware of the culprit.

Although the veterinarian literature on nightshade toxicity precedes that of man, humans are not exempt as thousands of poisonings have been documented, some leading to coma and death (Morris 1984). As in any sensitivity, it all depends upon the individual's genetic susceptibility, which can change over the course of a lifetime, leaving anyone vulnerable at any time.

The alkaloid solanine, from potato, is a drug just like the alkaloid nicotine from the tobacco plant, another nightshade. These nightshade alkaloids may explain why some individuals seem to have an **addiction** to nightshade foods as well as the tobacco nightshade. In fact, nightshade alkaloids are so potent that important and powerful drugs derived from nightshades for medicinal purposes include belladonna, atropine and scopolamine (Goodman 1975).

The nightshade glycoalkaloids interfere with the function of the enzyme that makes nerves and muscles work properly, *acetylcholinesterase,* much like organophosphate pesticides do (Roddick 1989, Abbott 1960, Orgell 1958, Harris 1959). In fact, Solonaceae sensitivity has been **misdiagnosed as pesticide poisoning** (Dawson 1990).

Solonaceae glycoalkaloids also destabilize and **destroy cell membranes** (Roddick 1988, 1990, Michalska 1985), analogous to the computer keyboard of the cell, and membranes of cell organelles, thereby producing seemingly unrelated symptoms. By disrupting chemical messengers contained in phosphatidyl choline/cholesterol liposomes, or damaging membrane hormone receptors or the detoxification membranes of the endoplasmic reticulum, nightshades clearly affect multiple aspects of the body's most critical chemistries. For example, nightshade alkaloids can damage the function of crucial calcium and sodium channels (Roddick 1988, Blankenmeyer 1995), which is a major problem in cardiology as judged by the number of calcium channel blockers and diuretics that are prescribed.

With 10 genetic variants for susceptibility, not all individuals are affected equally or at all (LaDu 1990), yet the manifestations of an individual's sensitivity to nightshade alkaloids are extremely varied. To complicate matters, the glycoalkaloids can bring about changes in gene expression (Layer 1991), including triggering cancer (Wasserman 1976).

In bones, nightshade alkaloids can cause inflammation and arthritis and many veterinarian books are replete with pictures of sheep and cattle brought to their knees in order to continue grazing with severe arthritis. But the Solonaceae (nightshade family) also contains a potent form of natural vitamin D3, which can reach such high levels as to cause toxicity (Childers 1993, Corradino 1974, Wasserman 1975).

By facilitating the removal of calcium from bone, this overdose of vitamin D3 can foster osteoporosis as well as abnormal reciprocal calcification of vessels and tissues like tendons and bursas, as well as blood vessels, plus initiate stones in the kidney and gall bladder. When vitamin D toxicity pulls calcium from bone, the calcium has to be deposited somewhere, and once it is taken from its natural reservoir, it lays down anywhere becoming an uninvited guest. Calcification of tissues other than bone signifies chemistry out of control. The number one cause of death and illness in the U.S. is the abnormal calcification we call arteriosclerosis: hardening or calcification of arteries. Dr. Childers theorizes that nightshades contribute to our epidemic of arteriosclerosis.

Many nightshade alkaloids that are used to make modern day medical prescription drugs like scopolamine, belladonna and atropine have such severe effects as to be able to cause hallucinations and death. Their main use is to dry up oral and intestinal secretions before surgery. And atropine, used to slow the heart rate, can even stop the heart. Essentially, the nightshade alkaloids are all potent in their ability to paralyze and even irreversibly poison selective areas of the autonomic nervous system.

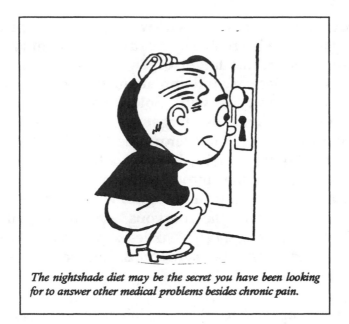

*The nightshade diet may be the secret you have been looking for to answer other medical problems besides chronic pain.*

In addition, the alkaloids of nicotine are potent enough to be used as commercial pesticides to kill insects. Probably the worst action is the ability of the Solonaceae alkaloids to mimic precisely the poisoning from organophosphate pesticides (Roddick 1989, Abbott 1960). Organophosphate (OP) pesticides work by poisoning acetylcholinesterase. Designed to break down acetylcholine, control over nerve muscle transmission is then lost. Since man can tolerate and accumulate an enormous amount before he reaches the lethal state, as compared with a bug, this accumulation in the nervous system can masquerade as many diverse symptoms as volumes of studies on OP pesticides attest. Two of the most commonly affected organs by pesticides are the brain with depression, inability to concentrate, migraines or schizophrenia, and the gut with all sorts of abnormal functions from spasm and pain to diarrhea (Hayes 1983, Rea 1993, 1995). Mysterious body pain is also a symptom.

The heart can also be affected with pesticide poisoning mimicking an acute heart attack or causing arrhythmia. If the skeletal muscles are the target organ, cramps, stiffness, incoordination, tenderness, inflammation, flu-like achiness or twitching occur, just as with Solonaceae. Pesticide or Solonaceae damage may also target the genetics resulting in teratogenesis and congenital deformities (Keeler 1973, 1978, 1990, Morris 1984, Pierro 1977, Renwick 1972, 1973, 1984), not to mention targeting the immune system, triggering many other diseases including auto-immune phenomena and cancer. Also, when the nervous system is affected, unexplainable paresthesias, weakness, paralysis, MS-type symptoms, Parkinson-type symptoms, bizarre pains, and more occur.

Of the many nightshade glycoalkaloids, 95% are either *a-solanine* or *a-chaconine,* both of which inhibit acetylcholinesterase (Nigg 1996, Orgell 1958, Harris 1959). Other saponic-like glycoalkaloids like capsaicins from cayenne are gastrointestinal irritants and can mimic ulcers and in Dr. Childers' own case produced diverticulitis. Because there is vast genetic or individual variation in degree of susceptibility to poisonings not only by pesticides but by nightshades in general, symptoms also vary tremendously from person to person. And they vary from time to time in the vulnerable individual, being subject to bioaccumulation and total load.

Since the nightshade alkaloids have tissue-binding properties as well as the ability to insidiously bioaccumulate and to eventually **alter genetics**, this leads to the notion that perhaps none of us, symptomatic or not, should be eating nightshades. But there are many cultures noted for their reliance on nightshades, as man has ingested them for over 200 years

(Ugent 1970, Spoerke 1994).    On the other side of the argument is the fact that the United States has over 80 million arthritics.    And many are elderly on fixed incomes, daily ingesting hamburgers with French fries and ketchup. And we have a concomitant record high sales of NSAIDs, whose side effects raise the chance of needing hospitalization 4-fold, and cause serious damage to numerous target organs (Gibson, Goodwin, Gutch, Guttman, Mamman, Murphy, Quiralt, Rogers, Shakel, Singh).    Congestive heart failure, one of the many conditions caused by nightshades in over 20% of cases, is more prevalent than and has a shorter median life span than the diagnosis of cancer (Page).

If the intrinsic properties of nightshades were not enough cause for concern as a public health problem in select individuals, genetic modification of nightshades poses even further problems.    For example, the gene of an unrelated plant species called snowdrops has been inserted into potato to make it express a snowdrop lectin that increases the potato's resistance to worms and insects.

Unfortunately this lectin binds to mannose on the surface of intestinal villi in animals stimulating mitosis and T lymphocyte invasion, the body's first sign of rejection, with carcinogenic potential.    They also had significantly greater mucosal thickness in the stomach and thinner caecal mucosa with shorter colonic crypt lengths with crypt hyperplasia (Ewen).    In humans, it also triggers mitosis.    In addition it is extremely resistant to mammalian digestion and causes agglutination or clumping of red blood cells, and binds strongly to white blood cells (Fenton).    Obviously this Frankenstein foods has no business on our plates.

Nightshades are difficult to avoid in processed and restaurant foods, both of which are on the rise.  As well, although the pain can occur within minutes of ingestion, in most individuals it takes 1-3 days to precipitously produce pain, by which time many have forgotten what they ate or are focused on more recent events as possible causes.

Furthermore, nightshade sensitivity often attacks areas of previous pathology (possibly due to damaged lymphatic flow), thereby causing former injuries to take the blame. Confusing also is the fact that the pain not only begins with usually no physical provocation, but leaves as precipitously as it started within 1-8 weeks. This can make the medical profession focus on hypochondriasis as a diagnostic possibility.

## Conclusion

Nightshade sensitivity can promote any symptom. With the ability to mimic calcifications including arteriosclerosis, osteoporosis, membrane ion channel damage (the basis of the specialty of cardiology), and pesticide poisoning (which in itself can mimic nearly every symptom), it is enticing to speculate that **nightshades might be an unsuspected source of chronic degenerative disease in general.** This opens up an enormous channel for therapy as well as prophylaxis.

Although the medical literature is full of other examples of fasting and changes in diet aiding various forms of arthritis (Kroker, Palmblad, Signalet, Skoldstam, Sundquist, Uden), manipulating the diet is not popular or common among rheumatologists.

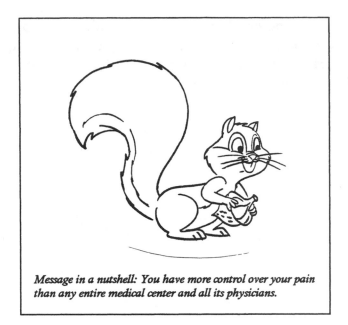

*Message in a nutshell: You have more control over your pain than any entire medical center and all its physicians.*

Clearly Solonaceae sensitivity is the cause of arthritis for many people, but no one knows how many are really affected. Whether there is an antigen-antibody complex that lays down on bone and other tissues or there is overt toxicity, both, or other mechanisms, certainly it deserves further investigation. In the meantime, just knowing what foods to avoid for total relief from pain in diseases where medicine has nothing more to offer, has opened up a whole new life of **freedom from pain** for an impressive number of people.

*(Remember, all references are in the back of the book in Chapter 10.)*

## Message in a Nutshell

Without strict avoidance of nightshades for 3 months, you may deny yourself access to one of the easiest and most common solutions for chronic musculoskeletal pain, anywhere in the body. Nightshades include tobacco as well as potatoes, tomatoes, peppers, tobacco, vodka, cayenne, chili, curry, paprika, pimentos, potato water, potato starch, modified food starch, eggplant, "spices" and "natural flavorings".

## Chapter 3

## CM: A Miracle in Medicine?

If anyone had told me there was anything that could turn off the pain of rheumatoid arthritis and osteoarthritis, I would have dismissed him as a quack. Billions of dollars have been funneled into research for decades to erase the miserable pain of this crippling arthritis. If such a drug existed it should make CNN and all international news services.

Given that absurd hypothesis, imagine
- if this product could perform this pain relief miracle in just *1-4 months*.
- Then imagine that after 4-6 months use, the pain relief was *permanent*. You read correctly; that you would never need it again and the pain relief would last forever. Do we dare even imagine a cure? Let's go one more mile.
- Imagine that this is an orphan nutrient that requires *no prescription*. That's right, anyone can buy it. And let's throw in one more dream cycle:
- it has *no side effects*. Wouldn't that just be too fantastic to be true?

Now you know exactly how incredulous I felt when I learned about CM, cetyl myristoleate. A list of serious rheumatoid arthritis sufferers flashed through my head that I couldn't wait to teach about it. These people I had come to love over the years and greatly admire for their ability to stoically endure pain without inflicting it on others. Their secret of how they were able to present the world with a continually cheerful countenance, was and remains a tribute to their

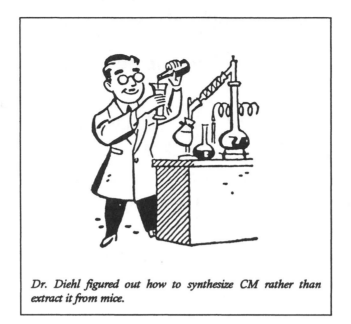

*Dr. Diehl figured out how to synthesize CM rather than extract it from mice.*

faith-driven fortitude. How excited and privileged I was to be able to share my discovery of CM with them.

But first we had better back up and learn how this was really discovered. Dr. Harry W. Diehl in 1962 was working at the government research laboratory, the National Institutes of Health. In fact he had just discovered and published 4 years earlier a method of synthesizing a special sugar (2-deoxy-D-ribose) used in the preparation of the oral polio vaccine of Dr. Jonas Salk.

His next assignment was researching drugs for arthritis control, yet as a prerequisite, he had to first create arthritis in the experimental rats. For researchers need a reliable animal model on which to experiment before giving a drug to humans. Actually creating arthritis in rats is pretty easy to do. You only have to inject them with a bacteria-like organism, *Mycobacterium butyricum,* to create little rats whose knee and elbow joints become so swollen, inflamed, and painful that the next morning they lay on the cage floor sprawled out, unable to support themselves.

But mice were resistant. Dr. Diehl could not give them arthritis. Curiosity peaked; he isolated the only compound that was different in the Swiss Albino mice that was not present in the arthritic rats, **cetyl myristoleate or CM.** He did the next logical thing, gave it to rats before he injected them with the arthritis-producing Mycobacterium. They did not get any arthritis. In other words, CM prevented rats from getting arthritis.

Further experiments in his own home laboratory, resulted in his first patent of CM for the treatment of rheumatoid arthritis in 1977, publishing his research in 1994, and the second patent in 1996 for osteoarthritis. Unfortunately as with many scientists, marketing was not his forte'. It never took off as it should, but many folks who did appreciate the discovery started to copy and modify the product.

## Government Research Has Curious Priorities

With scientific fervor rising, he next found he could relieve arthritis that had already started, and best of all, that he could do the same in humans. In fact, he was reportedly his first test case, having developed osteoarthritis. For many reasons, his government superiors did not deem this discovery worthy of further study. As often has happened in the history of medicine with items that are not patentable or that could produce a cure thus driving the research organization into extinction (as it could no longer justify its existence), such research is ignored, regardless of merit.

I do not want to get into the politics of medicine, so suffice it to say that for those interested readers there is a plethora of books documenting this recurring theme. When something is discovered that is inexpensive and effective as well as not able to be patented, it is soon abandoned for other efforts. It is a form of job security I guess. If you find it difficult as I did to believe, let me digress to give you one quick example out of hundreds.

Redux (dexfenfluoramine), the once popular "blockbuster" diet pill, had a few bucks behind it. As *The Wall Street Journal* touted in multiple articles, it took $25 million to develop it. So it should come as no surprise that in spite of being rejected initially for FDA approval, when a revote was done a mere month later, it somehow miraculously (and marginally) passed. This is in spite of the fact that decades earlier it was clearly shown that drugs of this configuration could cause serious cardiac abnormalities.

I guess they were hoping no one would notice if a few people died. For indeed they did. As one of many examples reported in *The Wall Street Journal*, one 30-year-old gal took it for a month just to lose a few pounds before her first wedding. She died (Assoc. Press 1997). It got so bad with people dying from the drug and the evidence mounting even in medical journals like *The New England Journal of Medicine* that the state of Florida had to preempt the FDA and ban the drug for use in Florida. They knew they couldn't wait for the government to protect their people; they had to do it themselves (Maremont 1997). I was proud of my adopted state for that move.

Meanwhile contrast that move with how something as safe, inexpensive and powerful as vitamin E is handled. A famous study in the 1993 *New England Journal of Medicine* was done on over 85,000 people to show that vitamin E in a low dose of only 100 mg a day, cut the number one cause of death and sickness, cardiovascular disease, in half. This is a monstrous saving in life and money. And vitamin E has no bad side effects. But the conclusion of the multitude of studies is that it is as yet premature to recommend folks take vitamin E until further research is done. There are now over 3,000 articles on vitamin E to support the life-saving benefits from higher doses (100-800 I.U.). Yet there are still no official recommendations, except that they just raised the RDA (recommended daily allowance) for vitamin E from 10 mg to 15 mg!

Or look at a government study by NIA, part of NIH (National Institutes of Health) which followed 11,178 seniors, aged 67-105 for 9 years. Those who took a mere 40 I.U. of vitamin E daily had a 41% reduction in heart disease, plus a 22% reduction in death from cancer and a 27% decrease in death overall from any cause (Losonczy). Yet rarely does any cardiologist in the country recommend it. And sometimes the excuse they use is that it could increase bleeding time, the very thing that they recommend folks take aspirin for! And contrary to vitamin E which has no side effects, aspirin can cause ulcers that have ended in fatal hemorrhaging.

The bottom line in these studies, which are confirmed in countless other papers, was that it is still premature to recommend to people that they take life-saving yet harmless vitamin E.

Compare this with Redux, that
- was tested on much less than 25% of that number of people,

- costs infinitely more,
- does not have 1/20$^{th}$ the number of research studies behind it,
- has not been proven to be of benefit in causing any lasting weight loss,
- and you can die from it, as it increases the chance of crippling primary pulmonary hypertension 45-fold (Langreth 1998).

Does a drug that pulls in $20 million a month (Langreth 1996) easily sway the FDA? It would appear so since it not only passed but stayed on the market in spite of urgings from 3 major medical studies as well as the reports of scores of people who died within less than a month of starting this drug (Langreth 1997).

I hope this tiny detour into the politics of medicine helps remove some of the incredulousness that you understandably have in learning that something so beneficial and inexpensive could be ignored. In fact, the inexpensiveness and non-patentable nature are the precise reasons that CM was shelved. Medicine is big business; and the more suffering people do, the more money they spend. Well people don't fuel the medical economy.

Meanwhile, you can be assured that if a major drug company had patented CM, it would be plastered all over the media, just as Redux was. Within 2 years Redux made well over a dozen issues of *The Wall Street Journal* and *USA Today*. You have never seen anything that is non-prescription, regardless of whether it is more effective, get that much "free" (?) press. Or look at Enbrel, a new arthritis drug that costs $12,000 a year, is not that great in improving rheumatoid arthritis pain, and usually still has to be taken with methyltrexate, a form of chemotherapy that can trigger cancer years later. And since the main mechanism of action of Enbrel is in suppressing your own manufacture of tumor suppressor factor, how much more should this contribute to your raised risk of cancer in the future?

## How Does CM Work?

Back to CM, the more I learned about it, the more excited I got. It turns out that as I would expect with any fatty acid that goes to literally every cell in the body, it would have a wide range of beneficial effects. For years we have observed that the correction of a fatty acid deficiency can solve a myriad of symptoms, all depending on the deficiencies of the person. And the scientific literature confirms, as I'll show you later, that one type of fatty acid, omega-3 oils, has improved many types of arthritis and pain syndromes. Also omega-6 oils provide marked relief in another subset of sufferers. And as a side effect the "oil change" has cleared other seemingly unrelated symptoms in these folks.

For the benefits of the essential fatty acids of the omega-3 class are not limited to merely arthritis. If you are deficient in a fatty acid, then correcting it may improve your disease, regardless of its label, from depression, learning disability, ADD, migraines, or eczema, to asthma, colitis, PMS, heart diseases lupus, prostatitis, MS, hypertension, diabetes, cancer. More importantly, being low in essential fatty acids can accentuate abnormal inflammatory mechanisms that underlie pain. And the reverse is true: being disease-free is dependent upon having normal fatty acid levels.

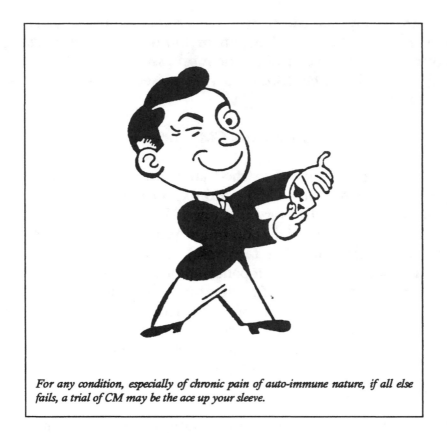

*For any condition, especially of chronic pain of auto-immune nature, if all else fails, a trial of CM may be the ace up your sleeve.*

Because CM is a fatty acid, that means it sits in cell membranes and regulates prostaglandin chemistry that in turn regulates inflammation and pain. That also means CM contributes to the structure of cell membrane receptors. Since the cell envelope is the docking site for allergens (like nightshades, as an example) that can turn on pain, they govern allergy through the release of cytokines and other chemicals from the cell that can cause pain. No wonder CM's uses were reported to extend far beyond arthritis to tough auto-immune diseases of a broad range.

Since this is not a book about other diseases, suffice to say that if I had any condition that had no known cause or cure, I would do a 2-3 month trial of CM, starting with one form and progressing every 4 months through a couple of different forms of CM, for they are not all equal.

## This Sounds Too Good To Be True

Since no one could show exactly how CM works, my skepticism was rising. So my next obvious step was to contact some purveyors of CM. I thought that with such an expensive product, they would not be willing to give me a few samples to evaluate on my patients, especially if it was not all it was cracked up to be. Not eagerly embracing the opportunity to show me how good it was would tell me in a flash whether the CM story was too good to be true. Also, I explained to them that I was writing my thirteenth book which was to be about pain. I rationalized that if CM was a hoax, they would not want the world to know about it nor to be part of any negative findings.

My fears were quelled when most companies I contacted enthusiastically embraced the opportunity to show how well their product worked and to get some free advertising. Most of the companies supplied me with product to evaluate on some of my toughest patients. They spent long hours explaining the products to me, pros and cons, and Mr. Klabin (CM Plus®), eager to reply, even returned my call from Italy. Convinced this was not a hoax, the fires of my enthusiasm were rekindled when the different products were sent to me to evaluate on a number of patients. Some companies were penny wise and pound foolish, only supplying a bottle or two. But CMO® and CM Plus® gave me enough to really evaluate a number of patients with severe pain.

As usual, God had provided me with a built-in Guinea pig system. Although I was more pain-free than I had been in decades due to the multitude of modalities I describe here, the fact is I had an underlying achiness that I had learned to tune out, since it paled in comparison to the intensity of pain I had endured in the past. Having broken or sprained my back over 6 times during 27 years of horse back riding, totaled 5 cars, plus dislocated my shoulder, breaking or spraining a few wrists, ankles 7 times, neck, knee, hand, fingers and toes, I had a bit of degenerative arthritis. Plus I was getting sloppy in my diet as I became healthier.

With much trepidation, I began to use the first product to arrive, CMO®. Slowly, but definitely within the first 3 weeks, my usual low level of stiffness and achiness that never left me for a moment, melted away. For example, when I got up in the middle of the night, my ankles were so stiff from so many previous sprains and daily pounding on the tennis courts, that I could barely walk. I looked like the Chinese ladies with decades of bound feet. I would stay up and work it out so there would be less to deal with in the morning. To my utter amazement, CMO® completely took this away.

Three months before I started the CMO®, I had had one of my worst ankle blowouts and fractured a foot bone as well. As fate would have it, 3 months after badly damaging my left ankle playing tennis, I did the same to the right (bowed legs, flat feet, improper technique and in need of lessons, playing with people more skilled than I, what do you want?). The amazing thing is that this 6th sprain was the fastest healing I had ever had in my life.

Granted, I was getting to be a pro at packing it in ice within 10 minutes of it blowing up, and having it up over my head for the rest of the day, immediate aspirin to reduce the inflammation, DMSO to improve the swelling distribution, detox enemas, carrot juicing, nutrients and more that you will learn about. But within 24 hours I was comfortably walking through airports with an Aircast Sport Stirrup® and in 48 hours was comfortably walking without anything on the ankle. This injury had resulted from the same type of torque as the others. Running backwards and jumping up for a high lob, I had literally come down with all my weight on a twisted ankle during tennis. I heard the machine gun-type rapid pops, snaps and cracks, and had an ankle three times its normal size within 5 minutes, which gradually turned various shades of blue and purple.

The only difference was this time I had been on CMO® for 2 months prior. By the second day of this break I had the usual black and blue discoloration of the whole foot where blood was spilled and leaked in between tissue compartments, but no where near the usual incapacitation. Within 4 weeks, I was playing tennis again (wearing the Aircast®), and regardless of residual swelling, had no pain (and, of course, was on no medications).

At the end of 2 more months of CMO®, my decades of chronic low-level back pain from perpetual over-doing was gone. You'll recall I had such enormous relief from the nightshade-free diet and other modalities you will learn about here, that I was able to tune out this residual pain. Compared with what I had endured, the residual was a piece of cake. Before the CMO® I was not even aware of it.... until it was gone! However this is not nearly as dramatic nor convincing as the results I have observed in others. Anyway, for me, as one person who for decades was accustomed to no days without pain, CMO® was 100% convincing.

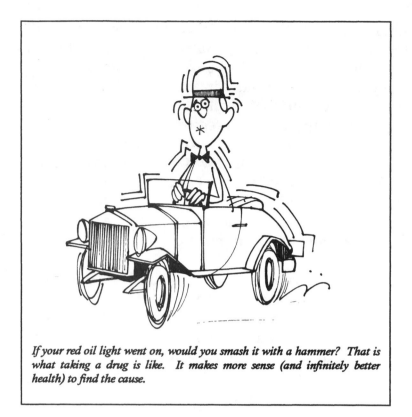

*If your red oil light went on, would you smash it with a hammer? That is what taking a drug is like. It makes more sense (and infinitely better health) to find the cause.*

Let's look at a few case examples. For my joy over what CMO® did for me pales in comparison to the thrill I had when it came through for one of my dearest patients. In her mid-seventies, she had endured the indescribable non-ceasing pain of rheumatoid arthritis for years. And although she was an extremely knowledgeable student of environmental medicine, she had no choice but to live on the chemotherapy drug used as last resort: methotrexate. She knew it would probably cause cancer one day, but the pain left her no choice. She began to use CMO® as well and within weeks was on the phone exuberant over the pain melting away.

A different CM product, called CM Plus®, produced equally impressive results. One middle-aged woman, a professional horse trainer, had much osteoarthritis from multiple injuries. Within less than a month she was already describing herself as having a vast 60% reduction in overall body pain for the first time ever.

Another young lady with decades of crippling rheumatoid arthritis and multiple surgeries to correct her deformities described herself as 95% pain-free after 3 months of CM Plus®. In fact the CM Plus® was a major factor in motivating her to endure further surgeries to improve her mobility, now that she had such surprisingly marked relief from her decades of pain.

Another older woman had had eleven years of a mysterious shoulder pain, that had stumped all of her specialists, disappear within weeks of starting CM Plus®.

There was no doubt in my mind that although not a cure for everyone, CMO® and CM Plus® had definitely worked their magic on over half the folks who had exhausted all that medicine had to offer. It got my attention.

Unfortunately, the field of CM is an unregulated jungle. There are products that contain no cetyl myristoleate and there are those that have no specified strength or assay on the bottle. There are formulations with intuited additions of other complementary fatty acids, and there are legal battles among manufacturers. But because there is definite benefit for the folks who need it, I cannot ignore it. And because all the CM products are different, and we are all different, I would evaluate several of the formulations if I had any condition that eluded cure. For the simple fact is that CM may turn out to be an unappreciated essential fatty acid deficiency for some individuals. And to go the rest of your life without correcting it when it has such enormous potential is silly.

## How CM is Supplied

Now comes the tricky part. When Dr. Diehl first discovered CM, he extracted it from the mice as the fatty acid differentiating the arthritis-resistant mice from the arthritis-prone rats. Obviously, it would be very expensive to consistently extract it from ground up mice. So he discovered how to synthesize it. This resulted in a pure CM (cetyl myristoleate) product, which was not actually pure CM, but a cetyl myristoleate fatty acid mix. When the patent for it expired, another company carried it on.

Now comes the tangled web. Currently over 25 companies sell CM. But they vary tremendously in source, dose, purity, additives, consistency of product, and method of synthesis or extraction. And many of the companies strongly disagree with the labeling claims of their competitors. It would take a giant research grant to untangle this web. CMO® and CM Plus® both had sufficient confidence in their products to send enough for multiple patients to evaluate. There is no question, they work dramatically for about half the people. In the other half it does nothing. But adding the nightshade-free diet, avoiding alcohol, and doing some of the many other things you will learn about here, should improve your odds even more.

The CMO® product does not state any milligrams of CM on the label (a major concern for me) and is supplied with a multi-digestive enzyme to facilitate the assimilation of CM. The Knollwood representative tells me that in spite of the

58

expense of the extraction procedure, if you say you read it in Dr. Sherry Rogers' book or newsletter, the price is discounted. As you will see, the prices and make-up of the CM products vary considerably and the prices are constantly changing. Check them out carefully.

CM Plus® is 12% CM. Cetyl oleate comprises 30-33% of the product and 10% of that has CM activity as well. CM Plus® contains 60 mg of CM in addition to other fatty acid esters, which might very well be synergistic with CM, meaning they do not dilute its effect, but make it stronger. It makes sense to keep a mixture of fatty acids with the CM as they occur in nature, as it would seem logical that they could contribute to its effectiveness.

CM Plus® is supplied with a bottle of synergistic factors to include glucosamine hydrochloride (not sulfate, the one that the actual double blind studies were done on), sea cucumber, hydrolyzed cartilage and MSM. These products are wonderfully synergistic with CM, as they further reduce inflammation and/or help to rebuild tissue.

CM Plus® has some other unique advantages that make it my number one choice. It has the benefit of a double blind study behind it. It also says "no solvents" on the label, and was better tolerated than other products by some of my extremely chemically sensitive patients. Some of the other forms did have an extremely noxious solvent odor and taste. The manufacturer states it is made from a vegetable (palm kernel oil) source and contains no animal products.

True CMO is labeled cetyl myristoleate extract (fatty acid complex) 760 mg and accompanied by an independent laboratory assay. It is a concentrated extract of the fatty acid cerasomal-cis-9-cetyl myristoleate from natural bovine source.

A fourth form of CM is inappropriately called CM-Pure®. It is made from a vegetarian source, and is herbicide and pesticide-free. This one actually does not contain any CM, but related fatty acid cetyl esters and myristic acid, instead of cetyl myristoleate. Although I did not receive enough to evaluate folks with arthritis, it has been particularly helpful for some tough asthmatics.

To complicate matters, another company, DNA Pacifica, says they had the original Dr. Diehl's product, which was backed by studies on rheumatoid arthritis. When the patent expired a few years ago, Dr. Diehl stopped contracting to have CM made for him, but they carried it on.

Dr. Diehl reformulated his original CM product, and applied for his second patent. This time through additional research, the product was passed not only for use in rheumatoid arthritis, but osteoarthritis as well, and he published a study on this. This is the most expensive form, sold as Myristin®.

Since his death in 1999, Dr. Diehl's daughter and son-in-law carry on distribution of myristin through EHP Products. Myristin® contains 260 mg CM, 260 mg cetyl oleate, and 130 mg of other esters. The purest and highest dose of CM is patented Myristin®. Because it is also the most expensive, you may elect to see if you are among the lucky ones who heal with the less concentrated forms first. Since it has a strong laboratory or solvent odor, I would not dare recommend it for my chemically sensitive patients and did not dare try it myself, although I am not even 1/100th as chemically sensitive as I was a couple of decades ago.

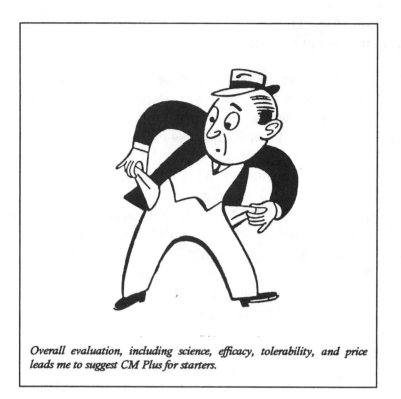

*Overall evaluation, including science, efficacy, tolerability, and price leads me to suggest CM Plus for starters.*

Chuck Cohran, D.C., who wrote the popular booklet about CM, recommends Everlasting® (by Integris) which is 275 mg of CM complex, not stating the breakdown of the complex.

Which one would I take? I took CMO® because the opportunity to evaluate that one arose first. It worked for me and many others. Then when I received samples of CM Plus® to evaluate on patients, I found this worked as well in a significant proportion of folks, and was more affordable. Interestingly, as different as the products are, they all have their share of very enticing successes. And I have not seen one side effect or adverse reaction. Does it work for everyone? No. Have I had an opportunity to try all of them on any one person? No.

But you can be sure that if I had serious problems, I would give several of them a solo 3-4 month evaluation, especially for pain unresponsive to the nightshade-free diet or for auto-immune disease. It makes sense to start with CM Plus®, hoping that your body also needs the accessory esters to compliment one another. The 3 forms, CMO®, CM Plus®, and TRUE CMO® are the ones that were most liberal with samples and eager to back up their products. As a result, I saw the most startling results with these diverse products. And when it works, be prepared to take it again in 2-5 years, or a small weekly maintenance dose indefinitely. For contrary to what some manufacturers claim, it does wear off in some folks, but they clear after taking it again.

The bottom line is that each of the products, as diverse as they are, in supplying a "non-essential" fatty acid to people with various "incurable" problems, has produced some very therapeutic results. This should not be ignored just because we cannot fully explain it. After all, for the majority of medications in the *PDR* (*Physician's Desk Reference*, a book of all prescription drugs), when it comes to the mechanism of action, most state "mechanism of action is unknown". So when potent, side effect-laden prescription drugs do not even require our understanding how they work, why should non-prescription nutrients derived from nature and without side effects be subject to more stringent requirements?

By the way I would love to hear the results that readers get from this interesting orphan nutrient, but please be sure to specify which product you used and where you purchased it. We are still in the midst of evaluating them, and results depend upon the biochemical needs and allergies of each individual. One aspect of it that makes comparative studies difficult it that if one form clears your symptoms, then you have annihilated any chance of seeing if another form would also have worked just as well or not at all.

Whichever products you try, be sure to do many of the other procedures that are written about in this book. I for one would not even think of putting someone on CM if they had not first been nightshade-free for at least one month. I would also assess their hidden nutrient deficiencies, leaky gut, and xenobiotic (foreign chemical) overload: all the things that you will learn about that could keep anyone from healing indefinitely. These products are not cheap, so you need to do as much as possible to assure their success.

I would try CM for any condition, especially auto-immune, diseases for which nothing else has worked, and arthritic diseases controlled by dangerous drugs, like methotrexate. I am amazed that many rheumatoid arthritis patients, do not know that methyltrexate, which they have been on for years, is a form of chemotherapy and has the distinct potential of causing cancer in them years down the road.

Meanwhile, I respect the reluctance of providers of CM-type products in providing more precise information about the exact nature of their products. For they do have their proprietary interests to protect. I do know they have enough belief in their products, as different as they are, to stand by them and allow them to be subjected to scrutiny. We have not yet finished evaluating all of them, but have enough patient feedback to know that the enthusiasm and claims are justified. The secret should be shared.

Having been impressed with the individuals from many of these companies and subsequently the uniqueness of their products, I look forward to reporting further details in our subsequent newsletters. For the fact is, an individual could require a nightshade-free diet (previous chapter) as well as CM to clear his arthritis pain. In addition, if he were only on one form of CM but really excelled on a different preparation, he might come to the erroneous conclusion that it did not work.

At the end of this chapter, I have spelled out the contrasting ingredient descriptions for the products, complete with the toll-free numbers.

### How to Take CM

As with anything new, start with one a day. Then in a day or two, take one twice a day. Then progress to two twice a day. You may even want to go to three twice a day. Some folks get just as good results within a month by cycling one week on the CM and 1-2 weeks off. It takes time and extra nutrients to incorporate the fatty acid into the body chemistry, so you might as well conserve money and let your chemistry catch up. And for this reason I would add a multiple vitamin-mineral like Tyler's Multiplex-1 Without Iron®. And as with all forms of CM, always have some sort of digestive enzymes (pancreatic especially) to facilitate digestion of the fatty acids. Some forms already have a companion enzyme preparation.

If there was no difference after 2-4 months, I would suggest you try another form or get the rest of your nutrient load and total load addressed (that I will explain later). For all diseases can potentially benefit from restoration of proper fatty acid balance.

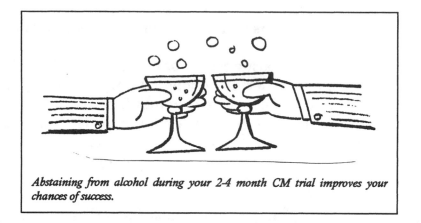

*Abstaining from alcohol during your 2-4 month CM trial improves your chances of success.*

It is important when using any nutrient that you have high hopes for, to maximize your success in as many ways as possible. In folks for whom CM did not work initially, but did later, they gave us clues as to what can be done to assure future successes. Some had insufficient pancreatic enzymes, others failed to avoid nightshades, or had interfering drugs, alcohol, undiscovered food allergies or liver problems. To maximize success, have no alcohol, junk foods, nightshades, foods to which you are allergic, tobacco, coffee, chocolate, citrus, and be sure to eat a healthful diet. In other words, when trying to heal the impossible why not maximize your chances of success by fostering healing in as many ways as possible?

Also take bone-building, inflammation-fighting supplements that will be discussed in later chapters that include some or all of the following: sea cucumber, Glucosamine Sulfate (Tyler or Enzymatic Therapy/PhytoPharmica or Thorne), hydrolyzed Bovine Cartilage (Klabin or Pure Encapsulations), MSM (Pain & Stress Center or Jarrow), detox enemas, and more. And have the CM on an empty stomach, with no food in the stomach that could compete with its absorption for 1 hour before or after. Some of the products also feature companion bone builders that include many of these agents.

Of note, there is an opposite school of thought for failures that says you would be better off having CM after a meal when maximum secretion of digestive enzymes has occurred, and a load of food would slow the transit time (impede whizzing it through the bowel too fast), promoting even more absorption. Obviously if you cannot tolerate it on an empty stomach, this would also be an option for you.

One other caveat: within 3-5 days there may be a worsening of pain. That is a good sign, although not a necessary sign. Try to stick with it; if you cannot, back off for a few days and restart. Aside from slight nausea (also possibly from the companion digestant), we have not yet seen adverse effects.

The good news is that after 3-6 months, folks who get relief from pain often no longer need any CM. It appears to be curative once the deficiency is corrected. However, I have observed that often folks need to take it again in 2-4 years; most likely it was metabolized out.

In order to further maximize the prospect of a CM product working for you, I suggest the following:

1.  Get a CDSA (Great Smokies Lab, see chapters 4 and 9). This test determines whether you have sufficient digestive enzymes. At the same time, you can get an Intestinal Permeability Test (also Great Smokies Lab, directions in next chapter) to determine if you have malabsorption or a damaged or leaky gut as commonly occurs from years of pain medications (next chapter). You will increase the chances of CM working for you if you make sure that you have a healthy well-functioning gut. If your digestive

system lacks enzymes or is leaky, you won't be able to assimilate CM, even if it might have helped you.

2. Do a nightshade-free diet before and during the time you are taking CM to be sure it is not an additional factor causing your arthritis. Most folks get better results if they also avoid citrus, alcohol, caffeine and processed foods. This can actually leave you with a very healing macrobiotic diet of whole pure foods.

3. If you postpone step 1, at least take 1-2 digestive enzymes like Biogest (Thorne), Wobenzyme (Pain & Stress Center), Total-Gest (Klabin, N.E.E.D.S.), InflaZyme (American Biologics) or Pancreatin (ARG, Klaire) with each dose of CM to facilitate absorption. Some products are supplied with their own digestives, in which case you would not need additional digestive aids.

4. Consider other supportive supplements like Glucosamine Sulfate and MSM, which I'll describe in Chapter 5. Some suppliers smartly supply these as a companion to CM.

5. Slowly build up to the maximum tolerated recommended dose of the product, preferably on an empty stomach if you tolerate it. If you cannot build, you may even benefit from a persistently lower dose. However, if you are stuck on a lower dose, you might decide to skip trying to save money with the "week on and 1-2 week off" cycle in order to bring yourself up to top corrective dose sooner.

6. As with everything in life, there is much variability when it comes to individual biochemistry. However, I definitely would not omit the nightshade-free diet.

# Are You Due For An Oil Change?

Trans fatty acids are hidden in foods as part of hydrogenated soybean or vegetable oils. No question we are part of the 3rd generation of man to have eaten a lifetime of trans fatty acids in the form of hydrogenated grocery store oils, margarines and shortenings. These oils have been exposed to abnormally high temperatures that have made them resistant to getting rancid. In the process, this chemical manipulation has stripped them of their beneficial vitamins that protect the cell membrane, like vitamin E. The reason this high temperature makes them resistant to rancidity and aging is because there is so little nutritional value remaining that it will not support fungal or bacterial life. If the bugs don't want it, should you?

Furthermore, this abnormally high temperature has caused a twist in the molecule that makes it behave adversely once it has been incorporated into cell membranes, making it a major contributor to arteriosclerosis, cancer, arthritis, accelerated aging and other diseases. And they are difficult to avoid, as it is a rare factory food or fast food that does not contain these trans fatty acids disguised as hydrogenated oils.

To determine if you have too many trans fatty acids damaging your membrane chemistry and promoting the chemistry of pain, have your physician order an essential fatty acid analysis (MetaMetrix or Great Smokies Diagnostic Laboratory). This test also shows whether you are deficient in other fatty acids, like DGLA. This can be supplemented with borage oil or Efamol's Evening Primrose Oil (Emerson Ecologics). And if you are deficient in omega-3 oil, Cod Liver Oil (Carlson), Eskimo-3 (Tyler, Prevail) or Flax Oil (Spectrum, N.E.E.D.S.) will correct this.

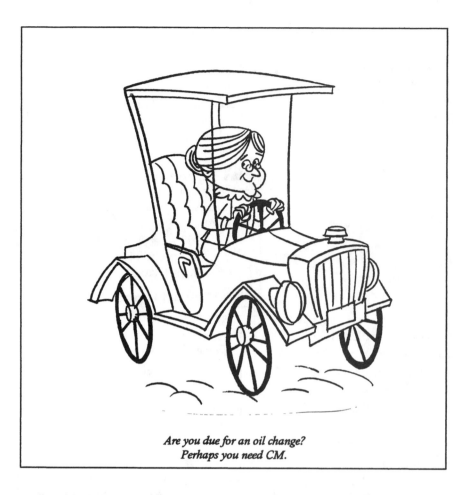

*Are you due for an oil change?*
*Perhaps you need CM.*

For many folks, an oil change to incorporate the missing fatty acid is what it took for them to correct and turn off the abnormal production of pain-triggering chemicals from the deficient cell membranes. And most important, incorporating cetyl myristoleate into cell envelopes has turned off enormous pain and disease.

# Cetyl Myristoleate Products

Longevity Science/
Klabin Marketing
2067 Broadway,
Ste 700
NY, NY 10023
1-800-933-9440
(212)-877-3632

**CM-Plus®**

60 mg cetyl myristoleate and cetyl oleate 125 mg, plus cetyl myristate 75 mg in a base of mixed fatty acid esters and olive oil; vegetable source, no solvents

**CM-Plus Support Formula**

Knollwood Inc.
2250 E. Tropicana
Ste 19-321
Las Vegas NV 89119
1-800-249-7816
1-800-829-1514

**CMO®**

100% cetyl myristoleate, but no precise number of mg specified)

**CMO Support Formula**

Jarrow Formulas, Inc.
1824 S Robertson Blvd
Los Angeles Ca 90035-4317
1-800-726-0886
fax: 800-890-8955

**True CMO**

cetyl myristoleate extract (fatty acid complex) 760 mg

EHP Products Inc.
P.O.Box 1306
Ashland KY 41105
1-888-EHP-0100
www.cetylmyristoleate.com
myristin@wwd.net

**Myristin®**

260 mg cetyl myristoleate, 260 mg cetyl oleate, 130 mg other oleates

**Myrist-Aid** (support formula)

Integris Corporation
Irving TX 75063
1-888-737-7307
www.integriscorp.com

**Everlasting®**

275 mg cetyl myristoleate complex

**Everlasting Support**

BioVita International
P.O.Box 768
Manson WA 98831
1-800-467-7810
also
DNA Pacifica
148-1 No. El Camino Real
Enchinitas CA 92024-2849
1-760-632-5382

| **Myristin®** |
|---|
| 265 mg cetyl myristoleate, 265 mg cetyl oleate, 110 mg cetyl esters |

## Mechanism and Science for Physicians

Unfortunately, no one knows precisely how cetyl myristoleate works. Because it is intimately intertwined in incorporating fatty acids into the cell membrane, I would strongly recommend 1 tsp. of Phos Chol Concentrate® a day (see *Depression Cured At Last!* for explanation and voluminous references on this unique and indispensable American Lecithin Co. product). In addition, include the associated nutrients outlined in Chapter 8 in order to assure best results.

CM is a fatty acid ester (actually the cetyl alcohol ester of the 14-carbon chain fatty acid myristoleic acid). Some of the CM products were cerasomal cis-9 cetyl myristoleate, an analog of cetyl myristoleate. Other manufacturers actually started with myristic acid, a saturated analog of myristoleic acid, which upon esterification with cetyl alcohol produces cetyl myristate, not cetyl myristoleate. Yet they are marketed as forms of CM.

To compound the issue, some lower percentage products worked better than those with higher percentages of CM, and some combinations of fatty acids are synergistic while others seem inhibitive. Furthermore, some reported analyses with GC-FID (gas chromatography-flame ionization detection) contained less CM than was stated on the label. And don't bother looking for a product that is 100% pure product, for no such thing exists, although, I'm not sure we need it anyway.

One of the products I investigated does not contain actual cetyl myristoleate and the others vary in the amount and quality they contain relative to one another. Yet all seem to share therapeutic benefits, although varying and unpredictable. Therefore, I suspect that myristoylation is only part of the mechanism. Being a rare but most likely unrecognized essential fatty acid for cell membranes, it has a seemingly infinite number of ways in which it can control cell behavior.

For example, the process of N-myristoylation is so important in anchoring proteins to cell membranes that the N-myristoyl group has been called **"the docking protein"**. Protein attachments to cell membranes are what membrane signaling transduction is all about. Cell membranes, analogous to the computer keyboard from which all cell communications emanate, control everything from the

- genetic messages from the intracellular **nucleus,**
- cellular communications from the **golgi apparatus**, and
- energy synthesis from within the **mitochondria** to
- synthesis and release of membrane extracellular chemical mediators that control messages governing inflammation and pain, as well as **hormone and antigen receptors** on the cell **surface membrane**.

Another interesting fact is that the N-myristyolation of some body peptides has reversed resistance to chemotherapy.
Because of its extensive effects on the body, the therapeutic benefits of CM, which extend to many conditions like auto-

immune diseases, may possibly include cancers. As an example, IP6 (Enzymatic Therapy), another cell membrane anchor, has caused cancer cells to stop growing and even to revert (redifferentiate) to normal cells.

## Message in a Nutshell

No matter what symptom you have, but especially if you have chronic pain, you may benefit enormously from "an oil change". By incorporating CM into cell membranes, along with a total load program, many have surprisingly terminated their pain within 3-4 months and no longer needed any further CM, at least for several years.

## Chapter 4

## Healing From the Inside Out

### Pain Medications Destroy Bone
### And Create New Diseases

When pain grabs your attention, your first response may be to "Reach for Aleve" as the TV commercial says. What medicine chest, gym bag or purse does not contain one of these magic pain relievers? And if pain reaches staggering heights, your doctor can then prescribe even stronger variations of the same family of drugs. For the number one drug for pain management is actually not one drug but a **category of drugs** called non-steroidal anti-inflammatory drugs or **NSAIDs** for short (pronounced as "en' sAyds"). These include over-the-counter medicines like Advil, Aleve, Motrin (ibuprofen), Naprosyn, Orudis and much more. They also include the prescription drugs of Indocin, Tolectin, Lodine, Feldene, Clinoril, Anaprox, Toradol, Nalfon, Voltaren, Celebrex, Vioxx, and much more.

How do these work? The same way that aspirin, the charter member of this category of drugs, works. In fact, some say with tongue in cheek that NSAIDs does not stand for non-steroidal anti-inflammatory drugs, but *"a new sort of aspirin in disguise"*.

Since aspirin is over a hundred years old, there is no patent on it. Hence, scientists have had to learn how to attach little chemical groups to the side of aspirin, creating synthetic mimics that automatically become "new" entities, patentable, and for which they can charge whatever the market will bear. Unfortunately on the whole, these *dressed up aspirin molecules* are often not that much more effective than aspirin, and most are much more toxic over the long haul. Some will brag that they do not cause as much gastric irritation as aspirin, but I consider the side effect a natural warning meant to urge us to limit our drug use and instead find the root cause of our suffering.

The NSAID category of drugs is what we call in medicine *cyclooxygenase inhibitors*. All that means is they turn down or moderate inflammatory chemistry so that we do not hurt so much. It is sort of like driving along the highway and seeing the red oil light of your car go on. If you smash it with a hammer that is analogous to taking the NSAIDs. You haven't done a thing to get to the root of your problem; you've done nothing to refill the oil reservoir, and so you are headed for disaster as the oil reaches an engine-damaging, fatal level.

The same thing happens with NSAIDs. They don't do a thing to restore function or enable you to find the cause of your chronic pain and inflammation, but they do have pretty nasty side effects. They can cause *fatal liver and kidney damage, fatal hemorrhage from the bowel, as well as irreparable damage to vision.* What is more astounding is that they **actually cause bone to deteriorate.** And the longer they are taken, the more bone they destroy, with the unsuspecting victim accumulating more *osteoporosis* and osteopenia.

NSAIDs can also *be addicting* and keep the pain cycle active. That has been shown in migraine cases where the more medication people used, the less able they were to discontinue it. So they were eventually always on pain medication and always in pain. However, four days after detoxifying the addicting NSAID medication (chapter 6), people got over the withdrawal and they astoundingly found that they no longer had as much pain.

Furthermore, NSAIDs have been implicated in promoting and accelerating a multitude of diseases, like **heart failure**. Over 20% of folks in heart failure have a long history of NSAID use for joint problems. The problem is that inflammation protects the heart from our daily chemical assaults in our air, food and water. If we turn it off, we allow the heart to burn out prematurely, which is exactly what occurs.

But it is assumed that heart failure is just something that happens to us without a correctable cause. In fact it is so under-recognized that if you were given a choice between cancer and heart failure, you would probably naively pick that over cancer any day. But as nasty as cancer statistics are (over 50% are dead in 5-10 years after diagnosis), heart failure is even worse. More people get it each year than get cancer and they die sooner from it (mean survival 5 years) (see article by Dr. Page, in reference section).

But what is worse is that studies also show that NSAIDs generally give their maximum relief from pain during the first 2-4 months of use. After that the pain relief dwindles off and in some cases disappears. This is what leads people to seek stronger doses, switch medications or resort to other medications and prescriptions of different categories of drugs.

## How the Sick Get Sicker, Quicker

One of the worst parts of the NSAIDs, however, is that they can cause the *leaky gut syndrome*. This causes large spaces to develop between the cells in the gut lining. These large spaces between cells inhibit the normal function of the gut.

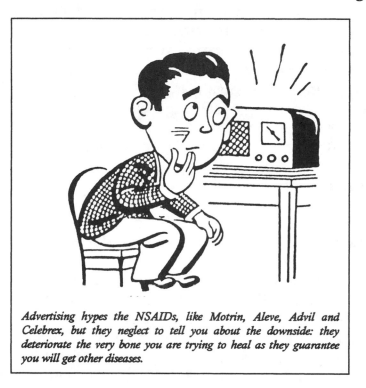

*Advertising hypes the NSAIDs, like Motrin, Aleve, Advil and Celebrex, but they neglect to tell you about the downside: they deteriorate the very bone you are trying to heal as they guarantee you will get other diseases.*

When the normal function of the gut is disrupted and damaged, one of the nasty results is that you no longer absorb the minerals and other nutrients you need to completely heal injured areas. Nor are you able to manufacture the chemistry of energy or synthesize enough of the "happy hormones" in the brain to make you joyful. For the inflamed gut or intestinal lining no longer produces the healthy carrier proteins that actively carry or transport crucial minerals across the gut wall into the blood stream, so necessary for health maintenance and healing.

## The Gut Leaks Toxins That Cause
## Fibromyalgia and Arthritis

If that were not enough, **the leaky gut** then leads to a landslide of symptoms throughout the whole body. First the leaky gut allows **nasty toxins** from the gut into the blood stream. These then **go to muscles** and cause achiness and pain, as seen in fibromyalgia. Or leaking gut toxins can damage the chemistry of cell organelles called mitochondria where energy is manufactured for the entire body and which determine the aging rate of the body. Hence, toxins from the leaky gut can cause fibromyalgia, chronic fatigue, and accelerated aging.

In addition, gut toxins overload the ability of the detoxification system to gobble up everyday toxins from our air, food and water, since these pathways are now busy dealing with the overload from bowel toxins instead. The result is the loss of the ability to detoxify everyday chemicals that never presented a problem before. Now suddenly the odor of perfumes, smoke, cleansers, new carpet or paints make the person sick. The innocent victim is labeled chemically sensitive by the knowledgeable and a neurotic hypochondriac by the unknowledgeable.

The problem is that this is only the beginning of chemical sensitivity, for **half of the detox capability of the body lies in the lining of the gut.** As it becomes progressively more inflamed and damaged from NSAID use, further detox capability is lost, so the victim is even less able to detoxify things that formerly never bothered him. He and his friends begin to doubt his sanity when they do not understand how he could have changed overnight. They are insulted when one day he tolerates their perfume or after-shave and the next day he is violently complaining about headaches and spaciness from it. And all the while he is setting himself up for an avalanche of symptoms that could result in chronic pain problems or even cancer.

## The Leaky Gut Causes Food Allergies

And this is far from the end of the damage that can occur from NSAIDs as they precipitate an avalanche of new symptoms, sometimes almost monthly. For the large spaces now allow large food particles access to the blood stream that were never allowed there before. Large food particles can slip through the leaky gut right into the circulatory system.

When the immune system's surveillance team sees these new food particles that it has never seen before, it launches an attack against these invaders by making protective antibodies to gobble up and destroy the food antigens. For after all, this is the reason for the existence of the immune system, to protect us from foreign invaders.

The problem is these food antigens are not virulent viruses or bacteria, but the building blocks of our bodies. And since these foods are the building blocks of the body, they have antigenic sites on them that also resemble antigenic sites on some of our body parts. So when the guard dog antigens (the police force of the blood stream) are flowing through the blood, they mistakenly attack our own tissues.

While searching for foreign invaders, our antibodies come across antigens they have been trained to attack like certain large food particles that leaked through the damaged gut. But they also stumble upon sites, for example, in our knee cartilage that resemble the potato and begin to attack that. This is one way that nightshade allergy can be borne overnight or insidiously sneak into your life over many years.

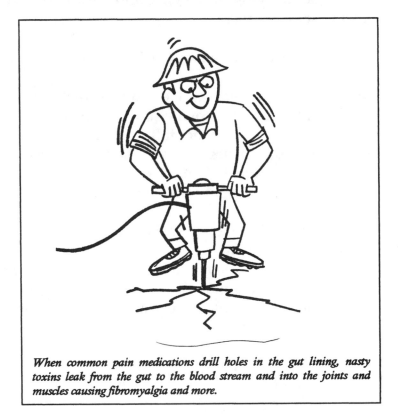

*When common pain medications drill holes in the gut lining, nasty toxins leak from the gut to the blood stream and into the joints and muscles causing fibromyalgia and more.*

To recap, larger than normal food particles pass through the leaky or damaged gut and float into the blood stream. Here the immune system police force, that makes antibodies against any foreign invaders, makes antibodies to latch onto invading food antigens. The antigen-antibody complexes lay down wherever they please. If the similar site is on the knee joint, the antigen (food) and antibody (immune system policing cell) join together forming an antigen-antibody complex. This then latches onto the knee tissue, and it turns on the chemistry of inflammation. Chemicals released into the knee tissue from this reaction result in a red hot, swollen and immensely painful knee.

Hence, we suddenly have arthritis resulting from the inflammatory reaction every time we eat potato. As you can begin to appreciate, **sudden food allergy can happen in any one at any time to any food.** But since potato never bothered us before, that is the last culprit we suspect as part of or all of the cause of our pain. And when the authoritarian physician tells us that everyone our age has arthritis, our sigh of relief at having no power over or responsibility for our pain ends the search for a cause.

## The Vicious Cycle of Escalating Diseases is Triggered by Medications

But the torture is hardly over. For the leaky gut does more than initiate arthritis; it can not only *perpetuate* it, but also *initiate* any *other disease* you can think of. For once the gut gets leaky, it can not only cause chemical and food sensitivity, chronic fatigue and fibromyalgia, but auto-immune diseases like lupus, thyroiditis, rheumatoid arthritis, diabetes, myocarditis, and multiple sclerosis. And recall that the more you hurt, the more NSAIDs you take; but NSAIDs are one of the principal causes of the leaky gut to begin with.... the very substance that initiated this *avalanche* of seemingly unrelated symptoms. No wonder *the sick get sicker.*

By continuing to take NSAIDs, you *perpetuate* disease and even stimulate the *worsening* of symptoms, which then necessitates stronger and newer medications to control the

81

pain.    Hence, once you begin medications, you begin a *downward cycle* of new symptoms and an ever-increasing array of medications; a veritable domino syndrome.

*For not only does the gut lining house half the detoxification system, but half the immune system.*    Since these are damaged, now you start having more infections, requiring more antibiotics that kill off the good bugs in the gut and cause even more inflammation in the gut lining through overgrowth of yeasts like *Candida albicans*.  This normally harmless yeast can cause any symptom you can think of from depression and brain fog to bizarre total body aches and pains as it further inflames the gut lining.

You soon have a pocket full of pills and a stable full of specialists, each vying for your medical dollar, but none helping you find the causes of your pain so you can be medication-free, symptom-free, and doctor-free.  And all the while NSAIDs are causing this relentless cascade of symptoms, they are also deteriorating your bones!

### Gut Level Medicine:
### The Leaky Gut Syndrome Triggers Depression

By now it should not surprise you to realize that if the colon or the gut is not healthy then the rest of the body cannot be. For this is where all food and healing nutrients are absorbed. Furthermore, if the gut becomes damaged or leaky, then it allows bacterial products of putrefaction and toxins to get into the bloodstream.  These not only make people achy with inflamed tissues and tender trigger points, but also tired and depressed.  These toxins can then leak into the brain and damage enzymes that would have made more happy hormones or neurotransmitters of upbeat mood.

In turn, these undetoxified chemicals back up in the system and can also lead to further achiness, fatigue and depression. So by having a sick or leaky gut, you accentuate not only pain but also depression by many different pathways or routes. You are on a roll; embroiled in the vicious cycle that not only perpetuates but escalates symptoms. But the unknowledgeable assume that the depression is just the result of hurting, or vice versa. They never connect the two as being the result of the same pathology or process in the body. To learn more about the depression, read my book *Depression Cured At Last!*

## The Gut Connection to All Disease

The purpose of the gastrointestinal tract (gut) is multi-fold.
(1) It digests food into small easily absorbed particles,
(2) *absorbs* small food particles to then be converted into energy,
(3) *attaches* nutrients like vitamins and minerals to carrier proteins which then transport them across the gut lining into the bloodstream,
(4) *detoxifies* the chemicals we daily imbibe through our air, food and water, as it contains a major part of the chemical detoxification system of the body which protects us from cancer and all other diseases, and
(5) *fights* off infection, as it contains over half of the immune system which synthesizes immuno-globulins or antibodies that act as the first line of defense against infection, cancer and other diseases.

The leaky gut syndrome is an extremely common problem, yet is seldom tested for. It can be asymptomatic with no intestinal symptoms, or cause any degree and combination of gas and bloating with alternating diarrhea or constipation, or just plain *mysterious body pain*. It is the reason that many will never heal any further. For if the gut is not totally healthy, you have no chance of healing anything else, regardless of the label on your condition. It doesn't matter what type of chronic pain you have, or if you have high blood pressure, multiple sclerosis, prostatitis, cancer, or merely accelerated aging. *You are stuck until the gut is healed.*

This leaky or hyperpermeable intestinal lining might sound like a good thing, that it would enable the body to absorb more amino acids, essential fatty acids, minerals and vitamins. Nutrients could slip right on into the gut. Sadly the opposite is true. For in order for the body to absorb a mineral, a carrier protein must be attached. This protein must hook onto the mineral that actively carries it across the gut wall into the bloodstream.

But when the bowel lining is damaged through inflammation, not only can nutrient **carrier proteins get damaged,** but **also** the finger-like projections that line the gut and allow us to absorb food. When these get destroyed, the result is **malabsorption.** So in addition to new food and chemical allergies and auto-immune diseases, the leaky gut victim may develop mineral and vitamin deficiencies, even in spite of taking adequate levels of them. He would be lucky to get away with only a symptom or two, for *nutrient deficiencies are at the beginning of all disease!*

### Bugs, Drugs, Food and Mood Damage the Gut

What can cause the inflammation that leads to the leaky gut syndrome? Examples include:

(1) Abnormal gut bugs, called flora (e.g., unwanted bacteria, parasites, and protozoa from contaminated food and water, and overgrowth of yeasts like Candida from antibiotics)

(2) Chemicals that irritate the gut (e.g. ingested alcohol and food additives or inhaled toluene or formaldehyde from that new carpet or paint, and of course, NSAIDs)

(3) Food irritants and allergens (e.g. eating things that you know bother you and processed foods with their long list of mysterious chemical ingredients)

(4) Emotions like anger and worry (which dump stress hormones into the system and cause loss of protective nutrients)

(5) Genetic and acquired enzyme deficiencies (e.g. lactose deficiency and celiac disease), and more.

You might say the causes are **bugs, drugs, food, and mood!**

For example, when people take antibiotics they are at risk of developing overgrowth of antibiotic-resistant yeast or fungi (e.g. Candida is one type that I'll tell you more about). In many instances of fibromyalgia, merely treating the Candida overgrowth has resulted in total clearing of disease that had existed for years.

Likewise, antibiotics can cause overgrowth of a bacterium, *Clostridia difficile* that can cause relentless colitis with diarrhea. This, too, can lead to inflammation and leaky gut. From the leaky gut you can get fibromyalgia, so in essence an antibiotic can usher in undiagnosable or seemingly untreatable and mysterious pain syndromes.

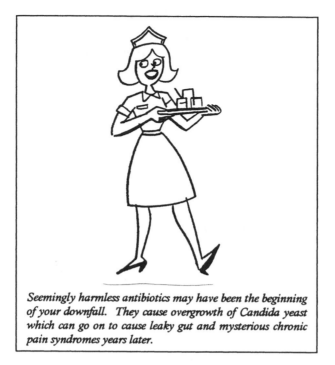

*Seemingly harmless antibiotics may have been the beginning of your downfall. They cause overgrowth of Candida yeast which can go on to cause leaky gut and mysterious chronic pain syndromes years later.*

And you can get nasty bugs from a myriad of sources. For example, many municipal or city waters contain Cryptosporidium, while eggs and any foods can be contaminated with a variety of bacteria from Salmonella, *E. Coli*, Listeria, or *Giardia lamblia* to Klebsiella, Citrobacter or *Helicobacter pylori*. Many more things cause leaky gut that in turn causes fibromyalgia and you can learn much more about the course, diagnosis and treatment from my book *No More Heartburn* (250 pg., 350 references).

**To review, the inflamed leaky gut:**

- does **not absorb nutrients** and foods properly, so fatigue and bloating can occur.

- allows large food antigens into the blood steam so **food allergies** and new symptoms are created (e.g., arthritis, fibromyalgia, etc.).
- results in damaged **carrier proteins,** so malabsorption and nutrient deficiencies occur. These can cause any symptom (e.g., magnesium deficiency-induced muscle spasms or body pain as in chronic back pain or angina, or copper deficiency-induced high cholesterol are just a few examples).
- overloads detoxification pathways, resulting in **chemical sensitivity** with brain fog, or feeling spacey, dizzy, dopey, unable to concentrate. Other times it can be other organ symptoms, including pain in places of previous injury. Undetoxified natural gas from the heating system or formaldehyde from the office carpet, for example, can back up and precipitate severe pain in old back injury sites. Furthermore, the leakage of toxins overburdens the liver so that the body is less able to detoxify all the everyday chemicals we breathe, encouraging their backlog and buildup in muscles and joints.
- damages the protective coating of your own gut antibodies, the secretory IgA. Once this is lost, the body is more vulnerable to **infections** in the intestines from bacteria, protozoa, viruses and yeasts (e.g., Candida). This overgrowth of unwanted bugs, called **intestinal dysbiosis,** further inflames the gut, creating a vicious cycle.
- allows translocation or passage of bacteria and yeast (there are hundreds of species in the intestine) from the gut cavity directly into the bloodstream where they set up infection anywhere, including muscles, joints, bones, teeth roots, coronary arteries, or even the brain.
- is responsible for **auto-antibodies.** Auto-immune diseases like rheumatoid arthritis, lupus arthritis, dermatomyositis,

multiple sclerosis, myocarditis, iritis, diabetes and thyroiditis are some of the members of this ever-growing category of mysterious "incurable" diseases.

Now you can begin to appreciate another mechanism for how the **sick get sicker** when the real cause of symptoms is merely masked by drugs and not looked for. For if the leaky gut is chalked up to *"irritable bowel disease"* or *"spastic colon"* or *"nervous colon"*, as it often is, the victim is on the fast road to further illnesses. And the last thing the person in pain needs is another disease. Clearly, years of pain that bounces from one joint to another, can all start with innocently taking NSAIDs for pain.

---

*CAUSES OF LEAKY GUT:*

- Intestinal dysbiosis (Candida, etc.)
- Medications (**NSAIDs**, antibiotics, etc.)
- Food allergy
- Chemical sensitivity
- Celiac disease, malabsorption
- Auto-immune disease
- Digestive insufficiencies
- Poor diet
- Nutritional deficiencies, and much more

---

BUT THE LEAKY GUT CAUSES:

- Food allergy
- Chemical sensitivity
- Brain fog/toxic encephalopathy
- Auto-immune disease (RA*, etc.)
- Nutritional deficiencies
- Labelitis (CFS*, FM*, etc.)
- IBS*
- Depression
- Chronic pain syndromes and more

  * RA = rheumatoid arthritis
  * CFS = chronic fatigue syndrome
  *FM = fibromyalgia
  * IBS = irritable bowel syndrome

## Common Scenario for Leaky Gut

An otherwise healthy person might take an antibiotic for a sore throat. The antibiotic not only goes to the throat, but also through the entire system, killing off beneficial bacteria that normally inhabit the intestines. When these bacteria are killed, the normally antibiotic-resistant fungi that remain in the gut have no competition. This uninhibited overgrowth results in an imbalance of yeast, which inflames the gut, producing the leaky gut syndrome.

From here, leaking food antigens can create new food allergies with arthritis, headaches, asthma or any symptom. Toxins leak in also, causing muscle and joint pain. The victim usually also starts having gas, bloating, pain, alternating diarrhea and constipation, which is often labeled "irritable bowel syndrome" or "spastic colon". In fact, it is actually a cover-up for the honest answer, "We don't know why you have gas, bloating, and indigestion, and we never look for Candida, leaky gut, or other environmental and nutritional causes". As the leaky gut progresses, the carrier proteins get damaged, there is poorer absorption of minerals, leading to fatigue, inability to concentrate, multiple chemical sensitivities, depression, more muscle spasms, more painful joints, and an avalanche of other symptoms.

So what do people do who have arthritis, asthma, brain fog, chronic fatigue, chemical sensitivities, headaches, depression, chronic sinusitis or asthma, irritable bowel, chronic pain and more? They usually go to various specialists, few of whom will ever test for leaky or hyperpermeable gut. Instead they prescribe more drugs to cover-up or mask symptoms, drugs that can cause or worsen the leaky gut. Always remember, regardless of the label of your problem, if the gut is not healthy, you may never get truly healthy (symptom-free and medication-free). You need to heal the gut first.

## Common Pain Medications
## Cause and Perpetuate Fibromyalgia

There are a variety of catch-all or cop-out terms that are currently used by lazy medicine as an easy way to label disease. Once all the symptoms are collected and given a mysterious new name, the case is closed. As a rule, the causes (the environmental triggers and biochemical defects) are not sought. In fact they are not even yet part of standard medical textbooks or medical journal protocol (but I have described them for you and your doctor, complete with what tests to order and their interpretations, in *No More Heartburn*).

Instead drugs are prescribed to mask the symptoms, as though the cause of the symptoms was a deficiency of some drug! A common cop-out term is *fibromyalgia*. It has "no known cause", "no curative treatments" and "no definitive diagnostic tests" to prove it.

Fibromyalgia is merely diagnosed by a history of bizarre aches and pains that can move over the body or stay in certain places. No amount of medication seems to help. Usually there are *tender trigger points* that are sensitive and out of proportion to anything that has happened to the body. These can be found by palpating different areas.

Obligatory diagnostic criteria for fibromyalgia are general aches, pains, or stiffness in 3 or more sites for 3 or more months, tender points, and no other explanation for the symptoms. Minor criteria include disturbed sleep, fatigue, paresthesias (bizarre numbness or tingling), pain, headaches, and irritable bowel (often the cause!). The conventional medical answer for fibromyalgia consists of non-steroidal; anti-inflammatory drugs (NSAIDs). Funny, I didn't know it was a deficiency of NSAIDs that caused it! In fact they make it worse, for they can be the very cause of it in the first place.

And as you have learned, **NSAIDs also accelerate the deterioration of the painful joints.** Ironically even though NSAID drugs do nothing to isolate the cause or get rid of disease, they are used as a **mainstay of masking,** or conventional medical wisdom and "treatment". And since they can actually cause or initiate fibromyalgia, they cause existing fibromyalgia to worsen. **In essence, the very drugs most commonly prescribed actually cause the disease; and they guarantee it will get worse. And what is even more**

91

**damaging, they guarantee you will soon get many other diseases.**

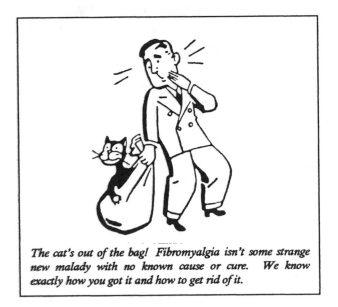

*The cat's out of the bag! Fibromyalgia isn't some strange new malady with no known cause or cure. We know exactly how you got it and how to get rid of it.*

People vary tremendously in the causes of their fibromyalgia. However, when looking at hundreds of cases of "untreatable", "incurable" fibromyalgia that I have seen improve, there is a common thread. Most people affected have had hidden dust, mold, and pollen allergies, as well as headaches, sinusitis, asthma or post nasal drip as milder symptoms for which they normally would not have consulted a physician. In fact, all of them, without fail, have had vitamin, mineral, or fatty acid deficiencies, as well as hidden mold, food and chemical sensitivities.

The bottom line is to remember that there are tools to diagnose and treat the causes of every disease or symptom, including chronic pain. No longer do you have to be a diagnostic puzzle, forever living on drugs. Fibromyalgia, chronic pain syndrome, arthritis, chronic fatigue, and the endless array of "incurable" diseases are now curable in the era of molecular and environmental medicine.

**The 8-R Outline:**
**How to Test and Treat**

(First an overview, then more details)

**The treatment of leaky gut syndrome is done in 8 phases:**

First you need to:

(1) **Recognize** or **diagnose** that the leaky gut is present. To diagnose leaky gut syndrome, one merely needs to do an intestinal permeability test, which is easily performed by doing a urine test at home. Your doctor merely writes a prescription for the "intestinal permeability test". Then you call the 800 number to have them send you the kit, put your urine in the tubes and return it in the mailer. What could be easier? (All the laboratories and their numbers are in resources chapter). Or you can just start treating it.

(2) **Remove** the cause of the leaky gut. To find what unwanted bugs (like Candida) might be lurking, your doctor can write a prescription to the same lab for a "comprehensive digestive stool analysis" (CDSA). This test will tell you if the cause of the leaky gut is overgrowth of the yeast Candida, poor digestive enzymes, abnormal bacteria, etc. For once you know you have the leaky gut, then it is imperative to proceed to a CDSA to find out **what is causing it to be leaky.** A good way to suspect that you have abnormal bacteria or yeasts is if you have very **foul gas**, or a lot of gas, or **bloating,** or indigestion, or alternating diarrhea and constipation. Or if

93

you are worse after sweets or ferments (bread, cheese, alcohol). A great start to kill unwanted bugs, and all that many need, is Kyolic (Wakunaga) and/or Paragard (Tyler; more detailed descriptions and references are in *No More Heartburn*).

(3) **Reinoculate** the gut by putting the "good bugs" back by using probiotics like *Lactobacillus acidophilus* and *Bifido* bacteria organisms. Having many beneficial properties in the gut, these promote healing of the leaky gut and provide competition to inhibit the return of the bad or disease-producing bugs. Start with Kyo-Dophilis (Wakunaga), 2 capsules twice a day with or after meals.

(4) **Replace** enzymes, as with Biogest (Thorne), Similase (Tyler) or Total-Gest (Klabin) 1-3 with meals. These promote better digestion, thereby improving nutrition as well as decreasing the allergenicity of foods.

(5) **Recall** the total load and how chemical sensitivity can keep the gut damaged. So rectify the gut overload of xenobiotics (foreign chemicals) by learning to reduce your total chemical overload in the diet as well as in the home and work environment (more described later and in *Tired or Toxic?* and *Total Wellness*).

(6) **Repair** the damaged gut with nutrients, like L-Glutamine (Pain & Stress Center), a nutrient important in healing the leaky gut wall in the small intestine.

(7) **Restore** function. This is done by increasing fiber in the diet, chewing thoroughly, and replacing digestive enzymes.

(8) **Repent** or **rectify** the causes.   For to resume your old dietary habits of sugars and refined, processed junk foods, the problem will invariably resurface. Remember, to return to your fast foods, gulping meals, resorting to NSAIDs and other damaging medications, alcohol, sweets, caffeine, and sodas, will bring you right back where you started from.

---

**So you might say the "8-R's" recipe for healing the gut is to:**

| | |
|---|---|
| Recognize | (diagnose) |
| Remove | (kill bugs) |
| Re-inoculate | (add good bugs) |
| Replace | (deficient enzymes, etc.) |
| Repair | (glutamine, nutrients) |
| Recall | (detoxification and the total load) |
| Restore | (function with fiber, chewing, and) |
| Repent or Rectify | (change your diet habits, stop NSAIDs , etc.) |

---

So a rational start could be to get:

1. The leaky gut test (also called intestinal permeability test) and CDSA (to determine why the gut is leaky, as from overgrowth of Candida).  These can be ordered from the Great Smokies Diagnostic Lab.   If you cannot find a doctor knowledgeable in the rationale for finding the causes of symptoms, check the organization addresses in the resources chapter.   Or you may just want to proceed with getting rid of the presumed most likely causes.

2. Begin with getting rid of the bad bugs with one of nature's natural antibiotics, *garlic*.  Not only is it an antibiotic for Candida, H. pylori and other unwanted intestinal bugs, but it lowers cholesterol, blood pressure, stimulates

natural killer cells which fight infection and cancer, and much more (Lau). Use **Kyolic** 2 capsules 2-3 times a day (Wakunaga; for free samples call 1-800-825-7888 and mention this book). You may also add or use separately ParaGard (Tyler) 1-2 with meals.

3. At the same time, put the good bugs back to promote healing of the gut lining as well as serving as competition for the bad bugs. Start with **Kyo-Dophilus** two capsules twice a day after meals (Wakunaga; for free samples, call 1-800-825-7888).

4. Next add chlorophyll which is healing and cleansing to the gut, as well as boosting detoxification: use **Kyo-Green** (Wakunaga) 2 caps or a heaping tbs. 2-4 times a day (for free samples, call 1-800-825-7888).

5. Use Super Glutamine 100 mg twice a day between meals to heal the gut (Pain & Stress Center, 1-800-669-2256) or Permeability Factors (Tyler; use N.E.E.D.S. 1-800-634-1380).

6. Similase (Tyler), 2-4 with meals or Biogest (Thorne) 1-2 with meals, or Total-Gest (Klabin) 1-2 with meals, to improve digestion.

7. Eat no junk food (packaged processed and fast foods) or sweets, which rob nutrition and irritate the gut while promoting the overgrowth of bad bugs.

8. Chew food 50 times a mouthful, eat mainly whole foods, to further improve nutritional status and digestion.

9. No NSAIDs (the most common cause of leaky gut).

10. See *No More Heartburn* for more details, especially for treating Candida, the leaky gut and fibromyalgia.

**Quick Start Yeast Terminator:** You may be able to heal Candida and the leaky gut in 3 easy steps, all twice a day (capsules for the first two and tbs. for the last one). Omit sweets, dairy, wheat and ferments while you quell the gut.

> 1. Kyolic
> 2. Kyo-Dophilus
> 3. Kyo-Green

If you are not improving within a couple of weeks, add Super Glutamine, a digestive enzyme, etc., as above. In many folks, the gut lining that houses the immune and detoxification systems is so damaged that a special boost is needed. Perfect for this is **UltraInflamX** (Metagenics) and **SeaVive** (Proper Nutrition).

### Healing With a Delicious Shake?

You've got it! Just when you might be feeling overwhelmed, along comes a malted milkshake-flavor packed with specially formulated nutrients to heal the 21st century gut. UltraInflamX (HealthComm, Metagenics, or N.E.E.D.S.) is quick, easy and surprisingly tasty. Fill the Easy Mixer ¾ full with water (N.E.E.D.S.), add 1-2 large scoops of UltraInflamX and press the button. What could be an easier way to benefit twice daily from a product resulting from a lifetime of study by one of the top nutritional specialists in the world, Dr. Jeffrey Bland, Ph.D (references for physicians in Chapter 10).

For an extra boost for the immune system, take 2-4 capsules of SeaVive (Proper Nutrition), 2-4 times a day. Each capsule contains quality colostrum to boost antibody levels, beta-glucan to boost infecting-fighting power of your white blood cells and a hydrolyzed fish protein to speed healing of the gut wall. Combined (as SeaVive) they not only protect the gut from NSAIDs damage, but more importantly accelerate healing once damage has occurred (Playford).

## Healing From the Inside Out

Clearly "modern medicine" overlooks this important and totally correctable cause of chronic pain, the Candida-laden leaky gut. The exciting part is that **if you are at an impasse** with chronic pain or any other symptom and cannot seem to rally, you may find that you now need to **heal from the inside out**. An undiagnosed leaky gut can be the reason why you are at an impasse and appear stuck with pain.

## Candida: The Major Cause of Fibromyalgia

Dan was a 46-year old professor who had been disabled for 3 years with total body pain. For lack of any better label, three physicians diagnosed him as having incurable fibromyalgia. When he came to the office we merely put him on the yeast program (detailed in *No More Heartburn*, but for milder cases, the steps above could suffice) to kill presumed Candida, since intensive questioning made me highly suspicious that this was the cause. His chronic sinus problems left him taking antibiotics 2-3 times a year. Within one month he was totally clear of all pain and back to work for the first time in 3 years. Now you understand my passion for getting this type of information and power into the hands of the consumer.

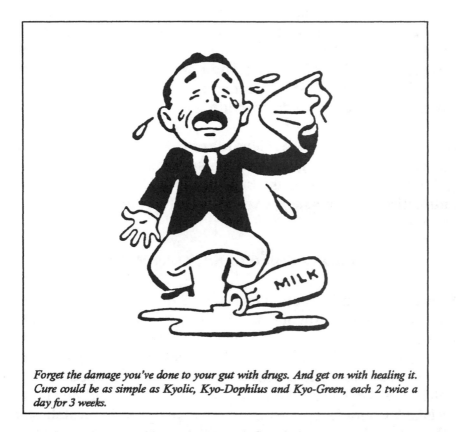

*Forget the damage you've done to your gut with drugs. And get on with healing it. Cure could be as simple as Kyolic, Kyo-Dophilus and Kyo-Green, each 2 twice a day for 3 weeks.*

I know we've thrown a lot at you, so let me recap some essential facts. Because you will most likely have to convince a physician who knows nothing about this to write your prescriptions, I need to make sure you are an expert in this big part of the picture necessary for healing chronic pain. So let's begin. First, at bare minimum, even conventional medicine knows that **one out of four people has the irritable bowel syndrome;** in other words, the gut is not healthy (*British Medical Journal,* Jan 11, 1992,304:87). Much of it can be due to the leaky gut, and in particular, Candida overgrowth.

Once leaky, anything and everything in the gut can make its way into the bloodstream, thus allowing these toxins to penetrate into other tissues, especially muscles and joints, causing a reaction of inflammation and pain. But ironically NSAIDs are prescribed which make it worse, setting you on a roller-coaster course of destruction.

If that were not enough, Candida, as one example of a bug out of control in the gut, becomes even more plentiful in the gut on a diet of sweets, breads, and alcohol as well as antibiotics, prednisone, cortisol, birth control pills, and estrogens.

### Don't Make Your Candida Drug-Resistant

**Caution:** If you happen to convince a physician untrained in environmental medicine to treat you with prescription Nystatin, he may treat you for several months, causing the emergence of resistant strains. Another common mistake that fosters drug-resistant Candida is to use it in conjunction with antibiotics, which select out the most antibiotic- and Nystatin-resistant Candida species. Also, treating with Nystatin or other prescription anti-fungals without the total program of diet, etc., easily fosters the growth of resistant yeast forms, like Candida tropicalis. For even more details on the diet, see *The E.I. Syndrome, Revised* and *No More Heartburn*.

Eventually Candida toxins can mimic anything from multiple sclerosis, arthritis, fibromyalgia, and depression, to migraines, chemical sensitivity, or colitis. A good clue to whether you might have Candida overgrowth is if gut or other symptoms are worse after ingestion of sweets. Surprisingly, medicine has staunchly resisted recognizing the importance of Candida, despite the fact that thousands of people have found relief from a multitude of pain syndromes once they cleared their Candida.

Perhaps one reason is that when yeast starts taking over or growing in the body, it does not do so in everyone. Instead it only happens in those who are not playing with a full deck of nutrients and therefore unable to defend themselves. In other words, it attacks those who are nutritionally deficient and therefore vulnerable.

For vulnerability from **attack** by any organism **depends more on the terrain or soil**, so to speak, on the resistance or integrity of health of the victim, rather than the virulence of the bug. That's why everyone does not get the flu when it comes around, but only **those who are vulnerable, who have a deficient terrain, or are not playing with a full deck of nutrients**. Drug-driven medicine has missed this concept.

One of the major clues to Candida, when a physical clue appears, is the growth of yeast on the tongue. It can be a white, yellow, brown, gray, or black growth, depending on which type of fungus it is. But realize that all coated tongues do not mean Candida specifically, but merely a toxicity of some sort.

Of course, when the growth of Candida is on the tongue, it signifies that most likely it is up and down the entire esophagus. This results in an undiagnosed cause of esophagitis or heartburn, for which H-2 blockers like Tagamet, Axid, Zantac or Pepcid are commonly prescribed. The irony is that these also make Candida worse. For they suppress stomach acid that is intended to inhibit or kill the yeast, and that is also needed for absorption of nutrients that boost your bug resistance.

101

Once you start taking H-2 blockers, this is like pouring gasoline on a fire, for you have turned off the stomach acid that was meant to kill Candida. Now the yeast can progress to growing throughout the entire gastrointestinal (GI) tract until you finally get the full-blown scenario. Again, **ignoring cause and suppressing symptoms with drugs makes the sick get sicker, quicker.** But the T.V. advertisements promote H-2 blockers as so safe that they recommend taking them in anticipation of a dietary indiscretion, even before you have a symptom. I can never understand how this pervasively destructive information gets by the FDA.

For example, Prilosec®, advertised on TV and medical journals says it is for heartburn and infections of *Helicobacter pylori,* an intestinal bacterium that can mimic heartburn, cause ulcers and even stomach cancer. And it can ride piggyback on blood cells to the heart arteries where it starts eating holes that have to be patched up with cholesterol. Once enough of a cholesterol Band-Aid accumulates, you can have a heart attack because no more blood can make it to the end of the artery. Prilosec (one of the leading drugs for H. pylori) is also like fertilizer to H. pylori, since it wipes out the acid that the stomach makes to fight Candida and H. pylori.

### We Are Full of Bugs
### With Ready Access to Our Muscles and Joints

People often wonder how so many abnormal bacteria can be found inside their intestines, and I wonder how we escape being chronically infected. For example, the Department of Agriculture (USDA) wants to define fecal matter as an acceptable part of the American diet. Even though it acknowledges the dangers of epidemic food poisoning, the "USDA pleads that condemning poultry carcasses

102

contaminated with fecal matter during processing would work an economic hardship on the poultry industry" (Leonard 1994).

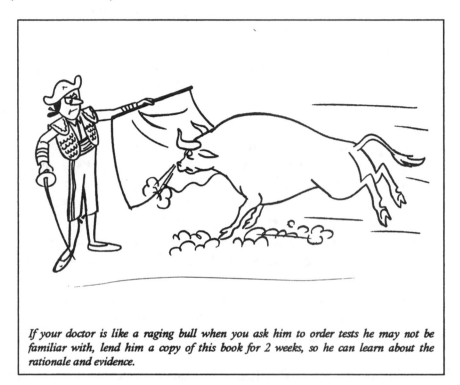

*If your doctor is like a raging bull when you ask him to order tests he may not be familiar with, lend him a copy of this book for 2 weeks, so he can learn about the rationale and evidence.*

In other words, because meat and fowl handlers lobbied in government halls, it is acceptable to offer us progressively more contaminated proteins. And with antibiotics fed regularly and prophylactically to farmed fish, fowl, and feedlot meat, more resistant bacteria emerge. Now that you appreciate how all bacteria and yeasts in the gut can translocate or migrate into the blood and penetrate into any organ, it is pretty scary. For the leaky gut makes this all possible. And hidden infection in joints can be another unsuspected cause of chronic joint pain.

Convincing statistics from government agricultural bureaus show that over 50% of fowl/meat/or fish are contaminated with unwanted organisms. Being fed to a nation of folks living on NSAIDs, guarantees the antibiotic manufacturers will never lack for business as these organisms journey from leaky guts with their once-protective acids turned off by Tagamet, Zantac or Prilosec, to race to every nook and cranny in the body. But when they get an infected tooth or inflamed knee, they never connect the two.

Since people make less hydrochloric acid in the stomach as they age, they lose another natural way to control unwanted bugs in the gut. In addition, with eating more processed foods that can irritate the stomach, they take more antacids to actually sop up any remaining acid. H2-blockers like Tagamet, Zantac, Pepcid or the prescriptions Prilosec and Prevacid even more effectively turn off acid. This further lowers the amount of stomach acid available to fight bugs. National newspapers regularly report on epidemics in our tap water of Cryptosporidium, Giardia, and more, providing an endless source of bugs to infect joints.

Furthermore, many unhealthful measures keep cropping up that contribute even more to the invasion of resistant bugs into the body, like the irradiation of food. For species of mold (Pullularia or Aureobasidium) and some species of bacteria (Salmonella) are resistant to food irradiation. So we have increased the likelihood of having these introduced into the diet as progressively more foods are irradiated. And once in the gut and on into the joints, these bugs can trigger unmerciful arthritis.

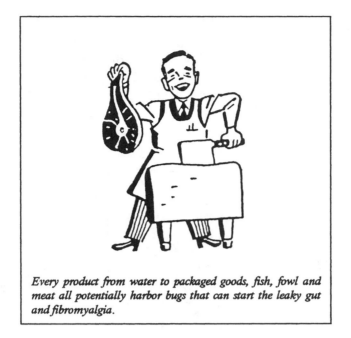

*Every product from water to packaged goods, fish, fowl and meat all potentially harbor bugs that can start the leaky gut and fibromyalgia.*

## Arthritis is Not an Advil Deficiency

So now that you know arthritis is not an Advil or Aleve deficiency, you still may have serious pain that needs urgent relief while you figure out the causes. So if you absolutely must take an NSAID, you might be coerced into taking one like Celebrex®, reporting that it spares the COX-1 (cyclooxygenase-1) enzyme that causes the leaky gut. Don't believe it for a second. Not only did it have over a dozen deaths attributed to it the first year on the market, it is not proven to prevent leaky gut.

The field of rheumatology is scaring me. Look at some of their other irrational recommendations. A year study of rheumatoid arthritics was done on those who had such severe disease as to be prescribed chloroquine, hydroxychloroquine, parenteral gold, D-penicillamine, sulphasalazine, azathioprine or methotrexate. These "second-line" (when NSAIDs fail to give relief) drugs are so dangerous that some of them are actually a form of chemotherapy and are capable of causing cancer. Others have side effects like aplastic anemia (you actually stop making blood cells), blindness and death.

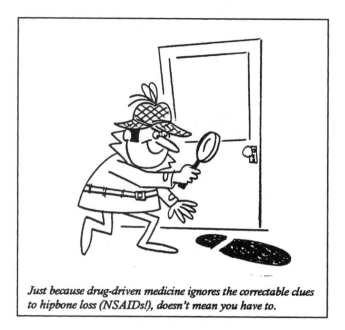

*Just because drug-driven medicine ignores the correctable clues to hipbone loss (NSAIDs!), doesn't mean you have to.*

The interesting part of the study was that 62% of 285 arthritis patients did just as well with a placebo (sugar pill) as they did with these expensive and life-threatening drugs. And they should have done worse just by the mere fact that withdrawing the real drug doubles the chance of symptoms returning more furiously (Woldes).

But this should not be too hard to fathom since the official management for arthritis promotes nothing but drugs and surgery. Nothing that you read in this book is part of a standard medical approach to arthritis, for cause is seldom a concern. It is almost as though they want to perpetuate the disease. In the American College of Rheumatology's medical journal article, "Issues and management guidelines for arthritis of the hip and knee", they never mention that the NSAIDs that they recommend so heavily actually cause destruction of the hipbone. Yet this is an example of one of the scariest and most disabling forms of arthroses (Acetabular bone destruction from NSAIDs, *Amer Fam Pract*, 33;3:320-321, 1985, Newman).

This type of drugs and surgery approach to pain pervades all of medicine as other articles limit their "treatments" to drugs and surgery, as though arthritis or chronic back pain or fibromyalgia were all an Advil deficiency (Gillette, Reiffenberger). Never once do these guiding articles for physicians look for environmental, nutritional or metabolic causes.

Yes, NSAIDs can not only cause leaky gut *syndrome*, which can mimic a multitude of diseases, but they can cause fatal liver and kidney diseases, not to mention blindness. And by lowering serotonin and melatonin they can cause depression; by other mechanisms they can cause colitis serious enough to warrant surgical removal of part of the colon, blindness, allergic pneumonia, heart failure, and death. You can find more extensive protocols for the entire cause-oriented work-up in *No More Heartburn* and *Depression Cured At Last!*. Meanwhile, let's look at some easier things you could do that have a big chance of being all you will ever need for pain relief.

## And Hold the Tylenol

If you are thinking, "No problem, I'll use Tylenol (acetaminophen) instead", don't. It has what is called a narrow therapeutic to toxic ratio. Translation? The dose that is used to kill pain is very close to the dose that can kill you. Many people have either taken a double or triple dose, or had alcohol or other medicines with it and killed their livers. They ended up with a very expensive liver transplant or dead. When J&J was interviewed in *Forbes* (T. Easton, 1998), they stated that it was better for business to pay for a few liver transplants and deaths each year than to put warnings on the product that would scare away users that make it the number one selling pain–reliever in the country.

## Quick Stop Summary

Now it should be clear to you that the very medications, over-the-counter or prescription, that are taken for pain actually deteriorate not only bone but hearts, liver, kidneys, eyes and more as well as usher in an avalanche of symptoms. WHAT CAN YOU DO?

(1)    First determine whether you have the leaky gut via the intestinal permeability test (Great Smokies diagnostic Laboratory).

(2)    Next you need to reverse the damage done by NSAIDs and **heal the gut**. Usually the avalanche of symptoms has already begun, with infections necessitating antibiotics that have caused an overgrowth of Candida. This in turn further inflames the gut and leads to general body aches and pains, as well as depression and fatigue. Use Kyolic, Kyo-Dophilus, Kyo-Green, L-Glutamine, Total-Gest plan as outlined above.

(3) Next is to find **safe substitutes for NSAIDs** that actually improve the function of other parts of your body as well, versus deteriorate it as the NSAIDs do.

(4) Last is to **repair the damage to bone and to the cell membrane** where the inflammatory mediators are released that causes all this pain to begin with (next chapter).

So what are we waiting for?

## Safe NSAID Substitutes

### *Lyprinol to the Rescue*

Now that you know how the primary drugs for inflammation and pain, prescription and over-the-counter, actually deteriorate bone and create new diseases, what can you safely take? Don't be hooked by the advertisements for Celebrex and Vioxx claiming sparing of the gastritis effect. Celebrex had over 8 deaths in the first few seasons, but as with any medicine whose sales exceed $88 million the first year, don't expect to see it whisked from the market. After all, there are over 5,800 NSAID deaths a year and you don't see any campaign to teach you that they deteriorate bone or cause death of kidneys, heart, and other organs. Just look at the newer drugs for rheumatoid arthritis, like Enbrel®. Not only does it cost $12,000 a year to take (yes, that's right $1,000 a month!) but it works by inhibiting the formation of tumor necrosis factor. This is a cytokine the body makes in order to kill cancer cells. Not a good thing to destroy. But never fear, Mother Nature to the rescue.

For centuries the Maori natives of New Zealand claimed that consuming the local mussel helped them stay healthy. But for decades men of medicine have assumed that anything other than prescribed medicines must be pure folklore with no underlying scientific merit. That is one reason I have such respect for the companies whose products I recommend, because they go to the science and find why and how natural products work. Then the part I particularly love, they show that natural products are not only devoid of the nasty side effects of drugs, but have additional good effects that further promote health, and are actually superior to the prescription medicines over the long haul.

A couple of decades ago, the green-lipped mussel, *Perna canaliculus*, was not only found to be effective in relieving the symptoms of rheumatoid arthritis and osteoarthritis, but without side effects. And if it has to be given with or after NSAIDs, it can heal or prevent the gastric ulcerations. Beyond the scope of this book, I feel it is important to nevertheless mention that it also inhibits the tendency for cancer to metastasize.

In studies throughout the world, Lyprinol (the lipid extract of the green-lipped mussel) has dramatically outperformed ibuprofen (Motrin, Aleve-type drugs) as well as omega-3 and –6 fatty acids. The bottom line is that the fatty acids in the New Zealand green-lipped mussel modulate the abnormal cell membrane chemistry (inhibit lipoxygenase and cyclo-oxygenase pathways) of pain and inflammation. But this is accomplished without interfering with normal "housekeeping" or healing functions that membrane chemistry is also responsible for. Contrary to the NSAIDs that destroy the intestinal lining, Lyprinol heals it.

The lipid extract of this marine animal can be purchased without a prescription in 100 mg capsules. The dose of

Lyprinol (from Prevail, Tyler, N.E.E.D.S.) is 2 capsules twice a day for 3-6 weeks, after which the dose can be dropped to 1-2 capsules a day.

### *Further Power Over Pain: Magnesium and Malic Acid*

In addition, if you still have pain, strange as it may sound, within hours of taking magnesium in a liquid form, the pain of old surgery, accidents, arthritis, lumbar discs, migraine and much more can melt away. I frequently get letters from our newsletter readers, physicians, dentists, scientists, and lay people, telling me how once they decided to do a trial of magnesium, literally years of pain melted away with hours or days. Yet it should not come as a surprise since the standard American diet provides 40% (less than half) the magnesium you need in a day. Furthermore, magnesium, needed in over 300 enzymes, is lost dramatically in sweat, with mental stress, alcohol and sugar ingestion, irritable bowel and much more.

The best test for magnesium is the magnesium-loading test that is in *Tired Or Toxic?* If you want to assay other nutrient levels as well, follow the plan for RBC mineral levels in *Depression Cured At Last!* Each tells what blood tests your doctor should order for you to assay your vitamin and mineral status, and then it shows how to interpret the tests and what nutrients to take.

Or have your doctor call either laboratory for ordering instructions for RBC (red blood cell) mineral assays: MetaMetrix, Great Smokies Lab, or Doctor's Data (all in Resources). Never settle for a serum magnesium (worthlessly insensitive, as less than 1% of the body magnesium is in the serum). The serum level can be normal even when you are low enough to have a sudden heart attack from undiagnosed magnesium deficiency, as famous athletes may have done.

Once an area becomes damaged, we expect to have pain there because of the old injury. But this dangerously erroneous thinking leads to a passive acceptance. Like I used to, you probably think if you eat a healthful diet, you could not possibly be deficient. But government studies show that the average American diet actually creates magnesium deficiency, which in turn commonly leads to muscle spasm, another reason why so much Advil is sold!

Normally magnesium is in happy balance with calcium. Calcium causes muscles to contract and magnesium causes them to relax. But if you are short on the relaxing mineral, then you are left with constant or intermittent spasm. If back muscles are the targets, you get spasm so painful that it can mimic a ruptured disc. Folks with auto-immune diseases have a different problem. They often get painful spasm in tiny vessels in fingers and toes, cutting off the circulation so well that blanching of fingertips can occur. Corrections of magnesium deficiency have relieved all of these symptoms of **Raynaud's** disease for many.

If the target organ for spasm due to magnesium deficiency is the brain blood vessels, you have migraine. If it is the lungs, you have asthma; if in the gut, you get spastic colitis; and in the heart vessels, you get angina or arrhythmia or sudden cardiac arrest. If you want to accelerate your loss of magnesium, just jog or do some other activity that makes you sweat like crazy. In fact, this most likely contributed to the mechanism of death for such athletes as Jim Fixx, Hank Gathers and Reggie Lewis.

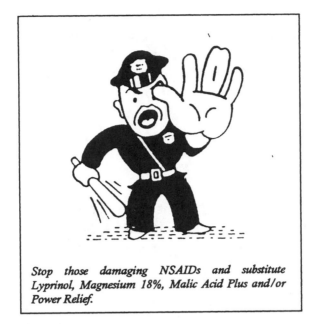

*Stop those damaging NSAIDs and substitute Lyprinol, Magnesium 18%, Malic Acid Plus and/or Power Relief.*

Start with one teaspoon (100 mg) of **18% Magnesium Chloride Solution** (Pain & Stress Center) in a large glass of water and total 4 times a day for at least a week, then you can back off to the lowest dose that keeps you spasm-free. You may want to add one Manganese Picolinate 20 mg (Thorne) a day, at it makes the magnesium work better. Be sure you don't take magnesium oxide, or tablet or capsule form when you are doing a trial to determine if you are deficient. The 18% Magnesium Solution is the best absorbed form. You can't beat it, and for such an important mineral, you can't afford to miss its benefits.

The fibromyalgia problem is a perfect example of needing to solve a total load of factors (as described in *Depression Cured At Last!*) in order to repair it. But malic acid gave subjective improvement within 48 hours in one study of this nutrient that fits neatly into the citric acid or energy cycle of body chemistry with magnesium. Two capsules of **Malic Acid Plus** (Pain & Stress Center) contain 800 mg of malic acid, 300 mg of Boswellia, an anti-inflammatory herb known for centuries to relieve pain, 100 mg of magnesium and some chromium, vitamin C and B6. Use 1-2 capsules of Malic Acid Plus 1-4 times a day.

## Take DLPA and Be Happy Plus Pain-Free

L-phenylalanine. Don't let it scare you. It is merely the name of an essential amino acid that we cannot make but we luckily get from foods. In the body it can be converted to tyrosine, the precursor to the adrenal (stress) and thyroid (energy) hormones. It also helps synthesize our endorphins, the neurotransmitters that make us happy and sometimes addicted. In fact the very chemistry of addiction to common foods like wheat and milk is that in some people, foods have become allergens for them and actually stimulate (addictive) opioid receptors and brain ("pleasure") endorphins.

Scientists found that somehow pain and happiness are tied together biochemically. In fact when you give a narcotic antagonist like Naloxone (used in the emergency room, for example to get an addict through withdrawal faster), it also increases pain. On the flip side, if we can keep those endorphins (brain happy hormones) hanging around in the blood longer, we have less pain.

And the natural compound that can do this is the biochemical mirror image (like a right and left-hand glove) of l-phenylalanine, d-phenylalanine. When they are coupled together, it forms d,l-phenylalanine or DLPA. It is the d-isomer that prolongs the pain-relieving, endorphin-

114

stimulating action of l-phenylalanine. Combining it with other natural helpers like the anti-inflammatory herb, Boswellia, has decreased pain even more.

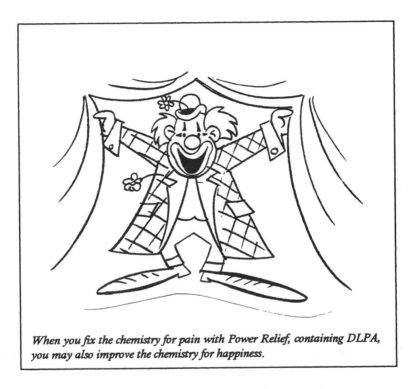

*When you fix the chemistry for pain with Power Relief, containing DLPA, you may also improve the chemistry for happiness.*

As far back as 1978 Dr. Ehrenpreis, and others from the departments of pharmacology and anesthesiology at University of Chicago Medical School, found that DLPA (d,l-phenylalanine) could relieve pain. The first patient was treated for 2 years for whiplash with Empirin and Valium with no relief. But in two days DLPA provided relief. This scenario was duplicated with chronic back pain and various forms of arthritis in other folks.

D,l-phenylalanine, an amino acid that has helped impressively down-regulate pain, comes in the form of 375-500 mg of DLPA, taken as 1-3 capsules 2-3 times a day with meals. Better yet, two capsules of **Power Relief** (Pain & Stress Center) contain 500 mg DLPA, plus 200 mg GABA, a relaxing amino acid, 300 mg of Boswellia, and some passion flower and a little magnesium and B6. What a dynamite combination for pain.

To recap, pain relief can come with one or more of the following, alone or in any combination: Lyprinol, 18% Magnesium Chloride Solution, Malic Acid Plus, and/or Power Relief.

### Message in a Nutshell

Unless you (diagnose and) heal the gut, you may never get well. The very drugs taken for pain actually assure that not only will your pain eventually worsen, but that you will develop new pain symptoms and diseases. Besides all the serious side effects from arthritis drugs like colon, eye, liver, heart, or kidney death, as examples, pain drugs actually destroy bone. If causing bone destruction and osteoporosis were not enough; they cause leaky gut, which can create an avalanche of auto-immune and other serious diseases.

Diagnose the leaky gut syndrome, find the underlying causes (Candida or whatever) and restore normal gut function via the program outlined. Substitute for NSAIDs, safe and more effective Lyprinol; and empower your program even further with, 18% Magnesium, Malic Acid, and Power Relief.

## Chapter 5

## Building Bone
## The Safer and Non-Prescription Way

### Glucosamine Sulfate Rebuilds Bone

Would you believe there is something that you can buy
without a prescription that has no side effects and that
actually rebuilds damaged or lost bone? The most convincing
type of medical studies (rigidly controlled double blind) have
shown that knee joints, backs, and other bone and cartilage
surfaces have been rejuvenated with glucosamine sulfate.

You just learned that NSAIDs generally lose their
effectiveness after a few months use and have a nasty effect of
slowly deteriorating or destroying bone. But glucosamine
does the opposite. Not only is it non-prescription and safer
than NSAIDs, but it builds bone, is less expensive and gives
better pain relief. It takes about a month or two for the pain
relief of glucosamine sulfate to reach its maximum and that's
just about when the pain relief of the NSAIDs has dwindled
away.

Glucosamine sulfate actually relieves more pain the longer
that it is taken, since it is anti-inflammatory as well as corrects
the problem by rebuilding bone and cartilage surfaces. So
there is no comparison about which item I would choose.
How about you?

There is frankly no contest. Certainly you may need to
continue your pain medications until you work through
identifying all the causes or triggers of your pain. To tide you
over until your glucosamine sulfate kicks in, which takes a

few months to reach its maximum benefit, you could use the remedies we've just described that benefit the rest of the body, versus fostering bone deterioration as NSAIDs do.

| Better Than NSAIDs in Every Way: A Safer, Cheaper, Non-Prescription Nutrient That Builds Bone and Relieves Pain | | |
|---|---|---|
| **Compare** | **NSAIDs** | **Glucosamine Sulfate** |
| Maximum pain relief in months | 1-4 | After 2-3 |
| Course of pain relief after 2-4 months | Dwindles | Increases |
| Side effects | Leaky gut, deteriorates bone; damage to liver, kidney, eye, gut, heart, and more | None |
| Builds bone | Never | Yes |
| Anti-inflammatory | Yes | Yes |
| Strengthens other Tissues like arteries | Never | Yes |

Regardless, remember that the longer you take an NSAID, the more bone you will deteriorate and damage, the more leaky gut you will get, the sooner the NSAID will stop being effective for pain relief, and the more you run the risk of developing other medical problems. Whereas the longer you take glucosamine sulfate, the more bone and cartilage you rebuild (as well as other structures like arteries), thus strengthening the area and relieving pain in an infinitely smarter way.

The dose for glucosamine sulfate is 500 mg, 2 capsules, 2-3 times a day.    Reliable sources include **GS-500**, the original patented form on which the research was done, by Enzymatic Therapy/PhytoPharmica, and **Glucosamine Sulfate 500 mg** by Tyler.    Some of the support formulas that accompany the various brands of CM contain glucosamine in a form other than sulfate.  Perhaps they work as well, but no studies have been done.  For that reason you may prefer to create your own support formula, as I'll show you later.

If you want an easy no-brainer (who doesn't in this complicated world?), use **Mobil-Ease** (Prevail, 1-800-248-0885).    Besides glucosamine sulfate 500 mg, it has white willow bark 100 mg (from which aspirin came, but without the aspirin side effects of leaky gut).    Other crucial and unique ingredients include Boswellia 50 mg (a potent anti-inflammatory), Turmeric (curcumin) 50 mg (another herb noted for centuries for pain relief and later found to be anti-inflammatory, anti-clotting, and to accelerate healing by triggering new vessel formation), and gamma oryzanol (a rice derived natural anti-oxidant).

If that were not enough, the enzymes protease and cellulase are there to promote nutrient penetration into the swollen areas as well as aiding in breaking down old diseased tissue. What a smart combination of the joint healer, glucosamine, with centuries old herbal anti-inflammatories, all without side effects.    And it combines beautifully with Lyprinol. Anyone doubting the ability of a non-prescription herbal compound to pack potent relief for pain, need only look at the references for the ingredients and their proven immunologic roles in the scientific references in chapter 10. In the meantime, take 2 capsules of **Mobil-Ease** 2-4 times a day for 2-4 months, then back off to determine what the lowest dose is you need for maintenance of pain relief.

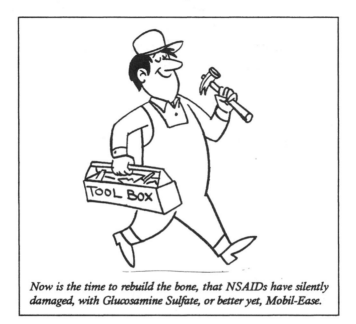

*Now is the time to rebuild the bone, that NSAIDs have silently damaged, with Glucosamine Sulfate, or better yet, Mobil-Ease.*

Glucosamine sulfate, as great as it is for eventual pain relief and building bone, works much better if it is combined with other nutrients to facilitate body repair. For starters, use a general multiple vitamin-mineral preparation, which contains minerals that are necessary for bone repair. Multiplex-1 without iron is one of my favorites (available from Tyler or N.E.E.D.S.), 1-2 capsules twice a day, or if you have much bone repair work to do, as with osteoporosis, use 2 twice a day of Osteo Complex Formula (Tyler, NEEDS).

## Other GAGs to Build By

GAGs? You'll be sorry you asked. It stands for glucosaminoglycans. It is merely the chemical category of substances that make up cartilage, connective tissue (including tendons, ligaments and blood vessels), and bone. It is the **gristle** of the body. There are many types and forms of GAGs. Sometimes it is also called ground substance or matrix or intercellular cement. You'll find products in all sorts of disguises from glucosamine sulfate that you just learned about, to shark cartilage, bovine cartilage, chondroitin sulfate, collagen, aloe, mucopolysaccharides, and sea cucumber.

And the GAGs all have their pros and cons. I have seen elevated mercury levels from the expensive shark cartilage and since I have found much more science behind bovine cartilage, that is one of my preferred sources to rebuild cartilage along with glucosamine sulfate. Glucosamine sulfate is the best-absorbed form of GAGs and has the best research behind it for rebuilding bone. But, whenever we use such a refined product, it makes me wonder how many ancillary ingredients were refined out of the pure product that nature deemed useful, even though their absorption is not so great. No one has answered this.

## Collagen Type II

Then there are products that combine glucosamine sulfate with other well researched GAGs, like type II collagen, along with magnesium, thiamine, carnitine and carnosine, all playing a role in rebuilding not only damaged muscle and bone, but blood vessels and cell walls. This particular formula, called **Fibromyalgin** (Ecologic Formulas or

Cardiovascular Research, Ltd) is taken as 2-4 capsules, 2-3 times a day. The same company also makes **Rheumatol Forte**, which contains collagen type II, chondroitin polysulphates, and hyaluronic acid. Collagen type II is particularly interesting as it has caused oral tolerization (Trentham). Translation: when given orally, it has down-regulated auto-immune diseases like arthritis where there is an antibody directed against one's own self or tissues, namely the joints. Collagen type II in essence makes the body stop attacking itself; it stops destroying its own cartilage.

**Point in fact:** In Barnett's and Trentham's (Harvard) study of children with juvenile rheumatoid arthritis, 80% of children had reduction in swelling and pain and increased mobility after 3 months of collagen type II. And these are kids, for whom methotrexate and prednisone were being considered, both of which significantly increase the chance of cancer in years to come. Giving collagen type II causes the body's attack on its own collagen to simmer down, much like an immunization. As you may know, not all immunizations need to be given by injection. Oral polio vaccine and many types of allergy injections can be given by mouth. Hence the term for the effect of collagen type II is *oral tolerization*. And this has no side effects, and requires no blood tests or prescription. It sounds like a win-win situation if it works for your pain. That is why I recommend **Rheumatol Forte®** (Ecologic Formulas) 2-6 capsules as tolerated 2-4 times a day as part of your bone and cartilage rebuilding program with glucosamine.

And don't forget that even though these results were great, they could have been better. For recall these kids did not have the benefit of a total load program, or even one that incorporates, for example, the nightshade-free diet. So if they can get that much benefit without, for example, the nightshade-free diet, think of how much freer of pain they could have been by implementing other treatments in this book. I readily recall three young kids all under 13 who were in chronic pain with a diagnostic label of juvenile rheumatoid arthritis from their local medical schools and rheumatologists. But since they began the nightshade-free diet, they have never had any more pain. And they take no pain medications what so ever. Yet their rheumatologists are still not recommending the nightshade-free diet to newly diagnosed JRA patients, or to the ones they have on chemotherapeutic agents, nor to those in agony for whom nothing works.

Now you are beginning to understand why the environmental medicine approach to pain can produce such astounding results in diseases that are supposed to have no known cause or cure. Whenever you hear that something is incurable, you know right away they have not used the environmental medicine approach to find the *total load* of causes and cures.

## Bovine Cartilage

As with any truly beneficial natural substance, bovine or cow cartilage's record is not limited to just improving one area of physiology, as in strengthening bones and supporting tissues like cartilage, tendons, fascia, and ligaments. Remember when your mother recommended Knox Gelatin for stronger teeth, nails and hair? That is a GAG. Anything that improves one body function is usually useful in other ways: Bovine cartilage is no exception, having, as an example, an interesting track record in cancer as well as arteriosclerosis. Although those subjects are beyond the scope of this book, you can find them in our monthly newsletter and other books. Chances are that if you have additional conditions besides your chronic pain, GAGs may help them, too.

The dose for **Bovine Cartilage** 500 mg (Pure Encapsulations, Klabin) for musculo-skeletal cases would be 1-2 capsules 2-3 times a day, in conjunction with other bone builders like glucosamine sulfate, a multiple vitamin-mineral or special bone-building formulas like Tyler's **Osteo Complex** (2 twice a day).

### Adjuncts to Rebuilding Bone and Tissue

## MSM

We are all always looking for shortcuts to vibrant wellness, some elusive, obscure natural factor that will be a landmark turning point, bringing us to newer heights of health. That secret surprise is what actor James Coburn found when he got relief from his 20 years of arthritis with MSM, making him the poster child for this nutrient. Depending upon your individual deficiencies, **MSM** could turn the tide for you, too. For MSM has improved chronic pain syndromes like arthritis, including rheumatoid and lupus, as well as other auto-immune conditions like diabetes and asthma.

You can almost bet that the name of a nutrient must be pretty bad when it is reduced to initials. But **methyl-sulfonyl-methane** isn't all that difficult to say. But what is difficult is understanding how one such fundamental natural chemical can do so much. However, it is by the very fact that it is so fundamental that it also provides such a wide range of symptom relief.

Unfortunately, whenever a nutrient is useful for several diverse conditions, it makes physicians untrained in

124

environmental medicine and unaccustomed to looking for the causes of symptoms very suspicious. They call it useless folklore and refuse to read the scientific proof. But remember, drugs usually axe or turn off only one biochemical pathway. So physicians wrongly assume that natural remedies work by the same mechanism. They don't think in terms of repair, but destruction.

For once the mind-set is in the destructive or turning off mode, it becomes all the more difficult to think that a remedy can not only bring about relief but aid many other symptoms and systems. They cannot understand how one item can effect so many beneficial functions in the body at once, because they have forgotten a vast amount of their biochemistry. And, as you know, when something is not understood, it is often labeled as quackery or at least unfounded in order to save face or cover up for lack of knowledge; a century old ploy not restricted to medicine.

Medicine almost exclusively uses specific chemicals to turn off specific poorly functioning pathways; a drug for every symptom. If your cholesterol is too high, for example, shut off the pathway that enables you to make it with Zocor or Mevocor. But don't look to see if the reason the pathway is no longer functioning normally is because of a copper deficiency, for example, after years of too many quick processed meals or taking too much zinc for infections or prostate.

Likewise, if you have high blood pressure, the medical mind-set dictates that you turn down the control that your nervous system has over the vascular receptors with beta-blockers like Inderal, Lopressor or Tenormin. Heaven forbid we should examine why the receptors are damaged and hyper-responsive, as often is the case from an accumulation of the wrong trans fatty acids from years of French fries, margarines and hydrogenated soybean oils in commercial salad dressings and processed foods.

Logically, since copper is in 21 enzymes, when you correct a deficiency that may be behind high cholesterol, as an example, it may also help something else, like your depression or ability to detoxify your co-worker's perfume without getting a headache. Likewise, when you correct a membrane deficiency of an omega-3 fatty acid via flax oil or cod liver oil, as another example, perhaps your dry skin, rash or energy will improve, as well as your joint pain, colitis and hypertension.

The point is that when you repair fundamental defects with natural medicine's techniques, many "side effects" of other symptoms improving are often part of the deal. For correcting a cell membrane defect that is severe enough to cause hypertension, is bound to improve other functions, including pain, since the cell membrane's functions are not only limited to blood pressure control. That is part of the fun of environmental and nutritional medicine because you never know what other benefits you will get.

This will help you understand the negative reactions you may get from docs unschooled in molecular biochemistry. To them, it appears like sheer quackery that a solo nutrient like MSM could have not one, not two, but many benefits and clear ferocious pain in the process, but only in those who need it. It also explains why when you resort to drugs to cover up or mask symptoms, that you also get a stable full of unwanted side effects.

But this ignorance is dangerous. For example, NSAIDs "harmlessly" inhibit cyclooxygenase, an enzyme needed to cause inflammation. Granted, it can calm that back muscle, but by not finding and correcting the cause for that muscle pain, it leaves you on Motrin indefinitely. This sets you up for any of the mountain of side effects from shutting down this God-given protective chemistry in the heart, which leads to congestive heart failure, to letting that undiagnosed magnesium deficiency cause a sudden heart attack.

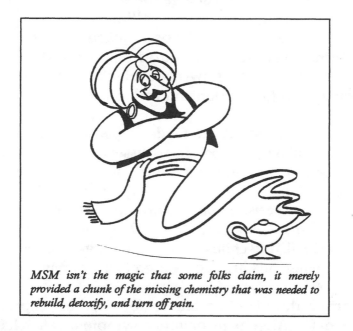

*MSM isn't the magic that some folks claim, it merely provided a chunk of the missing chemistry that was needed to rebuild, detoxify, and turn off pain.*

Three things make MSM potent in so many diverse and resistant conditions: (1) it is a great **sulfur donor**, used as a building block for structural support in collagen, bone, hair, plus bile, insulin and a scaffolding for our synthesis of proteins. It is crucial for building the many glucosaminoglycans or GAGs (like your own synthesis of glucosamine sulfate) for bone and cartilage repair. (2) As a derivative of DMSO and an **anti-oxidant mineral**, it is important in providing **sulfur groups** for detoxification in the body. In fact, sulfur forms great adducts or attachments for mercury and other heavy metals that get into our bodies from pollution, keeping them from damaging enzymes that then mimic any disease known.

MSM also known as dimethyl sulfone. (3) It is also a source of **methyl groups**, another conjugation group used by the body to detoxify toxins that cause pain. With so many properties, it is not a surprise that MSM helps to alkalinize the body and even neutralize pesticide exposures. No wonder it enhances blood flow, speeds the flow of nutrients to damaged areas, and promotes detoxification and collagen repair.

Although widely found in foods, especially onions, garlic, asparagus, cabbage, broccoli, Brussels sprouts and eggs, cooking reduces it, and our stores in our bodies tend to dwindle with age. Suffice to say that MSM should be included in any resistant pain, auto-immune, or inflammatory condition for a 1-3 month trial. Even recalcitrant dental, gastrointestinal, infectious, allergic and eye problems have improved when this has been added to a regimen.

The starting dose is often one to four 500 mg capsules, 2-3 times a day. After pain or other symptom relief has been achieved, then the dose can often be reduced to 250-500 mg, 3 times a day. I suggest **MSM 750 mg** (pure pharmaceutical grade from Pain & Stress Center). From the Pain & Stress Center you can also get 10% **MSM Cream, 5% MSM Lotion,** a booklet on MSM, as well as a tape on how it eases the pain of fibromyalgia, arthritis, leg cramps, and more.

## DMSO

DMSO is the parent of MSM, and for some folks DMSO can not be improved on, in spite of its garlic odor. Heel spurs, tendonitis, low back pain, injuries and arthritis, old or new, can benefit from topical DMSO. Although it does not rebuild, it is a great pain reliever to buy time while you do rebuild damaged bone and cartilage.

First do a test patch site first for 24 hours, then rub DMSO on over the painful area 2-4 times a day as needed. Also make sure that your hands are very clean and that nothing touches the area where DMSO is that you do not want in your blood stream, as it is a marvelous carrier. So don't put it on and then scrub the floor or work in the garden. DMSO Cream, 99% pure and the book, *DMSO Nature's Healer,* are available from the Pain & Stress Center.

If you were allergic to sulfur drugs, it does not mean that you would necessarily be intolerant of DMSO or MSM. However, I would always proceed with extreme caution. Usually sulfur intolerance means a reaction to sulfur-containing antibiotics. Often this intolerance really translates into an inability to metabolize or detoxify it. This often stems from a deficiency of the key mineral, *molybdenum, in the enzyme, sulfite oxidase* and it may mean that this needs correcting before you could tolerate sulfur. Since sulfur is almost as basic to the body as oxygen, and toxicity is relatively unheard of, it may be a vital adjunct to your current program.

## Taurine

**Taurine** is an amino acid-like compound that can stabilize cell membranes, especially those in the process of being rebuilt. As well, it is crucial in both the detox pathway and to attenuate inflammation, the underlying mechanism of bone destruction and pain. The dose is 500 mg **Taurine,** 1-3 capsules 2-3 a day (Pain & Stress Center).

## SAMe

Another nutrient that helps build bone as well as displace the need for NSAIDs for pain is **SAMe,** short for S-adenosyl methionine. In addition it can rev up the detox pathway. It is the activated form of the amino acid, methionine, and is a primary source of methyl groups which also underlie whether or not we get arteriosclerosis, accelerated aging, fatigue, depression, chemical sensitivity, and all sorts of diseases including fibromyalgia, osteoporosis and osteoarthritis.

In one study of 44 fibromyalgia patients who took 800 mg of SAMe for 6 weeks, they enjoyed reduced pain as well as reduced fatigue and depression. In the test tube, SAMe increases the number of chondrocytes (cartilage cells) and proteoglycans (GAG proteins needed to rebuild bone and cartilage). Take **SAMe** 1-2 once or twice a day as needed (Metabolic Maintenance, Jarrow, or Pain & Stress Center).

Since there are a number of ways of getting SAMe, which can be very costly, let's learn more about the scope before we narrow in on a prescription for you. Obviously where SAMe works, other methyl donors will benefit you as well, including choline, phosphatidyl choline and trimethylglycine or **TMG, 500 mg,** 1-2 caps 1-2 times a day (Klabin/Longevity Science, Jarrow). In fact, TMG is a less expensive alternative for the very expensive SAMe. As with another nutrient, MSM, the sulfur bearing and methyl donating adjuncts lead to many other unexpected healing benefits including revving up the detox system, which underlies healing of all disease, from chronic pain syndromes to cancer.

## Boron

After magnesium, boron is a very important mineral for relieving pain. English physician, Dr. Newnham, presented convincing evidence that boron, a mineral little heard of, has significantly improved arthritis of all types in large numbers of sufferers. In addition, it is especially important for rebuilding bone in post-menopausal women as it mimics estrogen's role in bone growth.

The dose for **boron** (Thorne, Bio-Tech, N.E.E.D.S.) is usually 4-6 mg, once or twice a day, balanced with other nutrients. Of note is that folks with rheumatoid arthritis who start boron often get worse initially, but usually get marked relief from pain if they continue. For **Boron Water** (Water Oz), an especially low dose, but well absorbed form, use 1 tsp. in a large glass of water 1-4 times a day.

## Silicon

And while you are at it, another forgotten mineral for healing painful body parts is silicon, crucial in building strong bones, blood vessels, tendons, skin, nails, hair and teeth. And silicon protects against aluminum toxicity that can lead to Alzheimer's, arteriosclerosis by acting like a Teflon coating to arteries, and makes the skin hold more hydroxyproline, an amino acid needed to prevent premature wrinkling and sagging.

But for our purposes here, you frankly cannot completely regenerate bone and cartilage without sufficient silicon. Lack of inclusion of silicon into bone-building formulations is a paramount reason for their failure. In fact, if you are at a standstill with trying to repair osteoporosis, a non-union fracture, or stabilize joints, remember to incorporate sufficient silicon into your program.

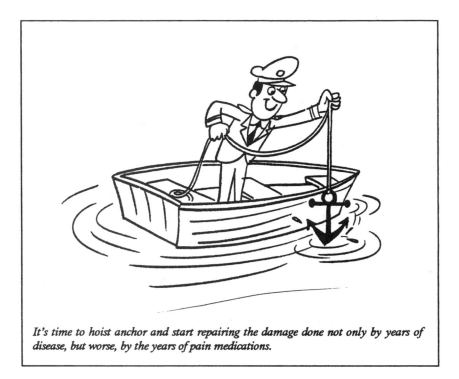

*It's time to hoist anchor and start repairing the damage done not only by years of disease, but worse, by the years of pain medications.*

Next to oxygen, silicon is the earth's most abundant element. By far the best-absorbed form of silicon is BioSil (Jarrow) which is a highly biologically active silicon as stabilized orthosilicic acid. In other words, you get about 250% more absorption than other forms. Use 10-20 drops in water once or twice a day.

So if you are intent on rebuilding damaged tissues, a quick start might include one or more of the following in any combination: Mobil-Ease, Rheumatol Forte, Osteo Complex, Bovine Cartilage, MSM, SAMe, Boron, BioSil, and more.

## The Niacinamide–Arthritis Connection

Niacinamide, a form of Niacin or vitamin B3 (but without the flushing of B3), has turned down arthritis and other forms of pain through a number of mechanisms. Like the $1,000/month prescription drug for rheumatoid arthritis, Enbrel®, it turns down the production of TNF-a (tumor necrosis factor) which is elevated in rheumatic joints. Coupled with this action is inhibition of a number of other sophisticated processes that also help to create inflammation and pain.

Because most pain stems from inflammation and inflammation produces oxidants that perpetuate the vicious cycle of inflammation and pain, it makes sense to combine niacinamide with a major anti-oxidant that can also beef up the detoxification pathways. Arthrogen combines 500 mg of niacinamide and 200 mg of N-acetylcysteine, which among other things, boosts glutathione for detoxification of free radicals that cause pain. Take **Arthrogen** (Metagenics) three times daily.

## Bone Soup

You know about taking glucosamine sulfate, minerals, other GAGs like bovine cartilage and collagen type II, sulfur, and/or methyl donors like MSM, SAMe, and TMG, plus minerals like boron and silica to rebuild. What else can you do on an everyday basis to repair and improve the strength of bone (and tendons, skin, vessels, ligaments and cartilage)? Make bone soup.

Bones are a superlative source of minerals, and the cartilage is the source of glucosamine sulfate. So save all your bones, gristle and cartilage, especially when you purchase any organic fish, fowl or meats.   Why would you ever want to discard the bones from an organic chicken? Freeze them in a baggie until you have sufficient to make soup.  Put in a large kettle of good water, add a little organic apple cider vinegar and sea salt to help release the minerals from the bones, bring to a boil, and simmer for a couple of hours.

Add your favorite herbs and spices, like basil, thyme, dill weed, garlic, or try pickling spice or bouquet garni. Incorporate left over vegetable scraps like celery leaves, broccoli stalks, onions, carrots, and cook an additional half hour or more, strain into jars filing them only ¾ full, and freeze.  Then when you are ready to make grain, vegetable, or bean soups, thaw your stock as you soak the beans.  All will be ready to cook into a nutritious soup.  The bone stock is the basis for not only soups, but also nutritious sauces or gravies. You should have bone soup daily if possible.  What could be easier and more basic to good health than recycling your GAGs the way our ancestors did?

### Now, to Repair the Source of Pain, the Cell Membrane

So you have great pain relief from one or any combinations of Lyprinol, Magnesium, Malic acid, and Power Relief.  But do you want to stay on these the rest of your life?  Of course not.   So the next step (assuming you already ruled out nightshades as a cause of your pain) is to fix the membrane. For each cell membrane can be thought of as a big fat envelope that keeps the cell from spilling its guts.   But more than a fence, the membrane serves many more functions. One is to release inflammatory mediators, chemicals that call up the forces of the immune system, like white blood cells to clean up after we have had an injury.  For you must clean up the old blood and debris so that a clean field is left in which new repair and growth can occur without infection.

The cell membrane is like a sandwich of many layers, with special nutrients that work in synergy to carry out this complex task. Unfortunately, if the wrong layers are in the cell membrane (usually because we have eaten too much junk food), the damaged membrane just shoots out these inflammatory messages willy-nilly any old time it feels like it. And you know by now, inflammation always means pain.

So the logical thing is to rebuild the membrane so it stops sending wrong pain messages. As with any natural treatment, you will benefit in many other ways once you have restored the membrane. You may enjoy more energy, clearer thoughts, happier thoughts, better memory, or unexpected relief of seemingly unrelated symptoms, because this chemistry affects all functions. So let's get busy and rebuild that fat sandwich.

You can read the biochemistry, reasons, and references for all this in my books and newsletters, so for now I'm just going to give you a formula that works for rebuilding many damaged membranes. The brands I recommend are particularly important for a number of reasons. In some cases, like **PhosChol Concentrate** (American Lecithin), for example, there is no comparison in the world, as this is the most potent source, necessary for this tough repair job. No wonder this is the most concentrated source and only brand of phosphatidyl choline that has studies at M.I.T. where they actually reversed early Alzheimer's. And not just for sick people, Boston marathon runners shortened their running times within weeks of taking it.

Or look at another unique product, Carlson's **Cod Liver Oil**, the only one that could send me an independent laboratory assay to show it was mercury-free. And don't forget another indispensably unique product for repairing cell membranes made by Enzymatic Therapy, the company that worked with the researcher who discovered the membrane-repairing and cancer-reversing properties of IP6. Would you want to use a product by a company that did not have this tight liaison and was merely trying to copy a product from afar? Not me.

### Membrane-Restoring Formula

- PhosChol Concentrate (American Lecithin) 1 tsp. a day
- E-Gems Elite (Carlson) 1-2 a day
- Tocotrienols (Carlson) 1-2 a day
- IP6 (Enzymatic Therapy) 4 twice a day between meals
- Cod Liver Oil (Carlson) 1 tsp. a day or 1 TBS twice a week; for this you can safely substitute Carlson capsules or
- Eskimo-3 (Prevail, Tyler) 2 capsules a day
- Efamol Evening Primrose Oil (Emerson Ecologics) 2 daily

Take this for 3-6 months, 2-6 times a week and feel what improves. Now you have some real power over pain!

### Message in a Nutshell

Any chronic musculoskeletal pain has to have nutrient deficiencies and/or damage to tissues, either as a precursor and/or result. Monumental healing requires rebuilding of tissues, and requires special nutrients not ever put into one compound, but mapped out for you here. And all the pain relievers in the world won't work if you fail to rebuild the membrane that is erroneously releasing all those chemical messages of inflammation and pain.

# Chapter 6

## Ultimate Healing From Pain

O.K., so you've done the nightshade-free diet, a trial of CM, healed the leaky gut, and tried many of the other corrective and temporizing remedies that have worked for thousands, but you still have pain? You have no choice but to get down to basics and get rid of the most likely remaining underlying cause of all pain, in fact of most disease: the **paradoxical plague**.

Paradoxical, incomprehensible, contradictory, that's what this plague is. For although it has swept the nation in epidemic proportions for decades, is responsible for nearly all disease, from chronic pain to cancer, from heart disease to mental disease, and is steadily gaining momentum, it breaks all the rules of epidemics or plagues:

(1) A plague visibly sweeps over a population, but this stealth plague is disguised as expected diseases of aging.
(2) A plague has one cause, but this one has hundreds.
(3) A plague kills its victims with the same symptoms, whereas this one produces a variety of symptoms.
(4) A plague kills quickly within a short period of time, but this one can take decades.
(5) A plague only takes out the weakest, whereas no one is immune to this one.
(6) A plague has one simple cure, whereas this one requires a total load of factors to conquer it.

The **paradoxical plague** is the slow but steady, pervasive, damaging accumulation of environmental toxins or poisons.

Hidden in our air, food and water, they come in many forms as pesticides, heavy metals, volatile organic hydrocarbons, and many other chemicals. I'll first show you that:

(1) You cannot escape environmental poisons. We all have them.
(2) Environmental toxins get into the body, and steadily accumulate with time, since the body does not have the chemistry to completely get rid of most of them.
(3) When they reach a certain level, they produce symptoms, sometimes seemingly overnight, that are assumed to have no known cause, no known cure. It can be as simple as high blood pressure or high cholesterol or as devastating as chronic pain or cancer.
(4) But getting rid of these chemicals has enabled folks to heal the impossible.
(5) And although the body does not have the chemistry to detoxify most of these chemicals, it can depurate or lose them through a God-given mechanism: sweat.
(6) The far infrared sauna is the most efficient, safest, most healing and the most well tolerated form of sauna. A tailored detoxification program can turn back the hands of time, giving the individual a body with the reduced toxic burden of yesteryear. This allows return to more normal function, as when the body was younger. It is the least expensive, yet logical and proven way of turning back the hands of time, which have brought on chronic disease. It is as close to the fountain of youth as man can realistically come.

# Environmental Toxins Are Everywhere

Pervasive poisons lurk in our air, food and water. Regardless of your commitment, you cannot avoid them, even if you live in a remote area inaccessible by 4-wheel drive, grow your own food and drink from a pristine mountain stream. For studies of just such areas have demonstrated the presence of PCBs and other nasty environmental chemicals, that are potent producers of cancer and other diseases. For example, water samples from remote areas of the Great Lakes and northern Canada, show deadly pesticides and PCBs.

And despite decades of overwhelming evidence of the hundreds of chemicals that the modern human body is exposed to and stockpiles, medical recognition is lagging pathetically behind. A perfect example is a front page article in the *Sarasota Herald-Tribune* (August 26, 2000) relating how government (CDC or Center for Disease Control, National Environmental Health Center) scientists are astounded that they have found "surprisingly high levels of phthalates from plastics" in the urine of ordinary Americans.

 They go on to affirm that these levels were "much higher than levels of (other) well-studied pollutants". The article acknowledges that scientists have known for years that humans harbor phthalates and that they cause birth defects, glandular and hormonal damage, and cancer. Yet it is ironic that the American Council on Science and Health (which the article admits is industry funded) claims that these chemicals are safe!

Where do phthalates come from? Every single plastic water and soda bottle, plastic baby bottles, plastic-wrapped food, PVC water pipes, and plastic machinery parts where processed foods are created, not to mention plastic computer housings, furnishings, out-gassing warm electronic wires and literally hundreds of other sources each day. And phthalates are just one of scores of chemical classes that cause bewildering diseases that outgas from plastics. There is even more danger in toluene, phenol, benzene, TCE, PCBs, vinyl chloride and others. And just think of the synergistic poisons they create, when you mix them together in one body!

As well, scientists have tracked wind-carried pesticides from huge African plains all the way to the U.S., industrial chemicals and radiation from smokestacks from other countries, and contaminated water from polluters hundreds of miles upstream. Since there are thousands of environmental chemicals, let's take a brief look at a few so you get an idea of how *pervasive* they are and what kind of symptoms they *insidiously* produce. Clearly, we will never run out of ways to poison ourselves.

## Stealth Poisons Lurk in Styrofoam Cups

Ah, the coffee break. You've worked hard all morning and you deserve a break today. But the Styrofoam coffee cup sends styrene and other plasticizers straight into your bloodstream. From here they are dispersed to every organ in your body to do their silent dirty work of damaging body chemistry.

The coffee break, practically a legal obligation, is one place you can unknowingly tank up on cancer-causing toxins.

Styrene cups, those crushable white "plastic" or "foam" cups in every office dispenser outgas toxic chemicals right into your coffee that are endocrine disrupters (damage the action of hormones). By either mimicking the action of hormones or blocking or stimulating receptors, they can trigger anything from breast and prostate cancers to thyroid and other glandular failures. And it is such a ubiquitous toxin that in an EPA study, 100% of fat biopsies from people contained styrene residues. Every single person had cancer-causing styrene residues stored in their fat that the body was unable to get rid of. No wonder cancer is the number two cause of death and illness!

You see, when the body meets a new-fangled chemical, synthesized in the laboratory, that has no business being in the body, often there is no metabolic mechanism with which to get rid of it. So *what the body cannot detoxify, it dumps into fat storage*. That explains why in this same government study 100% of the fat biopsies also contained dioxins (one of the most potent causes of cancer known). We get it from contact with bleached paper products (toilet paper, paper towels, disposable diapers, tea bags, milk cartons), incinerator air, water contamination from industry, and herbicides in foods.

Also present in 100% of the fat biopsies taken as samples from ordinary citizens were xylene from gasoline, paints and glues, another carcinogen, 1,4-dichlorobenzene from home deodorizers, mothballs, sanitizers in textiles for furnishings, bedding and clothes, and many other products. Let's face it. We are a cesspool. Our bodies continually stockpile nasty cancer-causing chemicals that we eat, drink and breathe each day that it has no other way of dealing with. And their harm does not begin and end with cancer. They can mimic or create

141

any symptom imaginable. It merely depends on the individual's unique biochemistry and genetic make-up.

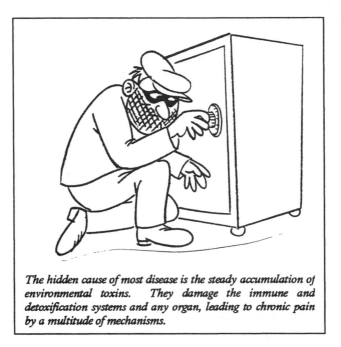

*The hidden cause of most disease is the steady accumulation of environmental toxins. They damage the immune and detoxification systems and any organ, leading to chronic pain by a multitude of mechanisms.*

As government studies suggest, there are very few uncontaminated or "normal" people left, as it is progressively more difficult to avoid these cancer-promoting chemicals in the modern world. We all silently stock-pile or bio-accumulate over the years a plethora of these toxins, which daily leach out to damage our genes and other proteins that regulate important functions designed to protect us from chronic pain and other diseases. When it takes a couple of decades to produce cancer or any of the other nasty chronic diseases, we chalk up the final emergence of symptoms to the normal consequences of aging. The only problem with that lame excuse is that the diseases of aging are clearly occurring at progressively younger ages... and they are curable!

The ubiquitous sources of the hundreds of unseen chemicals that we are all hoarding daily make them impossible to avoid. Dental fillings, called amalgams, contain mercury that poisons enzymes leading to anything from heart disease with angina to mood swings, depression or chronic pain. Cadmium from auto exhaust is a known cause of hypertension or chronic pain. Aluminum in foods can contribute to Alzheimer's or chronic pain. Pesticides in our air, food and water can trigger indigestion, angina, atrial fibrillation, mental diseases like schizophrenia or depression, fibromyalgia and a host of undiagnosable pain syndromes.

And all bets are off when you start mixing these chemicals and their unknown metabolites in any individual body. No wonder the cancer rate has so dramatically risen: from the tenth cause of death when I was in medical school 35 years ago to the second cause of death in adults now and the first cause of death in certain childhood age ranges.

### Cadmium, the Killer

O.K., so it's time to drive home and have a little relaxing cigarette on the way. Air pollution from auto exhaust and cigarette smoke (even secondhand) are some of the best ways to tank up on cadmium, another stealth chemical that can likewise mimic any symptom, including pain.

What does a woman with osteoporosis and back pain have in common with a man with hypertension and hip pain? And what do other people with other chronic pain syndromes, emphysema, chronic fatigue, protein-losing kidney disease, liver disease and prostate and lung cancer have in common with one another and with the first two? According to voluminous studies from the U.S. Department of Health and Human Services, they could all have the same cause of their symptoms, cadmium poisoning.

If you are like most people, you probably never even heard of cadmium, even though it is likely one of the myriad of environmental poisons you have accumulated over a lifetime. It is now clear that for most disease, 95% of the underlying cause is in the diet and the environment. But when a symptom appears, it is easier to plop folks on a drug to turn off the ailing, malfunctioning or *poisoned part* than to look for the *curable cause*. Pain medication is a quick and easy solution, and the patient goes away happy with relief, never dreaming that his prescribed medications are the cause of slow bone deterioration, heart, kidney, vision, and gastrointestinal side effects that will insidiously erode his health.

Sentenced to a lifetime of anti-hypertensive drugs, osteoporosis drugs or pain medicines, and considering that the underlying cause has neither been found nor corrected, the condition worsens, requiring more medications. As the toxicity spreads and other organs are damaged, new symptoms and new diseases arise, with no one the wiser as to the true cause. Medicine has done a great job at brainwashing the populace into believing that every disease is merely a deficiency of some drug.

# Cadmium the Cause of "Ouch-Ouch Disease"

So what is this cadmium and how would we ever get exposed to it in the sanctity of our clean homes and safe offices? As a silver-white lustrous metal, it is found naturally in the earth's soils. But man has concentrated it and dispersed it in a multitude of ways, contaminating his air, food and water.

Foods are the most important source, for the soils they grow on are increasingly polluted with cadmium-rich sewage sludge (actually sold as commercial fertilizer) and irrigated by industrially contaminated ground waters. Shellfish (clams, oysters, mussels, scallops) and other types of bottom-feeding fish effectively concentrate industrial contamination of streams and waterways feeding where they empty into bays. The typical daily intake of cadmium is 30 micrograms (ug) which seems small. But wait. The body has no way of getting rid of it, so it slowly accumulates (along with hundreds of other toxins) to accelerate disease and aging.

The greatest source of airborne cadmium contamination is the burning of fossil fuels like coal and oil, auto exhaust, and incineration of municipal wastes containing plastics and batteries. Smoking one cigarette provides 2 ug, giving a smoker more than double the average daily cadmium.

Drinking water is progressively more contaminated in our industrialized society, while softened water and acidic water hold even more cadmium, and can leach cadmium from old pipe welds and PVC pipes (since cadmium is a major stabilizer of plastics).

Occupations that increase cadmium accumulation include auto mechanics, engravers, glass makers, jewelers, lithographers, and those who work with solder, welding, plating, ceramics and pottery, porcelains, dental amalgams, electric instruments, electroplating, mining and refining, paints, pesticides, lawn and turf fungicides (golfers), pharmaceuticals, pigments, plastics, sculptors, textile printers, outgassing plastics, photographic materials, phosphorus fertilizers, auto exhaust, fungicides, x-ray fluorescent screens, instrument dials, second hand smoke, and more. In other words, you really cannot find a person without cadmium exposure. Many folks have it in their mouths in the form of porcelain crowns. And we are talking about only one of thousands of environmental chemicals.

No wonder we have so much disease, for this tiny example of chemicals that the body has difficulty detoxifying can mimic a multitude of symptoms and diseases. Meanwhile, unsuspecting physicians never seek it as a cause and medicines are powerless against it. Then as we age, we gradually accumulate higher levels of all these toxins. In fact the presence of cadmium and other heavy metals like aluminum, lead, and mercury stimulate the formation of metallothionein, a metal-binding protein, which concentrates cadmium three-thousand-fold in the body. No wonder we deteriorate as we do in exponential fashion.

For example, cadmium damages the kidneys and causes hypertension, one of the most common causes of cardiovascular disease. And cadmium not only interferes with the gut's absorption of calcium, but also increases the excretion of calcium in the urine. No wonder we have so much osteoporosis, spontaneous fractures, back pain, hip and knee replacements, neurological diseases and kidney stones.

Cadmium can lead to a simple anemia, poor sense of smell and yellowing of the teeth at the gum line or to a host of undiagnosable ills that baffle medicine. Or as a carcinogen, it can trigger cancer of the lung, prostate, testicles and more. Furthermore, cadmium spurs cancers to grow faster and metastasize if it is not removed from the cancer victim's body.

Often it takes a catastrophic spill to alert man to the dangers of an environmental toxin. In 1946 the Japanese residents at the mouth of the Jintzu River were afflicted with body pain and spontaneous fractures. They were in such pain that the disease name "itai-itai" translates as "ouch-ouch". The river, used for drinking and fishing, was contaminated with cadmium by an upstream mining operation.

Man has learned that cadmium is capable of not only chronic mysterious pain, but just about any symptom, from gastrointestinal hemorrhaging or hypertension to cardiomyopathy or cancer. And most often the diseases are bizarre, baffling physicians by having no obvious cause or cure, and are usually resistant to drugs.

### Arsenic, Another Hidden Cause of Pain

If you had burning, numbness and tingling from your fingertips to your forearm, what would you look for? Carpal tunnel syndrome, a spinal cord tumor? With a paresthesia occurring in a "stocking-glove" fashion, with or without a mysterious painful burning, probably the last thing you or your doctors would think of is arsenic poisoning. Where would you get it?  Cigarettes (even second-hand smoke, from being around smokers), paints, pesticides in homes, offices, schools and restaurants, fungicides in humid areas like boats, food, and southern climates, porcelain dental work, or wood preservatives are common sources.

Arsenic is a common industrial pollutant in ground water, in the air from burning fossil fuels (auto exhaust, industrial exhaust), in wine and grapes sprayed with arsenic-containing pesticides, and in shell fish which take it up from the bottom of rivers and bay basins.   It is a plywood preservative, and until the 1940s was used to treat syphilis, psoriasis, and is still used for amoebic diseases.  Gallium arsenide is integral in microwave devices and lasers, while meat, fish and poultry account for up to 80% of the source, due to their ability to concentrate it from contaminated air, food and water in the form of pesticides, herbicides, fungicides, and cattle dips.

Its symptoms can be anything from painful intestinal cramping and bloody diarrhea to death of the kidneys, cardiomyopathy, congestive heart failure, arrhythmias, *intense mysterious burning*, loss of sensation, weakness or paralysis, bizarre skin pigmentations, low white blood cell counts (leukopenia), anemia, or cancer.  Symptoms can be as obscure as headaches, brain fog, liver disease, or peculiar garlic odor of the breath and transverse white lines on nails.

### Polycyclic Aromatic Hydrocarbons

Polycyclic aromatic hydrocarbons is another group that is impossible to avoid and contains hundreds of chemicals. We are all stockpiling them, which inevitably leads to a point where the total body burden is more than we can handle and

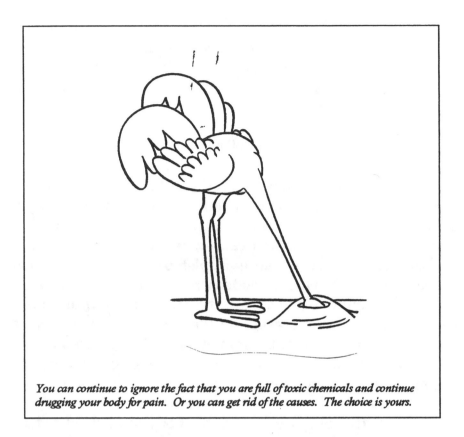

*You can continue to ignore the fact that you are full of toxic chemicals and continue drugging your body for pain. Or you can get rid of the causes. The choice is yours.*

disease results. Included in this group of modern chemicals present in every home, office and travel environment, plus found in most foods and water are the benzanthracenes. This group of chemicals is so potent in causing cancer that only *one* dose is given to animals in order to create research rats with cancer.

And when we mix pesticides, plasticizers and all the other everyday chemicals together, their carcinogenicity is synergistic. No longer does 1+1=2, but it is more like 10. In addition, once you get a pain syndrome or cancer, for example, having these chemicals still on board can annihilate any chance of recovery. On the flip side, once you unload the body of these unwanted burdens, it can leave the body so healthy that it becomes able to heal itself, regardless of how "hopeless" the diagnosis appears.

## No Toxin Pollutes Alone

So the bottom line is that we possess an overwhelming unseen burden of toxic metals and chemicals hidden in our major sources of food, air and water that can cause the top two diseases, cardiovascular and cancer, as well as chronic pain. In addition, they can cause a plethora of other serious diseases, none of which "modern medicine" considers as a possible cadmium toxicity. And the cadmium example is not alone, but one of scores of hidden environmental heavy metals that are all potent triggers of pain. And I haven't even begun to describe the thousands of other environmental chemicals that act similarly.

The half-life (the time with which the body can get rid of half of a toxin) of cadmium ranges between 25-30 years. Couple this with the ability of metallothionein (a protein we make in the body) to stockpile and concentrate it 3000-fold in red blood cells, liver, kidney, heart and other vital organs. Are we doomed? There is no drug, no medicine, to safely get rid of it along with all the other toxins, like the volatile hydrocarbons and pesticides. What could we do to get these toxins out, and turn back the hands of time? How can we bring disease to a screeching halt?

But before we go into the solution, bear in mind that no one gets a solo cadmium toxicity. Whenever you are exposed to cadmium, as one tiny example, most likely you are also tanking up on other metals (like mercury, aluminum, arsenic), pesticides, herbicides, and volatile organic hydrocarbons like formaldehyde, trichloroethylene, benzene, phthalates, PCBs, dioxins, hexanes, and a plethora of other chemicals that are more dangerous than cadmium. And like cadmium, the body has no way of completely metabolizing and detoxifying its total burden of these. Instead they accumulate day after day, year in, year out. The body attaches them to whatever it can to make them more stable to minimize their damage. But as levels and mixtures with unknown consequences increase, eventually the dam bursts and disease erupts.

## Toxic Teeth: The Hidden Health Hazard

"What are you doing? Just ask!"

My luscious husband is accustomed to my unbridled enthusiasm that uncontrollably (and impolitely) erupts when I try to sneak glances over his shoulder at his *Wall Street Journal*, or worse yet, tear out a portion while he's still reading it. But years ago on this flight when the headline "Heavy Metal Group Hits Moscow" caught my attention, I couldn't help myself. For I was smack dab in the middle of researching the best ways to help us all detoxify our mercury. I had no idea the Russians were right on target researching heavy metals.

Alas, my spirits plummeted, and I realized I was getting old when he had to affectionately explain, "Bunny, Heavy Metal is a rock group, not a delegation of environmental medicine scientists studying dental amalgams."

In medical school 35 years ago, as today, mercury was not a big subject. Rarely mentioned, it can nevertheless be a major reason why many will never get well. In fact it constitutes one of the big four that I see as precipitating the downfall of many: *Environmental chemicals, pesticides, hidden infection, and mercury.* And many individuals who developed over 20 symptoms, including severe chemical sensitivity (like myself and many of you), were burdened with all four causes.

Often people can give a concise history starting when they were last well, then recall every few years when they took another downslide and developed another handful of undiagnosable, untreatable symptoms. But then take them back down memory lane and have them factor into this time warp when they had their last dental filling, root canal, crown or major dental work done in the mouth, and it invariably starts to fall into place. Even extractions lead to a "dry socket" and infection. Likewise biting on a hard substance like a bone or nutshell can crack a tooth, and lead to a smoldering abscess that interferes with body function far from the tooth site. Months and years later this silent painless infection can cause mysterious pain in a joint far from the mouth.

The dental filling, also referred to as a silver amalgam, is actually 50% mercury. Root canals are even worse because they usually consist of a mercury plug deep in the old nerve trench. Bacteria can successfully hide here for years until there is a raging jaw abscess. Sometimes the silent infection smolders for years with just occasional sensitivity. But this metallic interference with normal body energy flows, coupled with the unsuspected infection, disturbs the function of organs that are in the acupuncture meridians or pathways that connect organs with each particular tooth. Suddenly one day a baffling symptom emerges relating to this organ. The tooth organ chart 2 pages ahead views the mouth as your dentist would, with your right side on his left of the chart. Let me make this difficult and new concept clearer.

## The Jawbone is Connected to Every Organ

Over a decade ago I broke a lower back tooth that had a big 25-year old mercury filling. Since I was still very chemically sensitive at that time, I dared not think of putting anything in its place, not knowing what I would tolerate. After months of my dentist's insisting, I decided that as long as I already had a mouth full of mercury for over 40 years, one miniscule piece more was not going to make a difference.

A few weeks later I let my baby sister teach me how to windsurf. That night, after having hauled up the blasted sail about 100 times (I did not have a very good teacher I found out later), my shoulder began to ache. No big deal, I thought; I guessed I deserved it. But day by day, then week by week it became more painful.

Six months and several orthopedic specialists later, I had not been able to use it for months to even pick up a medical chart. I called a colleague and explained the *mysterious incapacitating shoulder pain* and he wisely asked, "When did you have your last amalgam in your right posterior lower tooth?" He knew exactly what tooth was in trouble by knowing where my body pain was. For the tooth was in the acupuncture meridian of the shoulder and mercury was interfering with its energy pathway. He knew precisely what tooth was the culprit (#31) by following the area in trouble (right shoulder) back through the body's known electrical system (the acupuncture meridians) to the organ's corresponding tooth.

You see, the body has arteries, veins, lymphatics and nerves. And it has an unseen but proven additional circuitry, the acupuncture meridians. They can be thought of as an electrical system that ties the whole body together. The "wires" or meridians have been mapped out so that we know why kidney problems can lead to mysteriously painful soles of the feet or why a silent tooth abscess can lead to persistent angina, killer migraines or recurrent tennis elbow.

Luckily there are many ways to heal. At that point, I went on the strict macrobiotic diet (described in detail in *The Cure Is In the Kitchen*, but you need to read the primer first, *You Are What You Ate*). Within 4 weeks the pain was totally gone and I was wind-surfing, hauling up a 75 lb. sail in gusty winds. Months later as my chemical sensitivities also came under better control, I dared take the plunge and remove that mercury and a few, but not all, others.

# Tooth: Organ Chart

## Upper Teeth (Teeth 1–16)

| Row | Tooth 1 | Teeth 2–3 | Tooth 4 | Tooth 5 | Teeth 6–8 | Teeth 9–11 | Tooth 12 | Tooth 13 | Teeth 14–15 | Tooth 16 |
|---|---|---|---|---|---|---|---|---|---|---|
| **SENSE ORGANS** | Inner ear | Maxillary Sinus | Ethmoid cells | Eye | Frontal sinus | Frontal sinus | Eye | Ethmoid cells | Maxillary Sinus | Inner ear |
| **JOINTS** | Shoulder, Elbow; Hand, ulnar, Foot, plantar, Toes, sacro-iliac joint | Jaws; Front of knee | Shoulder, Elbow; Hand, radial, Foot, Big toe | Hip; Foot | Back of knee; Sacrococcyx; Foot | Back of knee; Sacrococcyx; Foot | Hip; Foot | Shoulder, Elbow; Hand, radial, Foot, Big toe | Jaws; Front of knee | Shoulder, Elbow; Hand, ulnar, Foot, plantar, Toes, sacro-iliac joint |
| **SPINAL SEGMENTS** | C8, T1 T5 T6 T7, S1 S2 S3 | T11 T12 L1 | C5 C6 C7, T2 T3 T4, L4 L5 | T8 T9 T10 | L2 L3, S4 S5, Coccyx | L2 L3, S4 S5, Coccyx | T8 T9 T10 | C5 C6 C7, T2 T3 T4, L4 L5 | T11 T12 L1 | C8, T1 T5 T6 T7, S1 S2 S3 |
| **VERTEBRAE** | C7, T1 T5 T6, S1 S2 | T11 T12 L1 | C5 C6 C7, T2 T3 T4, L4 L5 | T9 T10 | L2 L3, S3 S4 S5, Coccyx | L2 L3, S3 S4 S5, Coccyx | T9 T10 | C5 C6 C7, T2 T3 T4, L4 L5 | T11 T12 L1 | C7, T1 T5 T6, S1 S2 |
| **ORGANS** | Heart -R; Duodenum | Pancreas; Stomach -R | Lung -R; Large Intestine -R | Liver -R; Gall-bladder | Kidney -R; Bladder -R, Urogenital area | Kidney -L; Bladder -L, Urogenital area | Liver -L; Bile ducts -L | Lung -L; Large Intestine -L | Spleen; Stomach -L | Heart -L; Jejunum, Ileum -L |
| **ENDOCRINE ORGANS** | Pituitary, Ant. lobe | Para-thyroid; Thyroid | Thymus | Pituitary, Post lobe | Pineal gland | Pineal gland | Pituitary, Post lobe | Thymus | Thyroid; Para-thyroid | Pituitary, Ant. lobe |
| **OTHERS** | CNS, Psyche | Mammary Gland -R | | | ↙ midline | Mammary Gland -L | | | Mammary Gland -L | CNS, Psyche |

Upper teeth numbers: 1  2  3  4  5  6  7  8  9  10  11  12  13  14  15  16  (R … L)

## Lower Teeth (Teeth 32–17)

Lower teeth numbers: 32  31  30  29  28  27  26  25  24  23  22  21  20  19  18  17  (R … L)

| Row | Tooth 32 | Teeth 31–30 | Tooth 29 | Tooth 28 | Teeth 27–26–25 | Teeth 24–23 | Tooth 22 | Teeth 21–20 | Teeth 19–18 | Tooth 17 |
|---|---|---|---|---|---|---|---|---|---|---|
| **OTHERS** | Energy Metabolism | | Mammary Gland -R | | | | | Mammary Gland -L | | Energy Metabolism |
| **ENDOCRINE GLANDS / TISSUE SYSTEMS** | Peripheral nerves | Arteries; Veins | Lymph vessels | Gonad (Testes or Ovary) | Adrenal gland | Adrenal gland | Gonad (Testes or Ovary) | Lymph vessels | Veins; Arteries | Peripheral Nervous System |
| **ORGANS** | Ileum -R; Ileocecal region | Large Intestine -R | Stomach -R, Pylorus | Gall-bladder | Bladder -R, Urogenital area | Bladder -L, Urogenital area | Bile ducts -L | Stomach -L | Large Intestine -L | Jejunum, Ileum -L |
| | Heart -R | Lung -R | Pancreas | Liver -R | Kidney -R | Kidney -L | Liver -L | Spleen | Lung -L | Heart -L |
| **VERTEBRAE** | C7, T1 T5 T6, S1 S2 | C5 C6 C7, T2 T3 T4, L4 L5 | T11 T12 L1 | T9 T10 | L2 L3, S3 S4 S5, Coccyx | L2 L3, S3 S4 S5, Coccyx | T9 T10 | T11 T12 L1 | C5 C6 C7, T2 T3 T4, L4 L5 | C7, T1 T5 T6, S1 S2 |
| **SPINAL SEGMENTS** | C8, T1 T5 T6 T7, S1 S2 S3 | C5 C6 C7, T2 T3 T4, L4 L5 | T11 T12 L1 | T8 T9 T10 | L2 L3, S4 S5, Coccyx | L2 L3, S4 S5, Coccyx | T8 T9 T10 | T11 T12 L1 | C5 C6 C7, T2 T3 T4, L4 L5 | C8, T1 T5 T6 T7, S1 S2 S3 |
| **JOINTS** | Shoulder and elbow; Hand, ulnar, Foot, plantar, Toes, sacro-iliac joint | Front of knee; Hand, radial, Foot, Big toe | Back of knee; Jaws | Hip; Foot | Sacrococcyx; Foot | Sacrococcyx; Foot | Hip; Foot | Back of knee; Jaws | Front of knee; Hand, radial, Foot, Big toe | Shoulder and elbow; Hand, ulnar, Foot, plantar, Toes, sacro-iliac joint |
| **SENSE ORGANS** | Ear | Ethmoid cells | Maxillary Sinus | Eye | Frontal sinus | Frontal sinus | Eye | Maxillary Sinus | Ethmoid cells | Ear |

**Note:** When identifying teeth, this is how a dentist would view your mouth. So your teeth that are on the right side of your body are on the left side of the chart.

155

You might ask why I didn't take the mercury out right away. But realize that for every person who has their amalgams removed and gets great results, like major relief from pain, fatigue, chemical sensitivity, fibromyalgia, depression or the leukemia count goes down or MS or lupus symptoms improve, there is another person for whom it does nothing or they are worse. Often they cannot tolerate the new material. One major mistake I frequently see is that the detox system was not yet healthy enough for the overload of mercury that can be dumped into the system when mercury detox is begun. **It is a grave mistake that can end with disastrous results to remove any heavy metal or contaminating chemical until you are sure the detoxification system is healthy enough to complete the job.** More on this later.

Too bad life is not always this simple, because there are scores of other meridians that are not related to teeth. So although teeth are not always the answer for every malady, if you have resistant pain, investigate the teeth in that meridian. If there is an old root canal, filling, cracked tooth or it is the site of an extraction, there can be a painless festering abscess or a metal toxicity.

### The Many Disguises of Heavy Metal Toxicity

Most every doc has knowledge of lead poisoning. He knows how nibbling on woodwork and lead-based painted toys, or exposure to hair dyes, auto exhaust, drinking water from lead pipes or lead-based ceramic pottery pitchers, and the industrial contamination of the water table, living down wind from battery and painted object incineration, etc. can damage the brains of young children. And most appreciate how aluminum, another heavy metal, causes brain damage and

156

neurofibrillary tangles like those of Alzheimer's disease. Yet still there is an unaccountable gap between knowledge and the application of it, for there are more aluminum containers available now than ever before. Just look at the aluminum lining for children's juice boxes, thermos linings, coffee makers, and the aluminum desiccant in salt, flours and baking powders for breads, cookies, and biscuits.

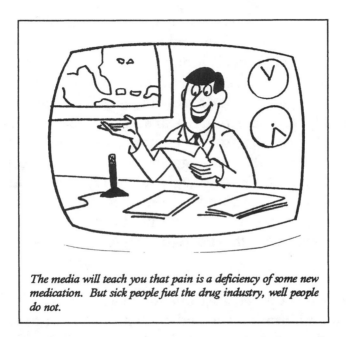

*The media will teach you that pain is a deficiency of some new medication. But sick people fuel the drug industry, well people do not.*

Likewise, dentists mask, gown and glove to work with mercury and pay exorbitant fees to have the tiniest amounts carried away by professional toxic waste haulers. Yet once it is in your mouth, it is considered harmless. But these heavy metals leak into the blood stream and sit in enzymes displacing minerals that must be there for proper function. Once heavy metals have kicked out the good mineral, they act like an anchor and severely dampen the action of the enzyme. No wonder scientists have found that mercury can even damage the ability of the body to fight off infection, leaving our resident intestinal bacteria and fungi (yeasts) resistant to treatment. And you have learned how the leaky gut can then initiate an avalanche of pain syndromes. It becomes a vicious cycle with no relief. You need to find the cause to get a cure.

Heavy metals can cause any symptom, like perplexing **peripheral neuropathy** (strange numbness and tingling, loss of sensation, loss of nerve control, unusual pain) in arms or legs. And heavy metals can mimic diseases that we call by other names, like carpal tunnel syndrome, shoulder tear, tennis elbow, or arthritis. The brain is a frequent target organ. Certainly our epidemic of depression, mood swings, brain fog with inability to concentrate, learning disorders, migraines, attention deficit disorder, memory loss, lowered I.Q., unwarranted irritability and aggression are all manifestations, at least in part, of the onslaught of heavy metals in our 3 environments, air, food and water. Yet each person carries his/her own unique total body burden of unwanted chemicals, which is why no two people get the exact same symptoms.

The sources are unseen and unavoidable. Cadmium in auto exhaust; aluminum in cans and cooking pots, not to mention antacids, baking powders, salt, deodorants, coffee makers and water heaters; then add lead in industrial and auto exhaust, seams in food cans, hair dyes; arsenic in cigarettes, pesticides, fungicides (mold and mildew retardants) and more.

What is worse is the powerful ability of heavy metals to mimic any symptom, and usually present as the most incurable and hopeless things like multiple sclerosis, manic depression, lupus, or chronic fatigue and chronic pain. Since mercury is one of the worst and most common of the heavy metals, let's look at that as our example, especially since the official position of the ADA (American Dental Association) is that it is not a problem, which is blatantly false.

---

## Case Examples

Kathy was chronically exhausted for months and had back pain, but all x-rays were negative. Her RBC (red blood cell) mercury was off the scale. She did not have even one amalgam. Her water was checked and found to be free of mercury. The source that took the health department's mercury meter off the scale? Her bedroom and basement paints that were at least a year old contained mercury as a mold and mildew inhibitor.

Mike was having memory problems and headaches in school. His mercury levels were markedly elevated in spite of no amalgams. He had the habit of downing a can of tuna fish after school sports. His level returned to normal with just a change to another snack and using the mercury detox cocktail for 3 months (in *Total Wellness* 2000).

Susan had over 40 different symptoms, and as many physicians, all of whom were stumped by her bizarre body burning sensation. She also had body aches that would migrate from one area to another, brain fog, exhaustion, and newly emerged heightened sensitivity to various foods and chemicals that never used to bother her. When I examined her mouth, her mercury had actually migrated out of the fillings into the gum tissues, staining them black, a condition we call *mercury tattooing*. Her RBC mercury levels were also off the chart.

---

You can experience a wonderful clearing of the cobwebs of years that you had become accustomed to in your head, depression can lift, or any number of pain symptoms melt away. As Dr. Stortebecker of the famed Karolinska Institute in Stockholm Sweden showed in his excellent book, *Dental Caries As A Cause Of Nervous Disorders*, the brain is the favorite place for mercury to hide out, especially in the pineal gland, a master gland which affects many others.

## Mercury a Common Toxin to Paralyze the Immune System

Although many countries like Sweden years ago banned mercury fillings for children and pregnant women, the American Dental Association still insists on the safety and harmlessness of silver (actually 50% mercury) dental fillings. These amalgams leach toxic mercury into the blood stream and impair the body's ability to fight off bugs in the gut like Candida. In fact, it is very common for mercury to poison the immune system. Whenever we see someone who is having a tough time getting rid of Candida or leaky gut, we usually find high levels of mercury in the cell lining, paralyzing the ability of the body to fight this "normal" fungus. If silently impaired immunity were not enough of a tragedy, mercury can damage any enzyme or regulatory protein or part of a cell, creating more mystery symptoms.

## Addressing the Total Load is the Only Way To Heal the Impossible

Let's look at one example of how you can pull parts of the total load of causes together in order to heal the impossible. Auto-immune arthritis, for example, can start with something as simple as Candida overgrowth after antibiotics, coupled with mercury toxicity from dental amalgams, paints or fish that impair the body's ability to fight Candida. From there you get a leaky gut from the prolonged inflammation of the intestinal lining caused by the Candida overgrowth. This leaky gut in turn impairs the carrier proteins in the gut lining that carry minerals and other nutrients across the gut into the bloodstream. With nutrient reserves dwindling, the ensuing cascade of symptoms makes drug-directed physicians doubt your sanity.

The leaky gut then can trigger auto-antibodies to your own tissues, leading to auto-immune disease like lupus arthritis. Depression, joint pains, and heart disease are only a handful of the other symptoms that drive folks to seek all that medicine can offer. Unfortunately, that merely means high doses of prednisone which makes the Candida grow even faster. When that fails, chemotherapy drugs are used that cause cancer years down the road. Now you can appreciate one reason why these folks have such misery, with the key prescription drugs actually making the disease worse. Using the currently recommended drugs for auto-immune diseases is like pouring gasoline on a fire.

### Is the Cause of Your Pain All In Your Head
### Or All In Your Mouth?

I don't want to leave you with the impression that all auto-immune disease is due to Candida, mercury and nutrient deficiencies, but rather to give you an idea of how these conditions commonly occur. For once you understand how we get disease, this will help you develop the thinking process that is required to unravel it and reverse disease.

Yes, you can actually reverse disease that medicine insists has no known cause or cure. I want you to have a strong sense that for conditions you have been told you have to live with, it just isn't so. I need to fuel you with enthusiasm to find and correct the causes of your pain. For it will be years before medicine grasps the environmental medicine **TOTAL LOAD** approach. It has already been around for 5 decades and look at how it continues to be ignored in favor of drugs that accelerate disease. Disease and drugs fuel the economy, not wellness.

You can appreciate how it warms my heart to see folks with chronic pain, thyroiditis, lupus, multiple sclerosis or other dead-end conditions begin to improve for the first time since their diagnoses were made. Luckily, if you need to heal now, you have a good chance of being able to pull it off. For always remember, the body was miraculously designed by the ultimate physician to heal against all odds, not to be chronically sick.

If you have a problem that defies cure, reconsider that the problem may stem from toxic teeth. And if you are well, bear in mind that this is one hidden threat that can suddenly reverse the tide and take you down at any moment. Alzheimer's, Parkinson's disease, cardiomyopathy, high cholesterol or triglycerides, ALS, heart attack, rheumatoid arthritis, stroke, cancer, auto-immune disease like MS, a chronic pain syndrome or anything you can imagine can be at your doorstep by morning.

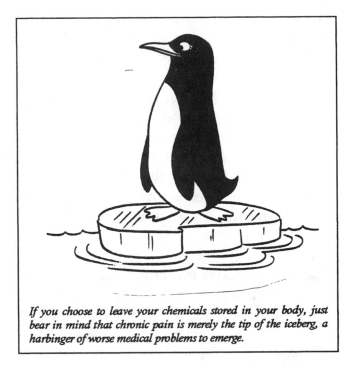

*If you choose to leave your chemicals stored in your body, just bear in mind that chronic pain is merely the tip of the iceberg, a harbinger of worse medical problems to emerge.*

And mercury is merely the tip of the iceberg when it comes to toxins in the teeth. The porcelain crowns contain cadmium, and the acrylic and methacrylate glues have caused heart attacks, cancer and more. *You have at some point in time probably been told the cause of your pain is all in your head. But now is the time to consider whether it is really all in your mouth.*

## Sauna, the Key to Dumping Stored Toxins

If I look at the last 100 people who were extremely ill, who have been everywhere, done everything, and are still sick, what caused it? What is holding them back from being well? The major demons are heavy metals (mercury leads the list), pesticides, and other environmental chemicals, like volatile aromatic hydrocarbons, that they had accumulated over a lifetime from their air, food, and water. Even the government admits that 95% of cancer is due to diet and chemicals.

How does the body normally get rid of toxins? It takes them through a series of chemical or metabolic reactions in the body to make them easier to expel. Then it boots them out into the stool, urine, and sweat. That is it. It has no other way of getting rid of toxins. Sure we find trace amounts in breast milk, tears, semen, vaginal secretions, saliva, and hair, but this is mere overflow and not a way designed to depurate or get rid of large amounts.

Since *the solution to pollution is dilution,* when you are acutely poisoned, drinking a lot of water is a great way to hurry getting rid of it. But once a toxin has firmly attached itself to body organs, it is no longer going to be merely flushed out of the body. The same goes for purging the bowel. But sweat is a different story.

The 1970's gave us a rash of drug addicts who needed *to detoxify or die.* Sauna saved their lives. Others reaffirmed the benefits of detoxifying saunas when, as a result of accidents involving pilots who did aerial spraying of pesticides, men were cleared of life-threatening symptoms. Likewise residents of Michigan gave us a huge amount of scientific information when a PCB-laden cancer-causing fire retardant was accidentally put into animal feed, contaminating their entire dairy industry for decades.

Studies six years and later showed that Michigan residents and folks from over 25 other states who also got the PCBs hidden in their dairy products just did not get rid of those nasty PCBs. The body does not have the chemistry to do so. But those who did saunas were able to eliminate the PCBs and other stored toxins. The truth is we have all eaten foods from there and have slowly bioaccumulated these and hundreds of other similar toxins that are known as some of the most powerful inducers of cancer and other diseases in existence. In fact, U.S. EPA studies show that 100% of human fat biopsies contain styrene (from plastic wrap on foods and plastic water and soda bottles, dioxins (one of the most potent cancer causing chemicals in the world), and many more dangerous disease-causing chemicals. More on all these in *Detoxify or Die*.

But the proof for the magic of sauna detoxification does not end there. In addition, other studies have shown that fire fighters, for example, who were toxic from the inhalation of burning plastic fumes (carcinogenic phthalates), were detoxified using the heat and sweating of sauna units. And workers accidentally contaminated from occupations as diverse as electricians to farmers, machinists to office workers had their lives saved as serious conditions that medicine was powerless to help were reversed through the use of sauna.

Then there are my hundreds of patients with severe chemical sensitivity, saddled with just about any symptom you can think of, who have traveled the world to find out how to get well. When exposed to simple everyday perfumes, fabric softeners, carpets, pesticides, malls or traffic fumes they were left unable to think or in total body pain, as examples of scores of symptoms. Some went to the specialized environmental units like the Environmental Health Center of Dallas, (Dr. William J. Rea, www.EHCD.com) or to North

Charleston, South Carolina (Dr. Allan Lieberman) and then returned home to continue saunas for life.

## The Superior Sauna —FIRS

What is the best way to get rid of toxic chemicals including pesticides, heavy metals and hydrocarbon residues? **The far infrared sauna**. It has been known for decades that sweating is a life-saving aid, and a natural way to get rid of stored chemicals, including heavy metals. But many people, myself included, never could tolerate a sauna. We felt weak, sick, fast heart rate, faint, dizzy, panicky, crampy, headachy, or just miserable. Thanks to improved technology, the far infrared sauna is tolerated much better, because it uses a heat energy that penetrates the deeper tissues, triggering mobilization of chemicals from fat storage and into the blood stream, then finally into the sweat. This activating penetration allows for a much lower overall temperature to be used, one that is very enjoyable and not torture nor is it contraindicated for even heart patients.

Another thing I always worried about in a conventional sauna, even for the few brief moments I could stand one, was the fact that my eyeballs burned so much. I couldn't believe that intensive heat on my corneas was good for them and feared triggering cataracts. No studies have ever been done on this. Anyway, I don't get that type of eye pain in the infrared sauna, only profuse sweating. And that is just the effect you want in order to release toxins from body storage.

The body gets rid of stored mercury and other chemicals in stool, urine or sweat. The sweat route is drug-free and the most efficient and natural (man used to physically work before computers were invented). I used to hesitate to recommend something as expensive as a home sauna. But when you realize the lifelong incapacity and expense of diseases such as chronic pain syndromes, heart disease, chemical sensitivity, chronic fatigue, fibromyalgia, migraines, neuralgia, Alzheimer's, cancer or others caused by chemical toxicity, a sauna is very inexpensive.

We are continually being bombarded by new chemicals every day. As a tool to keep you "cleaned out" for life, it is a win-win situation. I'm convinced that the **far infrared sauna** is something that everyone should do to restore health, and then continue to do on a less frequent basis to maintain the "cleaned out" state for the rest of their lives.

I hope this brief introduction gives you an idea of how prevalent toxins are in the 21st century in the industrialized world. We are clearly the first generation of man ever exposed to many of these chemicals. For many of these chemicals, the body just does not have the biochemical pathways with which to detoxify them. So they accumulate. But they do not sit harmlessly in storage, but leak out and damage tissues and regulatory genetics and other proteins. They cause chronic disease.

For further information about chemical sensitivity, how to diagnose it and how to avoid it and how to treat it with measures in addition to what is presented here, consider some of my other books, *Tired Or Toxic?*, *Chemical Sensitivity*, *The E. I. Syndrome*, *Wellness Against All Odds*, *Depression Cured At Last!*, and *No More Heartburn*, plus the monthly newsletter. And for much more details on the far infrared sauna program, read *Detoxify or Die*.

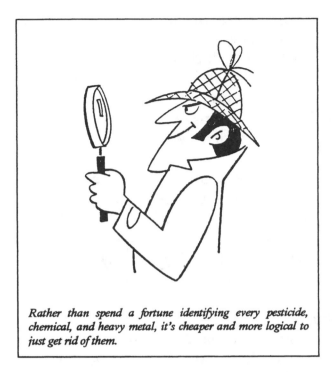

*Rather than spend a fortune identifying every pesticide, chemical, and heavy metal, it's cheaper and more logical to just get rid of them.*

## The Hot Solution for Body Pollution: FIRS

How can we bring illness to a screeching halt? Better yet, how can we turn back the hands of time by booting these nasty disease-causing chemicals out of the body? Sweat out the poisons is the answer, but not any old sauna or sweating program will do, in fact some are dangerous.

Many people who are sick, like heart patients, would never tolerate the extreme temperatures of regular saunas. In fact it would make them worse, raising their blood pressure and heart rate, while triggering arrhythmias and shortness of breath. Clearly heat is contraindicated. But in a man with cadmium-induced arthritis and hypertension, or a woman with mercury-induced shoulder pain and angina, or toluene-induced migraines and arrhythmia, as examples of environmental chemicals that create pain and cardiovascular disease, what is the heart patient to do?

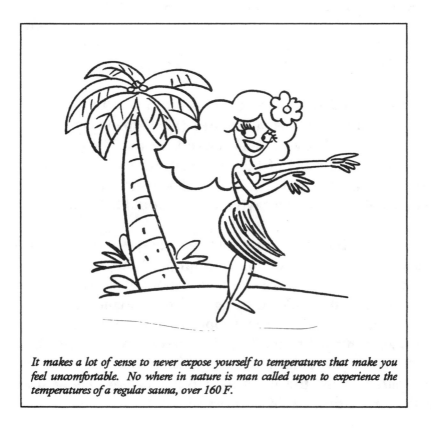

*It makes a lot of sense to never expose yourself to temperatures that make you feel uncomfortable. No where in nature is man called upon to experience the temperatures of a regular sauna, over 160 F.*

## What Makes the FIR Sauna Unique?

How is the far infrared sauna different? Let's look at the energy that comes from the sun. Responsible for photosynthesis, the process by which plants make energy to grow, solar energy is responsible for all life (since animals must have plants to eat or there are no animals).

The spectrum of energy from the sun is classified according to the length of the waves. The shortest (and most damaging) rays of the solar spectrum are *gamma rays*. Think of a gamma gun in a sci-fi movie that vaporizes assailants in an instant. The next longer rays and a little less destructive are *x-rays* (carcinogenic), then *ultraviolet* (causes sunburn, corneal and lens damage and skin cancer), and then *visible light*. After that is the *infrared* spectrum, then radio waves.

At the far end of the infrared spectrum are the longest and most healing rays, the *far infrared* (FIR), spanning from 1,000 to 4 microns. Between 4-14 microns in the FIR (far infrared) spectrum, falls most of the rays that are the safest and most vital to health and healing. They are responsible for photosynthesis, without which there would be no life.

In fact, our bodies radiate infrared energy through our skin between 3-50 microns, mostly around 9.4 microns. This is the basis for infrared glasses allowing Special Forces to see the enemy at night. Palm healing and other hands-on therapies are based on the healing properties of natural far infrared rays, with our palms emitting infrared energy at between 8-14 microns. Our bodies absorb 93% of the infrared waves presented to us, the basis for similar heaters being used to warm premature infants in nurseries.

The FIRS uses a patented zirconia ceramic infrared heater, emitting between 2 and 25 microns, with a third of the output in the 2-5.6 micron range for deepest penetration, about 1.5 inches. Patented in 1965, it was used extensively in Japan, and then extended to the U.S. in 1981. Being safer and more economical to operate, lower in EMF, it induces 2-3 times the sweat volume, while allowing a much more tolerable and safer operating temperature. This makes it my preferred tool for purifying and detoxifying the body. Naturally nothing stands alone, and a clean diet, environment and soul are, of course, crucial components to healing the impossible.

The far infrared wavelength has other beneficial properties; it lowers lactic acid (the acid that accumulates and causes *pain in muscles* when you have overdone during exercising), stimulates endorphins or happy hormones of the brain, and kills organisms like bacteria and parasites. More important, it penetrates tissues, detoxifies cells by vibrating ionic bonds, stops swelling, improves lymphatic flow and blood circulation, and attracts calcium to cell membranes where it is needed for healing. The far infrared wavelength also decreases the size of water clusters, giving them greater mobility and penetration in and out of body tissues. And it is when these hyperactive or energized water molecules move in and out that they also carry toxins that were not mobilized before.

The lungs, urine, stool, breast milk, and sweat are the main vehicles the body has for getting rid of nasty chemicals. But by far sweat is the most efficient. And as Mayo Clinic studies demonstrate, FIR is the safest way to induce healing sweat, using the most heat-sensitive cardiac patients as proof.

### FIRS Cures Pain In the Most Mysterious Cases

The bottom line is that folks with the most severe forms of heart disease, resistant to all medications, not only tolerated the FIRS, but it improved their heart health within 3 short weeks. Of course, it is recommended to continue longer, say a year of daily or every other day saunas to completely get rid of stored chemicals causing disease. Then it is necessary to do them at least twice a week for life, since the world will never run out of ways to poison us.

It should not surprise you now that mysterious joint pain in war veterans exposed to Agent Orange also disappeared, as did a host of other pain syndromes. Schnare of the U.S. EPA (Environmental Protection Agency) also showed that not only did sauna reduce HCB (hexachlorobenzene) and PCBs (polychlorinated biphenyls) in electrical workers, for example, but even though the men were continually exposed at work, it keep their total body burdens reduced. This is important because it means that if your livelihood depends on an occupation that continually exposes you, you still have a chance of being able to tolerate it safely, as long as you are getting rid of the chemicals faster than you are tanking up on them.

Schnare also reported on different types of workers, drug users, victims of accidental ingestion, and those who were poisoned by a variety of environmental chemicals, who recovered with sauna detoxification. And scientists from the Tokyo Medical and Dental University and others explained in various studies how the FIR is superior to just plain old heat in regular saunas. There is no lack of data on this subject that has remained a *secret cure* for decades.

There are a few places that sell far infrared sauna, but the only one I know that makes them of poplar wood for chemically sensitive folks is High Tech Health of Boulder, Colorado (1-800-794-5355). You see the terpenes of cedar smell great, but saunas were originally made from cedar because it was native to Sweden. And because they usually had their saunas outside as a separate building, they wanted them bug-proof and mold-proof, as they were perpetually creating steam by pouring water on the hot rocks (don't worry, no mold or steam in FIRS). But for an in-home unit and the need to avoid terpenes, poplar is ideal. Furthermore, there are lower electromagnetic fields (EMF) generated in a FIR sauna than in a conventional electrically heated one. This is important because it reduces the chance of becoming EMF sensitive.

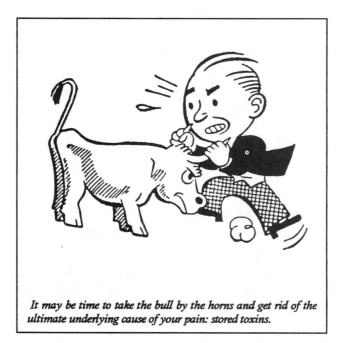

*It may be time to take the bull by the horns and get rid of the ultimate underlying cause of your pain: stored toxins.*

Sweating is a God-given mechanism, but it must be done properly and safely to be successful. The infrared sauna is something that you and your family would use for a lifetime, for the world will never run out of ways to poison us. It should be a *major tool* not only in your *pain program*, but also in your *anti-aging program*. Because it is a major expense, you might want to figure a way to put it in a garage, basement, game room, patio, lanai or porch to share it with neighbors, or have your church, physician, chiropractor, gym, or organization buy one, for example. You could use the insurance company letter (in future book in progress) to try to persuade your insurance company to cover this medically necessary expense. For the evidence bears out the facts: FIRS will save untold lives and dollars. But remember, many insurance companies are resistant to logic and tightly wedded to the pharmaceutical industry.

## What Exactly is FIR?

If you are like I was, you may not be exactly sure what infrared is or if it is even safe.

---

### *Solar Waves or Energy*

➤ Gamma, shortest rays, most destructive to life
➤ X-rays = penetrate tissues, carcinogenic
➤ Ultraviolet = sunburn, corneal and lens damage
➤ Visual wavelength
➤ Infrared: contains at the lowest end of spectrum, far infrared (FIR); Far infrared = lowest = 1000-5.6 microns; the rays most vital to healing are 4-14 microns, also are the majority of sun energy or photons (safest and most beneficial) responsible for photosynthesis; lowers lactic acid, stimulates brain, kills organisms, penetrates tissues, stops swelling, improves lymphatics, attracts calcium to cell membranes; detoxifies by vibrating ionic bonds and reducing the size of water clusters; by creating a resonance dance between water and chemical molecules, it facilitates water in removing stored toxins from the cell.
➤ Short wave radio
➤ Broadcast radio

---

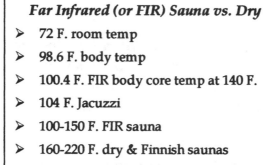

*Far Infrared (or FIR) Sauna vs. Dry*

➤ 72 F. room temp

➤ 98.6 F. body temp

➤ 100.4 F. FIR body core temp at 140 F.

➤ 104 F. Jacuzzi

➤ 100-150 F. FIR sauna

➤ 160-220 F. dry & Finnish saunas

➤ 212 F. boiling water!

## Is Your Detox System Ready For a Sauna?

The chief caveat to assure success in the sauna to be sure your detoxification system is ready to handle the onslaught of chemicals that have been silently stored in your body over the years. For you can get much worse if these are mobilized from storage and dumped into the blood stream. If in doubt, get the detox panel measured, assessed and corrected by your doctor (or see phone consults in Resources chapter).

### Centigrade-Fahrenheit Conversion Chart

Centigrade = 5/9 (Fahrenheit – 32)
Fahrenheit = 9/5 (Centigrade + 32)

| Centigrade | Fahrenheit | Centigrade | Fahrenheit |
|---|---|---|---|
| 0 | 32 | 50 | 122 |
| 5 | 41 | 55 | 131 |
| 10 | 50 | 60 | 140 |
| 15 | 59 | 65 | 149 |
| 20 | 68 | 70 | 158 |
| 25 | 77 | 75 | 167 |
| 30 | 86 | 80 | 176 |
| 35 | 95 | 85 | 185 |
| 40 | 104 | 90 | 194 |
| 45 | 113 | 100 | 212 |

# How to Use the FIR Sauna

**General rules:**
Start using the sauna in short 10-20 minute increments at first, 100°F. building up a feel for your body's tolerance. Older or sicker folks should proceed at a much slower pace. Also before chemicals are excreted in the sweat, they are pulled out of safe storage and into the blood stream. If you suspect you've had severe poisonings that may create serious repeat symptoms as you mobilize chemicals, go at a slower pace. If you are pregnant, have metal parts in your body, a pacemaker, take important medications whose levels should not change, or are within 48 hours of an acute injury (still in the swelling phase), definitely do not do it until you check with your doctor. In fact anytime you embark on a health program, his input should be included in your decision-making.

It is a good idea to get a complete physical from your doctor and discuss your sauna plans with him/her. If you are on any medications, sauna may help you detoxify and get rid of the drug too quickly, thereby changing your blood levels. For some drugs this is not desirable, or you may need to have blood levels of the drug drawn or other parameters affected by the drug monitored.

I suggest you take your blood pressure, pulse rate and assess its regularity, respiratory rate, temperature and weight before and after a sauna. It is just good medical practice to have a blood pressure cuff (sphygmomanometer), stethoscope and thermometer around the house anyway. There are digital ones available at most drug stores. Any neighborhood nurse, local firehouse or ambulance personnel, your doctor's nurse, etc., can show you how to use them.

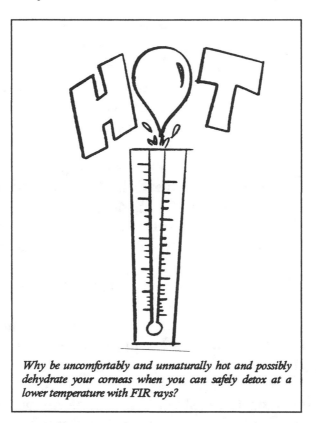

*Why be uncomfortably and unnaturally hot and possibly dehydrate your corneas when you can safely detox at a lower temperature with FIR rays?*

If your blood pressure, pulse or respiratory rate increase or decrease 10 points, or your pulse gets irregular, get out. Next session use a shorter time and lower temperature as well as you increase your pre-sauna minerals and water. If your temperature goes over 100 F., stop for the day. If you weigh less after a sauna, you did not drink enough water to compensate for the loss. Also document any symptoms. If you get exaggerated withdrawal symptoms, it could be magnesium or other mineral deficiencies (see emergency measures below).

You may start with 10-20 minutes daily at 100-110 F. Then slowly over several days or weeks advance to an hour at 130 F. If you cannot attain that in one session, no problem. You may leave at any time, shower off toxins, and sauna again in the same or next day. Sometimes just opening the door for a bit or turning down the temperature is enough to allow longer exposure. Some folks (as I was) are so severely pesticide-poisoned that their sweating mechanism is damaged. They just don't sweat. In this case, you need to be absolutely sure that you and your doctor have corrected your detox panel findings first. You must be able to immediately detoxify old chemicals as they are brought out of storage.

You should stop at any time that you feel increased headache, nausea, vomiting, diarrhea, forceful pounding heart, fast heart rate, irregular heart rate (if this is not a symptom you normally have), shortness of breath, dizziness, disorientation, weakness, muscle cramps, muscle spasms or twitching, or any adverse symptom. Use a tepid shower to cool down slowly without shocking the system. The symptoms of heat stroke (dry and/or cold skin) are more dangerous and require immediate removal and Tri-Salts with plenty of water. Include a retention water enema (with 1 tablespoon of Tri-salts in 2-4 cups of water) as well. Unless you had a mineral and fatty acid analysis before you entered, no one knows what nutrient deficiencies you started with. Anything borderline can be accentuated or made dramatically worse with the losses sustained with sauna.

**Before the sauna:**

Your goal at this phase is to cause vasodilatation or an opening up of channels to improve outflow of chemicals from tissues. This can be accomplished with one or more (they are not mandatory but do improve the effectiveness of FIRS) of the following:

- Exercise for 10-30 minutes prior improves circulation and mobilization of chemicals from the fat. It can be jogging, calisthenics, jumping rope, or whatever you choose.

- If you cannot exercise, a massage or a loofa sponge or natural bristle body brush stimulates skin circulation.

- Taking niacin (vitamin B3) to tolerated dose is another option. Start with 50-100 mg before the sauna. Each day the dose is the same until the flushing, redness, burning or tingling from histamine release stops. Then advance by 50-100 mg every day as long as you have stopped burning, and tingling with the previous dose. You are able to advance the dose much faster if you take it 3-4 times a day. This forces the histamine out of storage in your cells, allowing you to tolerate a higher B3 dose without adverse symptoms. Some folks can get up to 1000 mg or more (as 250 mg 4 times a day): others are forever stuck at 50-300 mg total. If you accidentally push ahead too fast and take too large a dose, you may get a niacin flush reaction. If you miss a dose for a few days and forget to back down and slowly build up again, this may also precipitate the temporary flushing reaction. If you find the burning, redness or tingling unbearable, over-the-counter Benadryl® (diphen-hydramine) 50-100 mg will shorten the reaction (it also makes you sleepy. Do not drive until your reaction time is normal).  You may prefer to skip the niacin option.

- Take an enzyme like Wobenzyme (Pain &Stress Center, Carotec), Bromase (Bio-Tech), Bromelain (Jarrow, Pure Encapsulations, Thorne) or Total-Gest (Klabin, N.E.E.D.S.). Enzymes clear sludge, encouraging mobilization of chemicals from fat more easily.  Use 1-5 of any form, as tolerated.  It is preferable to have no food in your stomach so the enzyme is working in the blood stream, not on digesting your food.

- Take ginkgo in the form of Ginkgo-Go (Wakunaga), 1 or 2 a day for its vasodilating properties.  This will help improve circulation and toxic mobilization.

Mandatory before each sauna session totaling half an hour is to drink 1-2 quarts of water (alkaline water is preferred, available from High Tech Health) and take one or two chelated Liquid Multiple Minerals (Carlson), 1-2 teaspoon 18% Magnesium Chloride Solution (Pain & Stress Center), ½-1 teaspoon Coral Calcium (Premier Neutraceuticals), and one teaspoon of Tri-Salts (Bio-Tech or American Environmental Health Foundation). This step should not be an option, since you want to get a head start on correcting the fluid and mineral losses that inevitably occur along with loss of stored chemicals.  For every additional ½ hour segment that you may stay in the sauna, repeat this protocol when you get out. For example, if you stay an hour, do this before and after the sauna. If 1 ½ hours, do it before, after, and somewhere in the middle of the session.

**Take into the sauna:**

- Whatever you need to entertain yourself. Some folks set a TV outside their sauna, others listen to tapes or CDs or read or meditate. The time is never wasted.
- A large clean bath towel to continually wipe the sweat from your body to prevent it from being reabsorbed.
- Other towels for the floor and to sit on to absorb the sweat
- Water to drink

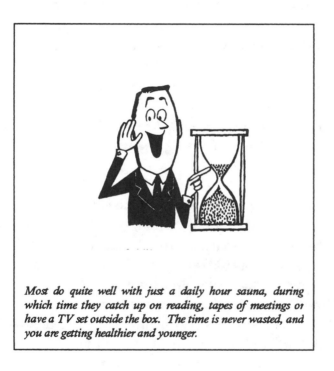

*Most do quite well with just a daily hour sauna, during which time they catch up on reading, tapes of meetings or have a TV set outside the box. The time is never wasted, and you are getting healthier and younger.*

**Emergency Measures:**

- Bare minimum you must have on hand a very inexpensive product, **Tri-Salts** (Bio-Tech, or American Environmental Health Foundation), to replace potassium.

• Also you must have **18% Magnesium Chloride Solution** (Pain & Stress Center, N.E.E.D.S.), for the first sign of muscle cramp or twitch most likely means you have sweat out too much. As well, magnesium deficiency can mimic drugs, medicine and toxic chemical withdrawal. Although this tastes dreadful, it is so imperative that you should never begin a sauna without it. The 18% solution is the best absorbed form next to an I.V. For some, the capsules are not sufficient. Since enormous amounts of life-saving magnesium are lost in sweat, you should use this form until you never get magnesium deficiency symptoms. Then you can try to switch to capsule equivalents. In the meantime, you can dilute 18% with as much water as you need to mask the taste.

• You must also have immediately available a cool shower. In fact don't even think of doing a sauna until you have these three available.

• In case of feeling lousy, weak, woozy, exhausted, muscle cramps, spasms, cardiac arrhythmia, or other symptoms, you should have on hand extra water, Potassium Citrate (Pain & Stress Center) or Complexed Potassium (Carlson), Calcium Citrate 225 mg (Metabolic Maintenance or Pain & Stress Center), Zinc Picolinate 30 mg (Pain & Stress Center), Premier Coral Calcium (Premier Neutraceuticals) or Calcium Citrate 225 mg (Metabolic Maintenance), Multiplex-1 (Tyler), your detox enema and detox cocktail, sea salt, and Bragg's Apple Cider Vinegar (health food store or N.E.E.D.S.).

Without ready availability of tests to measure what you are depleted in, you need to make some educated guesses. This is not as far off the mark as it may sound, for even if you went to the hospital emergency room, they would not do the tests with the precision you need. They would measure serum potassium or serum magnesium. But since only 1% of these is in the serum, the serum assay is too insensitive. You need the RBC (red blood cell) values. I repeat (not because I fear you don't get it, but because medicine has persisted in making this fatal mistake for over a decade): only 1% of the magnesium in the body is in the serum. This means you can be so low in magnesium, for example, that it triggers a heart attack, yet the serum test will look perfectly normal. The RBC magnesium is much more sensitive (but takes longer to perform) and gives a much more accurate picture.

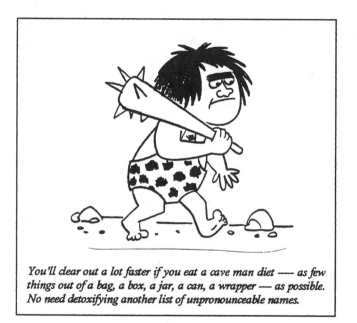

*You'll clear out a lot faster if you eat a cave man diet — as few things out of a bag, a box, a jar, a can, a wrapper — as possible. No need detoxifying another list of unpronounceable names.*

The first thing you do with any adverse symptoms is lie down and get your feet up and drink 2-4 large glasses of water with ½-1 tsp. of Tri-Salts (Bio-Tech, AEHF) added.

## CAUTION: All Tri-Salts Are Not the Same.

Tri-Salt powder from the American Environmental Health Foundation or AEHF (Dr. Rea's environmental unit in Dallas) contains 329 mg calcium (from calcium carbonate), 687 mg sodium (from sodium bicarbonate), and 652 mg potassium (from potassium carbonate) per teaspoon. This is a superior product as far as I am concerned, because you can easily get more calcium from Coral Calcium and more magnesium from the 18% solution, both superior forms. But it takes over 6 capsules of potassium (99 mg each) to equal one teaspoon plus the salt loss needs to be compensated for. Bio-Tech Tri-Salts is very similar with 362 mg calcium (carbonate), 738 mg sodium (bicarbonate), and 701 mg of potassium (bicarbonate). There are other products called Tri-Salts but they only have 99 mg of potassium with 450 and 250 of calcium and magnesium respectively. In this case, it takes a totally different approach to adjust or compensate.

If you use AEHF or Bio-Tech Tri-Salts, one chelated Multiple Mineral, 1-2 teaspoons of 18% Magnesium Chloride Solution, and ¼-½ teaspoon Coral Calcium with 2 large glasses of water, may be all the correction you need before a sauna. And it can be repeated after as well, if need.

If you use another Tri-Salt form with calcium 450 mg, 250 mg of magnesium, and 99 mg of magnesium per ½ teaspoon, then you still need more of each, magnesium, calcium, and potassium, plus the salt, but you are particularly low in potassium and need 5-6 capsules of Complexed Potassium (Carlson). AEHF and Bio-Tech Tri-Salts may be more expensive, but are easier because they are more chemically complete. It is important to be sure of what you have.

It need not be tricky figuring out what you need. If you have been low in magnesium in the past with atrial fibrillation or muscle cramps, for example, and it was a magnesium deficiency symptom, take that first: 1-3 tsp. of the liquid 18% Magnesium Chloride solution (Pain & Stress Center) will confirm this. And remember that everything should be with 1-2 large glasses of water. If, on the other hand you suspected that calcium was your deficiency, use ½-1 tsp. of Coral Calcium, in a large glass of water (Premier Neutraceuticals). If you are older, on heartburn medications, or have poor acid or faulty digestion, you may want to add ½ tsp. of Braggs' Organic Apple Cider Vinegar (health food stores, or N.E.E.D.S.) to improve assimilation. If your sweat is particularly salty or you crave salt, sodium chloride may be what your body is hungry for; so take ½-1 tsp. of sea salt in water.

Some people lose a disproportionate amount of potassium and feel restored with Potassium Citrate, 99 mg, 5 capsules 2-6 times a day (Pain & Stress Center) or Complexed Potassium (Carlson). Again, lots of water is imperative as well as evaluating a different mineral if the one you are correcting does not do the trick within a few hours, or in a day at most. And do not ever do another sauna if you have not yet recovered your prior status. For a fast fix, you could take all of the above, but stretch it over an hour or more to avoid nausea, diarrhea, stomach cramps or ill feeling.

And if you cannot figure out how to correct an ill feeling from doing a sauna within 24 hours, by all means get your RBC minerals assayed through your doctor (MetaMetrix 1-800-221-4640). MetaMetrix is the only lab I know of that provides RBC

185

calcium, magnesium, potassium, vanadium and chromium as well as manganese, copper, zinc and molybdenum.

For most folks, a good diet of whole foods, 2-4 quarts of water, a tsp. of Tri-Salts (AEHF), 1-2 tsp. of Magnesium Chloride 18% Solution, ½ teaspoon Coral Calcium, a chelated multiple mineral and a multiple vitamin-mineral (see specific recommendations below) will balance them out per every 45-60 minutes of sauna time. This may be the slow boat to China, but it requires less adjusting of minerals that were sweat out.

### The sauna program:

The most important part of a safe sauna program is to remove mobilized toxins from the body as quickly as possible, while restoring the nutrients that have been lost in sweat. The five important aspects of a nutrient program include:

(1)     Penetration: This is done with either exercise, message, skin brushing, niacin, and/or enzymes like Bromelain (Jarrow). The purpose is to vasodilate and/or cut through the sludge to improve removal of toxins stored in tissues. Do this before the sauna.

(2)     Detoxification: This involves revving up phase I and phase II of the detoxification pathways to accelerate getting rid of  mobilized toxins, once they have been pulled from storage. Use any one or more of the following, depending on your needs.

For **phase I,** Vitamin C (Klaire) and glutathione (in the form of Recancostat, from Tyler) make up the **detox cocktail.** This may be all you need with the above. Further phase I help comes from 1-2 Lipoic Acid 300 mg (Pain & Stress Center or

Metabolic Maintence), and CoQ10 in the form of 2 Q-Gel (Klabin or N.E.E.D.S.), or one 200 mg CoQ10 (Carlson) or 1 tsp. Opti-Q100 (Phillips Nutritionals) and 2 twice a day Kyolic (Wakunaga). All are great heavy metal detoxifiers, as well as anti-oxidants. Also important to boost phase I of detoxification are any combinations of IndolPlex (Tyler), Microhydrin (Feidler), Ginkgo-Go (Wakunaga), Non-Hydrolyzed Whey (Thorne), L-Arginine (P&S), Carnitine (Pure Encapsulations), Thisylin (Bio-Tech), ThioNAC (Jarrow) Alpha Keto-Glucaric Acid (P&S), ImmPower (Klabin Marketing), ImmunoPro (N.E.E.D.S.), SeaVive (Proper Nutrition), Taurine (P&S), PhosChol (American Lecithin), OPC (Thorne, Primary Services International, Jarrow) and many others. Use as directed later on. **Mandatory: Detox Cocktail.**

For **phase II** help use one or more of the following: Recancostat (Tyler), IndolPlex (Tyler), TMG (Klabin), Calcium-D-Glucarate (Tyler), Glycine (Pain & Stress Center), MSM (P&S, Jarrow), DHEA (Premier Neutraceuticals), CoQ10 (Carlson, N.E.E.D.S., Klabin), DGL (Rhizinate: Enzymatic Factors), Detoxification Factors (Tyler), Cyto-Redoxin (Tyler), and more.

(3)     Restoration: Putting back the minerals and other nutrients lost in the work of detoxification and in sweat is crucial. Water, multiple minerals, multiple vitamins, fatty acids, phosphatidyl choline, CoQ10, carnitine, and others are important, depending on the individual's diet, environments, diseases and other parameters.

(4)     Intestines: Because the gut houses half the immune and detoxification systems, special nutrients and

procedures play a decisively beneficial role in gut health: the detox enema, Kyo-Green, SeaVive, Kyo-Dophilus (with meals), Kyolic, Carlson's Cod Liver Oil, vitamin C powder, PhosChol, and UltraInflamX are a few examples. **Mandatory: Detox Enema.**

(5)   Maintenance nutrients for every day health: B Compleet 100, Cod Liver Oil, E-Gems Elite, Heartbeat Elite (as your general multiple vitamin-mineral), Liquid Multiple Minerals, and Tocotrienols (all 6 from Carlson), Pure Ascorbic Acid Powder (Metabollic Maintence, P&S, Klaire) 1-4 tsp. a day as tolerated. Rinse your teeth after vitamin C to avoid dissolving enamel. As well, it is recommended to take 2-3 times a week additional zinc picolinate (25-60 mg) selenium (400 mcg), chromium (400 mcg), vanadium (400 mcg), iodine (400 mcg), molybdenum (400 mcg), and lithium (400 mcg), as well as boron 4 mg, manganese 4 mg and copper 4 mg (all from Pain & Stress or N.E.E.D.S.), 1 tsp. of PhosChol (American Lecithin) and 20 drops a day of BioSil (Jarrow). These will further replenish trace minerals and phosphatidyl choline, most often to a better state than you have ever had before.

Many of these supplements overlap from one category to another, so don't be scared off. And no one needs all of these. The frequency and amount of these will depend on individual chemistry, diet, current diseases, medications, environmental chemical overload, and intensity of sauna. For example, if you do a slow steady sauna program of an hour or less a day, you may not need to take extra nutrients until your total sauna time finally reaches one hour. It may take 1-3 months to use up one order of some nutrients (a bottle of 100, used as one capsule a day lasts 100 days).  You may, for example, with a good diet and sleep schedule, get away with just AEHF Tri-Salts, 18% magnesium, Coral Calcium, a multiple mineral with saunas, and the detox cocktail and detox enema in addition to your usual nutrient program, or just a multiple vitamin-mineral.  Sweat studies show that water, magnesium, salt (sodium chloride), potassium, calcium, and zinc plus body fats (e.g. replaced with Cod Liver Oil and Phos Chol) are the main losses in sweat.

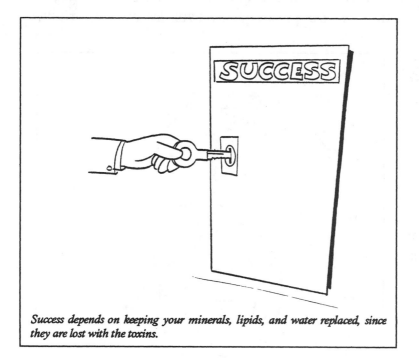

*Success depends on keeping your minerals, lipids, and water replaced, since they are lost with the toxins.*

The best prevention of deficiencies is to have a RBC mineral analysis (MetaMetrix).  Also desirable would be heavy metals to determine what metal toxicants (MetaMetrix) you started with, fatty acids (MetaMetrix) to determine what is deficient and needs correcting, and a detox panel (Great Smokies Lab) to determine where your detox deficiencies are. The labs in resources can guide your physician and the tests and their interpretations are described in more detail in *No More Heartburn, Depression Cured At Last!,* and *Detoxify or Die.*

Do you need all of following? No. They merely give you an idea of part of the spectrum of nutrients that could be used, for many people are so sensitive to nutrients that they need a wide variety from which to choose. The once weekly boost of solo minerals as suggested, however, is very important.

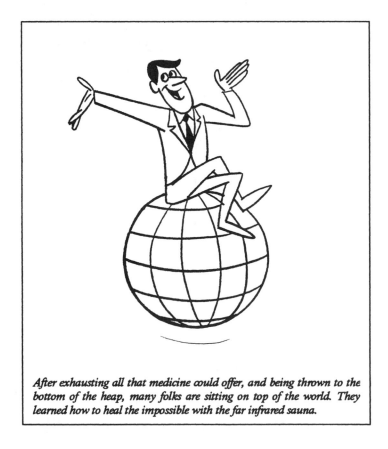

*After exhausting all that medicine could offer, and being thrown to the bottom of the heap, many folks are sitting on top of the world. They learned how to heal the impossible with the far infrared sauna.*

For **starters,** you could use the following example as an approach to restoring your nutrient status while doing an hour sauna a day. Again you need not use every suggestion in each category, but the more you do include, the better your program results. Any duplication from one category to another should be omitted, being there just so you can see that some items are important for more than one process.

1) To **open channels:** (P&S refers to the Pain & Stress Center)

- Take Ginko-Go (Wakunaga) 1-2 before
- Exercise, yoga, massage or skin brushing
- Enzymes like Wobenzyme (P&S) or Organic Pancreas (ARG) or Bromelain (Jarrow)

2) **Daily Maintenance:** (easy, top 6 all available from Carlson)

- Heartbeat Elite, 2
- Cod Liver Oil, 1 tsp.
- Tocotrienols, 2
- Liquid Multiple Minerals, 1-2
- B Compleet 100, 1
- Vitamin C Crystals, 2-6 gm
- PhosChol 900 (American Lecithin) 2-3 a day

3) **Restoration.** Additional supplementation after every hour of sauna, especially if you have any symptoms: (P&S refers to the Pain & Stress Center, AEHF is American Environmental Health Foundation.)

- Tri-Salts, 1 tsp. (AEHF, Bio-Tech)

- Potassium Citrate (P&S) or Complexed Potassium (Carlson), 5-10 capsules
- Magnesium Chloride 18% Solution, 2-3 or tsp. (P&S), or 1-3 Magnesium Citrate 170 mg capsules (ARG) or 150 mg (Pure Encapsulations) once you no longer get magnesium deficiency symptoms.
- Extra Liquid Multiple Minerals (Carson), 1-2, or Mineral Complex (Tyler)
- Coral Calcium (Premier Neutraceuticals), ¼-1 tsp.
- And more water (whenever you are hungry, drink water first to rule out hidden thirst, getting at least 4-6 quarts a day). You may add a half-teaspoon of sea salt, if need.
- Zinc picolinate 25-30 mg

4) **Detoxification** help could come from one or more of the following:

- Detox cocktail (1-2 tsp. of Vitamin C powder (Klaire) and 400-800 mg of Recancostat (Tyler) in a large glass of water, 1-4 times a day. This as well as everything in (3) Restoration (above) and detox enema are mandatory.
- Detox enema (see chapter 7), highly recommended daily
- Lipoic Acid 300 mg (P&S, Metabolic Maintenance), 1-2 twice a day
- Detoxification Factors (Tyler) 1-2 caps of each 1-3 times a day between meals
- CoQ10 200 mg(Carlson, Klabin, P&S), 1 cap 2-3 times a day
- MSM 500 mg (Fiedler, Jarrow, P&S) 1-2 caps 1-2 times a day
- Phos Chol Concentrate (American Lecithin), 1 tsp. a day
- Cyto-Redoxin (Tyler) 1-2 three times a day

- Silymarin as Thistle Rx (Enzymatic Therapy) or Thisilyn, (Bio-Tech) 1-2 twice a day

5) And attending to the **gut**, for it houses half the detoxification system:

- UltraInflamX (Metagenics, HealthComm) 1-2 tbs. twice a day
- Kyolic (Wakunaga) 2 twice a day
- Kyo-Dophilus 2 caps twice a day (with meals) (Wakunaga)
- Kyo-Green (Wakunaga) 1 tbs. in water 2-4 times a day
- Oils and fiber can be taken as a raw salad containing a cup of raw veggies with 1 tbs. organic extra virgin olive oil and/or flax oil
- Additional Vitamin C (Klaire), 1-10 tsp. in addition to the vitamin C in your detox cocktail above. If you get diarrhea, cut back until you do not. The key is to keep vitamin C powder as high as you can without side effects, because it is such a wonderful detoxifier of blood and bowel, as well as having over a dozen other benefits in the body. **Caution:** Every few months you will need to recalculate your top tolerated dose, for as you begin to heal, it will change. Never use off white or yellowish vitamin C; it should be pure white. Off-color means it is old and oxidized and will not help.

I've put the sources of nutrients in parentheses and their usual doses. The 800 numbers so you can compile your shopping lists easily are in the resources.

Above all, be sure that you have medical guidance, for you can also sweat out medications, hormones, and a multitude of nutrients for which we do not yet have readily available tests, like phosphatidyl choline, silica, CoQ10, lithium, carnitine, tocotrienols, etc. Further more, FIRS can speed the absorption of injected medications, like insulin. As well, you need someone to counsel you if you react to the mobilized chemicals as they are passing through the blood stream on their way out. Or if you do not have sufficient ability to completely detoxify them, they could become stuck or sent to another target organ. An undiagnosed absorption problem, as from the leaky gut could lead to mineral depletion that could trigger cardiac arrhythmia or even a seizure. Having an initial assay of your detox capability, and later monitoring your minerals certainly makes life a lot easier. Sure, many people have successfully done a program by themselves, but no one knows what surprises lurk underneath your skin.

**In summary:**
Pardon me if I sound hooked on the far infrared sauna (FIRS). But after 30 years of struggling to help poisoned people get well, it is pretty clear.
- Toxins are everywhere, in our air, food and water.
- The nastiest, most common toxic causes of disease that have dramatically destroyed lives have been the heavy metals, pesticides and hydrocarbon derivatives.
- The body does not have the mechanism to detoxify or metabolize many of these man-made chemicals, plus it can be easily overwhelmed by the combination of the hundreds that exist in our everyday air, food and water.
- The result is that the body stores them in the fat and other tissues.
- These bioaccumulated chemicals slowly leach out of storage and damage body systems, producing what we know as chronic disease. In fact, these chemicals stored in the body

are a major cause of all illness including pain, cancer and accelerated aging.

• Fortunately, removing them turns back the hands of time and erases diseases that were labeled as incurable.

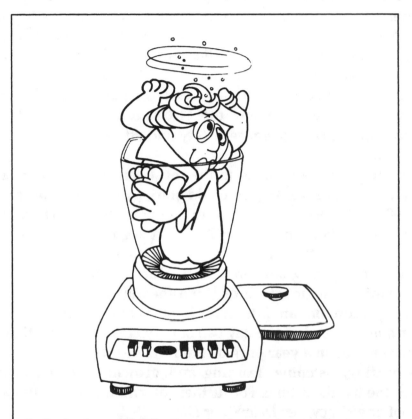

*Confused and overwhelmed? Remember that most do very well prior to one hour of sauna a day, with just a multiple mineral, Tri-Salts, 18% magnesium, coral calcium, weekly individual boosts of zinc, selenium and other nutrients, and lots of water. All the other things can be once or twice a week, or for the remote occasions with emergence of disagreeable symptoms. For no one knows your particular chemistry and harbored chemicals. Most important, don't forget your detox cocktail and detox enema.*

At the far end of the infrared spectrum are the far infrared (FIR) rays that are the safest and most vital to health and healing, responsible even for photosynthesis, upon which all life depends. They decrease the size of water clusters (a quantum physics phenomenon) which translates into giving water higher mobility, easier penetration into cells, and increased ability to mobilize toxins. Numerous government, medical center and other studies throughout the world have proven that sauna is the only way to reverse otherwise impossible diseases, including resistant pain. Furthermore, Mayo Clinic studies show the FIR sauna is superior to all saunas in terms of tolerance, safety and efficacy.

It is completely adaptable to the most sensitive persons, and to the most poisoned. You could start with 10 minutes a day at 100° and work up by weeks to one hour at 110-130° F. You can fool the body by having 2-6 short segments a day if you can only tolerate a short time at low temperature. Or you may go for getting out some heavy-duty toxins with multiple 30-60 minute segments throughout the day at 100-140° F. The busy person on an intensive 45-60 minute session at the beginning or end of the day can slowly clean out a lifetime of stored toxins in a year or two. And the beauty of it is you can be reading, listening, learning and growing while you roll back the hands of time. For further information on its use and proof of efficacy, see *Detoxify or Die*.

There is no question in my mind that the FIR sauna is a crucial tool that enables the average person to help heal the impossible. It is the closest thing to the elusive **fountain of youth** that I have seen in 35 years of medicine. Chronic pain is merely an overload of undiagnosed toxins. Once they have been sufficiently unloaded from the body, the body becomes healthy enough to once again heal itself as nature designed it. And the pain ceases.

## Chapter 7

## Picking Out the Remaining
## Pieces of the Pain Puzzle

There is a rule in medicine, as well as in other parts of life, called the 80/20 rule. What it means is that 80% of the people are going to heal with only 20% of what we have to offer. This is great because it saves them time and money. Only the super resistant cases will need to explore the other 80% of our armamentarium. And this holds true for people with chronic pain syndromes.

Regardless of the cause or type of pain, the vast majority of people have substantial or total relief from pain if they abstain diligently from the nightshades, heal the leaky gut and correct its underlying causes (like Candida overgrowth). Others need to add enzymes to dissolve the antigen-antibody complexes and improve circulation to the swollen inflamed areas. They also need to correct nutrient deficiencies (including fatty acids, like CM), rebuild their bones and detox their diet (from arthritis-triggering foods other than nightshades). In addition they should detox their lifestyle (reduce chemical load as I'll show you here). The problem is no one has a crystal ball to know how much work you have to do.

So for those who need the rest of the story, let's get started to see what some of the other missing parts might be for you.

### Fast Yourself

Many times I awoke encased in that unbelievable pain, only to be baffled about its cause. Screaming in agony, I would be lovingly helped out of bed in order to make it to the bathroom. These episodes could last for days and weeks, so I consider myself extremely blessed to have been able to figure out how to end this misery sooner. There are in fact many things you can do to get yourself out of a reaction sooner. But nothing takes the place of FASTING. And let's face it. If you are bedridden in that much pain, you do not need to eat.

If you restrict your intake to **glass-bottled** spring water, and lots of it, you will clear your system quicker, and even force the antigen-antibody complexes off the joints and cartilaginous surfaces faster. For if the steady flow of antigens from the gut ceases, there is nothing to hold the complexes on the joint as you change the equilibrium kinetics of the reaction. You actually make them drop off, although it can take 2-21 days or longer of a complete water-only fast to accomplish this. But if you are in that much pain you are most likely bed-ridden and not going anywhere; so you might as well fast. Even if you cannot fast the whole time, several days may provide significant improvement, accelerating recovery and getting you out of pain faster.

Fasting means no food. If you think you cannot do it, your pain must not be severe enough. For when it is, you can do anything. And the beauty of being in bed is that you have no worry about being hypoglycemic or light-headed. You cannot fall down if you are already prone. You may go through some wicked withdrawal symptoms if you are addicted to cigarettes, coffee, sugar, wheat, alcohol, NSAIDs, or whatever. Withdrawal can masquerade as any symptom, although headaches, mood swings, nausea, diarrhea, sweats or chills, and body aches head the list. Regardless, dig in and get it over with as quickly as possible. It is a miracle cure when you are at your lowest. Take it from someone who has had unlimited free access to doctors and drugs and has been to the depths of despair with pain.

If you need something other than water, use Kyo-Green® (Wakunaga, 1-800-421-2998) 1 tbs. in a large glass of water 1-8 times a day. If you suspect gluten-grain sensitivities or need additional potent gut healing, use UltraInflamX® (HealthComm, N.E.E.D.S., Metagenics) one scoop in water three times a day. If you absolutely cannot fast (diabetic on insulin, need food to buffer important medications, etc.) consult with your doctor about a carrot juice "fast" or a simple diet of brown rice and steamed kale.

It boggles my mind that rheumatologists generally ignore the many scientific studies (don't forget to consult your scientific references in chapter 10) demonstrating relief from pain with just fasting. It's almost as though they don't want you to get better. It costs nothing to at least mention it and give you the option.

### Feed Yourself

Vegetarian diets have been proven in the literature to help people in pain. The problem is that the definition of vegetarianism is too broad. Many will include the deadly nightshades, which can defeat any benefit from the diet. The ultimate and most thoroughly healing form of vegan diets is the macrobiotic diet. It caught my attention when I read of and later met people who had literally been at death's doorstep with metastatic cancer and rallied. In spite of having been given mere days to live, they had healed the impossible. Then when I saw the x-rays, specialist reports and the robust people for myself, I realized this was something too important to ignore and furthermore, I owed it to myself and to others to explore it.

I'll give you one example, as many others are in our books. Elaine Nussbaum was a New Jersey housewife when she got cancer of the ovaries and uterus in 1980. After a hysterectomy, the cancer relentlessly spread to her lungs and liver. After maximum chemotherapy and radiation, the cancer continued to metastasize throughout her body. It spread to her backbones, which then became mush and collapsed. At this point she was bed-ridden, racked in pain, bald, 78 pounds, and the cancer was still viciously spreading. Doctors gave her 2 weeks to live and apologetically said they could not even give her an antibiotic for her current pneumonia, since she was so frail they thought the antibiotic might prematurely kill her.

It was at this lowest possible point, when you could not find a physician who would bet a nickel on her survival, that she began the macrobiotic diet (this program is described in *The Cure Is In The Kitchen,* but you need to begin with the primer, *You Are What You Ate*). She not only totally healed all of her cancer including the metastases, but also is exuberantly well. It is over 20 years later and I lecture with her about every third year in Vermont and usually she is just coming in from jogging when I see her. When I had dinner with her a couple of years ago, I couldn't help but marvel at how anyone would guess that this vivacious, perky, attractive young woman who appears to be only in her early forties is actually a mother of 4, a grandmother of 7, and a decade older. Her autobiography, *Recovery From Cancer,* is available from this publisher.

Needless-to-say there are many other cases. I know 5 people who healed inoperable brain cancers with the same program

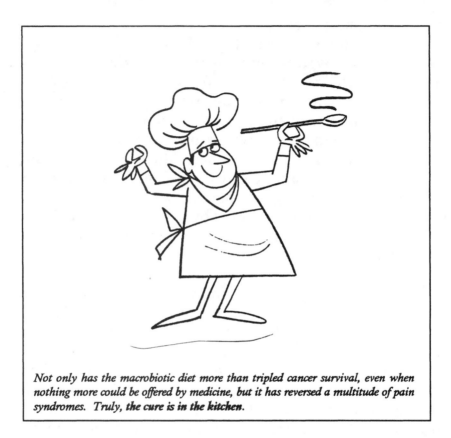

*Not only has the macrobiotic diet more than tripled cancer survival, even when nothing more could be offered by medicine, but it has reversed a multitude of pain syndromes. Truly, **the cure is in the kitchen**.*

and many other seemingly unbelievable cases. At this point you are asking for the medical backup, which is also there. Epidemiologist, Dr. James P. Carter of Tulane Medical School in New Orleans, published a study showing that if you do everything that American medicine has to offer for cancer of the prostate, as an example, the median survival is 6 years. But for those who did the macrobiotic diet, the median survival was 18 years, and some of them are still alive. Eventually the researchers just had to end and publish the study before they themselves died! They couldn't wait for the macrobiotic cancer patients to die off or the researchers might never get to publish their life-saving results.

And in order to qualify for the macro study group, folks only had ·to do the diet 3 months (those participants were guaranteed not to succeed) and there was no monitoring of how accurately the diet was followed by those who did do it. So the deck was stacked for failure, as these less than serious participants severely brought down the statistics. Regardless, it was still a "no contest" win. For the diet group (in spite of having included in it the people who foolishly only did the diet for 3 months, not long enough for them to heal their cancers) **more than tripled** their survival against the best of what modern medicine has to offer.

So here you have it: the average survival in the U.S. from cancer of the prostate, when absolutely everything available has been done, is 6 years. But for those on the macrobiotic diet, many of whom refused surgery and other conventional treatments, it was over 18 years. In other words, they more than tripled their survival with diet (in spite of having those who did not follow the diet seriously included in their statistics).

To give you an idea of the potency of this diet for chronic pain, remember my wind surfing episode in Chapter 6. That evening I had right shoulder pain, but to me pain is something you learn to tune out. The next day it was measurably worse, and the subsequent day unbearable. As the weeks progressed, it got unimaginably worse until it was way out of proportion to what should have happened with my little sports activity.

I had had enough experience with specialists to know that I would get an x-ray, nothing would be found, and it would suddenly become a deficiency of some NSAID. I would be told of all the possible differential diagnoses and that if it was not self-limited we could do tests where a dye would be injected that I could die from, just to diagnose a tear in the rotator cuff. So I figured I would just let it heal itself. Five months later, it was so bad I could not even open a door or pick up a patient chart using that arm. My right shoulder was chronically in pain without a moment's relief and useless.

At that point, I decided to act like the environmental physician that I am trained to be and stop tuning out the obvious. Just to confirm my hypothesis, I called a colleague and told him the story without giving him a clue as to my suspicion. He hit it right on the head when he asked out of the clear blue "And when did you have something done to the right lower posterior jaw?" "You got it, Tom!" I announced, "Exactly 3 weeks prior to the onset of pain." You see, mercury (in our "silver" fillings) leaches at varying rates into the body. And its first stop for causing disaster can be anywhere along the acupuncture meridian from that tooth to the nearest structure. Add a little stress or injury, and you get a condition way out of proportion, that baffles medicine.

The problem was, his solution involved removing the amalgam, something I was not prepared to do at that time because I was still too chemically sensitive in those days to tolerate the acrylic substitutes much less the glues used to adhere them. Having no other options, I bit the bullet and went full steam ahead on the macrobiotic diet to detoxify.

After meeting so many people who had been given as little as 2 weeks to live who had gone on to completely clear their cancers, I figured a little mercury toxicity was a piece of cake. And how right I was, for within one month I was wind surfing in the ocean picking up a 70 lb. sail in gusty winds. Plus the diet cleared my years of allergies: asthma, sinusitis, migraines, and eczema. I no longer needed allergy injections, which had been my lifeline for over 15 years. Luckily, there are many roads that lead to wellness.

Do I still do the diet? No. I can go out and have a steak dinner, wine, etc. (but no nightshades, to this day) with no problem. But if I ever awoke not feeling 100% well, vivacious and happy, or if I had ever had even one tiny symptom, including a cold, flu, ache or pain, I would return to it until well. It is not a life sentence, unless you have cancer, in which case I would never go off (see *Wellness Against All Odds*, and our monthly newsletter, *Total Wellness*, including back issues for further vital information on that subject, all of which is very crucial if you have cancer).

One gal in her forties with rheumatoid arthritis had been on methyltrexate, strong prescription NSAIDs, and prednisone for eight years. Within 3 months of the macrobiotic diet as described in the books below, she was medication-free and pain-free. That kind of power over pain no one can give you but yourself.

So for those who are serious about healing the impossible, you should start with *You Are What You Ate*, which is a primer showing you how to start the macrobiotic diet. Then proceed to *The Cure Is In The Kitchen* which tells you in expanded detail the strict phase healing diet that people with cancers and other impossible to heal conditions like chronic

205

lupus, rheumatoid, and other pains cured themselves with. For those who need to know why and how it works, *Tired Or Toxic?* is the first start, then proceed to *Wellness Against All Odds* for further healing advise, as well as being a "must read" book for anyone with cancer or "impossible to heal" diagnoses.

In a nutshell, the macrobiotic diet consists of grains, greens and beans, seeds and seaweeds, roots and fruits. These are merely whole, highly nutritious, unprocessed foods. While on the strict healing phase, there are no flour products or broken grains, no frozen, canned or microwaved foods, no dairy or meat, no additives, colorings, preservatives, and minimal pesticides. I've watched documented nutrient deficiencies heal with only this diet in diseases as diverse as rheumatoid and lupus arthritis to MS, migraines, and cancer. The label attached to the symptoms is inconsequential. The key is how much do you have to do to revitalize the body so that it is now capable of healing itself!

For those who do not choose to make the time to do the macrobiotic diet, you may prefer a live food diet. To get started read Elizabeth Baker's *The Gourmet Uncook Book* (1-800-846-6687) and Rita Romano's *Dining In the Raw* (1-800-846-6687), Rev. George Malkmus' *Why Christians Get Sick* (1-800-722-6774) and see Dr. Lorraine Day's excellent video, *Cancer Doesn't Scare Me Any More* (1-800-574-2437). For this diet also enjoys as impressive a track record for cancers and other recalcitrant conditions, again documented by physicians, lay survivors, and molecular biochemistry, and for some it is an easier diet to do. But statistically speaking, the macrobiotic diet, with more easily digested cooked food, has the best-documented overall track record.

206

Whichever program you choose to accelerate your healing, I would read the macrobiotic books because they form the foundation of food preparation and cooking that will be used for good health regardless of which plan is chosen. Eventually, many people switch between different diets as their health condition, environment and nutritional status undergo metamorphosis.

Whichever plan you chose, it is often just as important what you omit from your diet (like the nightshades as a shining example) as what you include in a specific diet plan. Obviously the body has delayed and imperfect healing with a diet of fast foods, convenience foods, restaurant foods, processed foods, and the standard American fare. If neither healing diet is for you, or you are a carnivore who just does not feel good without meat, I would highly recommend Sally Fallon's cookbook, *Nourishing Traditions* (ProMotion Publishing, 1-800-231-1776), to give you a foundation in more nutritional food preparation. Also read Dr. Mary Enig's *Know Your Fats* (301-680-8600 or bethesdapress.com or knowyourfats.com).

Many pain syndromes like lupus, rheumatoid arthritis, and vasculitis involve immune (antigen-antibody) complexes. There is no question that most immune complexes (antigen-antibody reactions) are triggered by foods. So even when the leaky gut syndrome is healed and the nightshades are avoided, still food allergy can play a critical role in perpetuating the pain of most arthritics. And in concert with the right diet some need the addition of enzymes to dissolve the immune complexes. Both the use of digestive enzymes as well as adding back good bugs (probiotics, like Kyo-Dophilus®) has caused many to lessen or lose their food allergies.

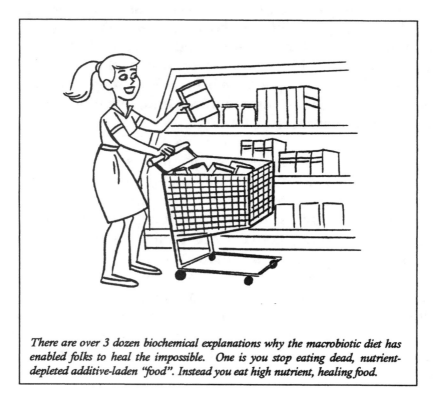

*There are over 3 dozen biochemical explanations why the macrobiotic diet has enabled folks to heal the impossible. One is you stop eating dead, nutrient-depleted additive-laden "food". Instead you eat high nutrient, healing food.*

Clearly, it is a total load phenomenon where each person must find the components to his total load before he is free of pain. And in 30 years of medical practice, I have never seen 2 people with the same food allergies. For beginners needing to figure out what foods are triggering their symptoms, the simplest approach would be to do the rare food diagnostic diet as described in *The E.I. Syndrome, Revised.*

Meanwhile, there is a plethora of cases of all types including rheumatoid arthritis, chronic back problems with deteriorated discs and sciatica, scleroderma, polymyositis, fibromyositis, bursitis, dermatomyositis, tendonitis, lupus, vasculitis, fibromyalgia, and many more, that cleared chronic pain with a macrobiotic diet. And this list omits the cancer patients that had failed surgery, chemotherapy and radiation who went on to totally heal with macrobiotics.

There is overwhelming evidence in the biochemistry literature explaining how the phytochemicals in plain ordinary foods, like quercetin in cabbage or flavonoids in tangerines, for example, down-regulate and even inhibit cyclooxygenase and other mediators of pain and inflammation. The answers are all there. It never ceases to amaze me that when all the high tech bologna of the medical world has failed, that a return to God-given whole foods, taking responsibility for our health, and a respect for the environment and our role in it can enable us to heal the impossible. "For has God not made foolish the things of this world?" (1COR1).

As you will learn in the two recommended macrobiotic books, as pain syndromes are healed with the diet, symptoms often start to melt away in the exact opposite order in which they first appeared. For example, rheumatoid arthritis frequently starts in the feet, then over months and years progresses upward to the other joints. The last joint affected is usually the first one to clear on the diet. On the diet, symptoms melt away week by week in reverse order. If you cheat on the diet, they start piling on again.

## Hydrate Yourself

When in severe pain, get as comfortable as possible with cotton pillows to gently support your back and legs or whatever joints are involved, and drink 1-2, 8 oz. glasses of pure water every 1-6 hours. You have this much leeway because in the beginning the pain can be so severe that you do not want a reason to have to get up any sooner than you must. But as the pain begins to get more bearable and you can get to the bathroom without such intense agony, increase the water so you can accelerate your improvement.

Water is the most fundamental detoxifier and healer of all. You need plenty of it to carry away those enzyme-dissolved antigen-antibody complexes and to float toxins out of the body, to promote the healing response. And water even provides electrons to facilitate the body's detoxification and reparative chemistry; for **the solution to pollution is dilution.**

The quality of water is important. Mountain Valley in glass bottles, available from the health food store is one of the best. Avoid plastic bottles as the toxic and carcinogenic plasticizers or phthalates outgas into the water and add more of a load to your already-overburdened liver to detoxify. Most plastics also contain xenoestrogens, or chemicals that mimic estrogens. They leach into the water and can turn on estrogen receptors in the breast, for example, triggering precocious puberty in children or cancer in anyone.

If you have neither bottled water nor a kitchen tap filter, distiller or reverse osmosis, you can at least boil the tap water to remove some of the chlorine and foreign chemicals, 500 of which contribute to the pollution of most municipal or city water supplies. Do not boil it in aluminum pans.

There is also a machine that makes alkaline water, called Singer Spring. The Japanese have used alkaline water to accelerate healing of a variety of chronic pain conditions from diabetic neuropathy to arthritis. Pain is invariably associated with acidity, and acidity invariably uses up calcium and other buffers to neutralize it. Since the pH of most tap and bottled waters is around 5.5 or very acidic, this would compound the stress to your system, forcing you to deplete more calcium. It makes sense to drink alkaline water.

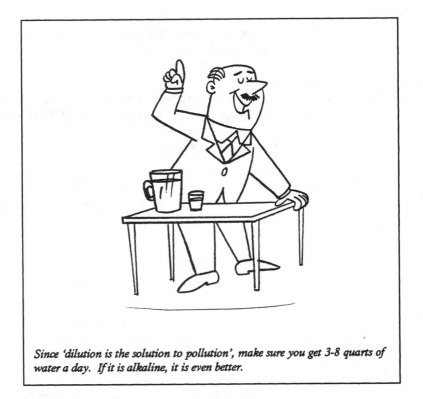

*Since 'dilution is the solution to pollution', make sure you get 3-8 quarts of water a day. If it is alkaline, it is even better.*

The Singer Spring alkaline water machine easily attaches to your faucet. Complete with carbon filter, it also ionizes the water creating a large number of electrons that act as free radical quenchers, and creates structured water by clumping the molecules of water, making them more permeable to the cell. I'll tell you more about that in the next section.

Meanwhile remember that when you hurt the most, your repair chemistry has become over-burdened with pollutants. Since the **solution to pollution is dilution**, and that goes for the inside as well as the outside of your body, drink away as soon as you can reasonably make it to the bathroom.

**Resources:**
**Alkaline water, micro-ionized, restructured, filtered**
Singer Spring from High Tech Health, Boulder Co, 1-800-794-5355

**Glass-bottled spring water**
Mountain Valley bottled spring water from Mountain Valley Spring Co., PO Box 1610, Hot Springs National Park, Arkansas 71902, 1-800-643-1501

## Alkalinize Yourself

In the 1950's a country doctor, Dr. Jarvis, put out a little paperback about a Vermont folklore treatment for human arthritis that was successfully used on domestic and farm animals as well. It involved a tablespoon each of vinegar and honey several times a day. The vinegar should be organic apple cider vinegar containing the "mother" culture, such as Braggs', which is found in most health food stores. The grain-distilled form from regular grocery sources is not desired, nor is grocery store honey, which can be cut with corn syrup and has no freshness dating.

How did it work? It merely is a fast way of alkalinizing the blood, which serves several purposes: it promotes the dissociation of immune complexes, revs up detox capabilities, down-regulates inflammation, promotes healing, and more.

You can also measure your own first morning urine pH (acidity/alkalinity level) and compare when you are in pain versus out of pain. Most people who are in pain are also acidic with a urinary pH under 6.4 and a salivary pH of 7.0 or less. In fact, the sicker they are the lower the pH can get. Just as a diabetic in acidosis has a low pH, so do many in pain. The quickest way to alkalinize yourself is with the macrobiotic diet or the live food diet. For both are rich in alkalinizing (non-nightshade) vegetables, which, of course, is one of the mechanisms of why the macrobiotic diet helps so many conquer not only arthritis and other forms of pain, like metastatic cancer, after medicine has failed.

How do you know when you are sufficiently alkaline? A good start is to purchase pH paper with a range of about 4.5 to 8.5. Tear off a tiny strip of pH paper, dip it in the urinary stream of your first morning urine, and the color chart will tell you the pH. For the more fastidious, urinate into a cup and dip an end of the paper in. Match up the color with the interpretive color guide on the side of the pH strip dispenser and you have the pH. Your goal is a pH between 6.4 and 7.4. If it is less than 6.4 (more acid), increasing calcium is one way to supply buffer and spare your body the work of stealing the calcium form bones. If it is above 7.5, consult your doctor, for there are a number of alkaline conditions that are beyond this book that deserve immediate medical attention if this is from a fasting first morning urine.

*Calcium is one of the main buffers the body uses to turn it from acidic to alkaline.* Start with ½ teaspoon of Coral Calcium Legend® each morning (this and pH paper available from Premier Neutraceuticals) in any amount of water. If after 3-6 weeks the first morning fasting urine pH is still below 6.4, increase the calcium to one tsp. a day. It takes several months for many people to restore the pH. Calcium, in addition to being the main buffer for an acidic body, is the membrane gatekeeper that allows many other minerals access to the cell. So as the pH raises, there are often many other health benefits noticed as the cell membrane and internal cell have restored their calcium reserves.

Vitamin C Power (Klaire, Metabolic Maintenance) is also a great way to alkalinize, working up gradually from usually 1-10 teaspoons. Once you find the dose that causes diarrhea, cut back a teaspoon to a dose that does not. That dose can be split into 2 doses if it is too much to take at once. That is the dose you need twice daily to alkalinize. Be sure to brush or rinse your teeth after, as the acidity can dissolve tooth enamel. Once in the body, ascorbic acid becomes an alkalinizer to buffer pH, sop up free radicals, increase cancer fighting natural killer cells, boost detoxification, and much more. It is one of the best bargains in medicine.

One caveat for the beginner is very necessary. Just because the body heals best in a slightly alkaline environment, does not mean all alkaline conditions are good. The pH (whether it is in urine, saliva or blood) must always be correlated with how you feel to be properly interpreted. Two simple examples are that you could be very alkaline after days of vomiting up all your acid, or overdosing on antacids. This could cause serious heart arrhythmia from low potassium. In other words, you could feel dreadful but have an alkaline urine simply because you had depleted your acid reserves. So if you are ever worse, stop the calcium and find what else is wrong. Likewise there is a natural alkalinity after meals (called the alkaline tide), which is why it is generally not a good time to measure pH.

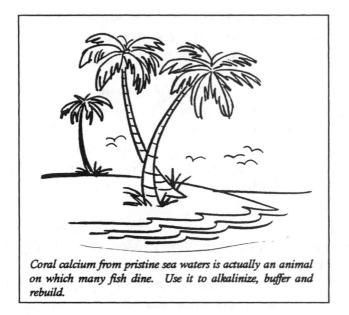

*Coral calcium from pristine sea waters is actually an animal on which many fish dine. Use it to alkalinize, buffer and rebuild.*

You can also use pH to assess the effect of various diets, determining their correlation with symptoms. Do you hurt more when you are acidic? Acidity correlates with more junk food, coffee, alcohol, sodas and sweets. Many derive gradual relief from symptoms by alkalinizing themselves with diets of grains, greens and beans (macrobiotic) in addition to using an especially well-absorbed form of calcium like Coral Calcium Legend®, ½-1 tsp. once or twice daily.

You could also measure your urinary pH before dinner and do a second dose of Coral Calcium here if the pH is not between the 6.4 and 7.4 range. Again, for the second dose of the day, start with 1/2 tsp. and move to a whole tsp. in a few weeks if the pH is still below 6.4. *A bad diet is chief among causes for failure.* Often the answer can be as simple as fresh carrot juicing 2-8 times a day. It is a great alkalinizer like calcium and vitamin C. You really need the help of a physician trained in acid-base balance to assess your total responses and program if your results are not within range. Once you are well, you can drop back to whatever dose maintains your pH in the favorable range.

Correcting a calcium deficiency doesn't just help one symptom, but many other areas of the body benefit. One for example, is preventing osteoporosis. For when the body has enough extra calcium to make up for the buffering action of our indiscretions, it stops stealing it from the bone. For it is only when the bone bank is depleted that osteoporosis rears its ugly head.

Another way to alkalinize the body, used successfully by the Japanese for chronic diseases from diabetes, cancer, chronic infections, to hypertension, arthritis or speeding recovery from surgery is with **alkaline water.** The machine that alkalinizes water has a pre-filter before the water is ionized. Not only does the charge create a large number of electrons that become free radical quenchers, but also the water molecules or clumps actually become smaller and more **compact.**

Structured water is able to permeate and penetrate areas of previous poor perfusion. Since dilution is the solution to pollution, proper water is the first phase of detoxification. The best machine is Singer Spring (High Tech Health), with an ultraviolet light and carbon pre-filter. It also has adjustable pH for alkalinization of the microionized water, yielding two processes to help it better penetrate the cell.

With your pH paper you can measure the acidity of tap water then your current water filtration system. You will be surprised that they are most likely pretty acidic (pH under 7, the pH of "real water" without a lot of chemicals). With microionized water, you can adjust to the desired amount of alkalinity. It is really foolish that we try to hydrate the body with acidic water that uses up even more of our dwindling buffer reserves, especially calcium. When the body is slightly alkaline, all its functions, from detoxification to healing, work optimally.

Like any water system, this is a sizeable investment in your future. But certainly once you have purchased one you will be sure to drink plenty of water. It is small enough to attach to the kitchen faucet so that you have alkaline drinking water constantly available. If you are at a healing plateau, this just might be a turning point. Check it out, compare prices; see if any might rent it for a month or two trial.

**Resource:**
**Singer Spring Microionized Alkaline Water,** High Tech Health, Boulder Colorado, 1-800-794-5355

## Dissolve Yourself

What is arthritis? It is an attack of the body's own cells against cartilage and bone. Instead of making antibodies to streptococcus or other bugs, our mechanism goes awry and we attack ourselves using our own inflammatory defenses to destroy our bones and bodies.

When doctors want to confirm their diagnosis of rheumatoid arthritis, they measure the antibody level or titer in the blood of the patient. Some forms of arthritis have no identifiable antibody test yet, but that does not mean it is not an antigen-antibody reaction. It merely means science has not yet identified that particular antigen.

One thing that makes arthritis go away is for the antibody to stop attacking the joint. There are many ways to foster this:

(1) By not eating a food that forces the body to make destructive antibodies, such as the nightshade-free diet.

(2) Once food has been ingested, not eating or fasting shifts the body's antibody balance, so the antibodies drop off the joints.

(3) And last but never least, enzymes have been used for decades to rip antibodies off from joint spaces. The enzyme dissociation of the antigen-antibody complex is dose dependent, however. Sometimes you just could not take enough enzymes, in which case you must look at the rest of the total load.

## Enzymes Dissolve Destructive Antibodies

Long before you can rebuild bone, you have to turn off its daily destruction. Luckily enzymes do two important services: (1) By dissolving sludge, they improve the actual circulation to bone, cartilage, tendons, ligaments, and muscles, so that all your great nutrients can get to them. (2) Enzymes rip the antigen-antibody complexes from bone. For the antigen-antibody combination or complex is what directs the chemistry of not only pain, but also the inflammation and ultimate destruction and demise of bone. And when enough bone is chewed up by these complexes, it's reconstruction (artificial joint) time.

Let's back up and look more closely at the first task of enzymes, that of improving the circulation to bone. Often because of years of inflammation and poor bone alignment, there is scar tissue and stagnation from plugged or blocked lymphatics that supply circulation to the areas that need it the most.  Enzymes can break through this stagnation and improve blood flow to damaged areas.

Next, enzymes do even more as they weaken and break down the antigen-antibody complexes that actually attach to and attack joints.  It is the attachment of these complexes to joints that cause the release of chemicals from the cell, called inflammatory mediators; the stuff that actually causes the chemistry of pain, and later the destruction of bone and cartilage.

Why isn't our own supply of enzymes enough?  Because there are many lifestyle factors that can serve to weaken and deplete our natural pancreatic enzyme production and reserves.  The mere escalating dietary choices of sugars can stress the demands of the pancreas.  Add to that the high amounts of dietary fats requiring pancreatic lipases and you begin to appreciate factors that strain the productivity and deplete the reserves of the pancreas.

 Furthermore, such common deficiencies as zinc can jeopardize pancreatic enzyme output.  Even the mere elevation of calcium to current recommendations can severely lower zinc levels within months, slowly ushering in silent enzyme deficiencies.  In addition, everyday home and office chemicals and pesticides can act to damage pancreatic enzyme function.

Enzymes forge the road through vessel and tissue sludge to the bone, cleaning out smaller nutritive vessels necessary for good circulation.  Otherwise all your money spent on nutrients is wasted if they don't get to their chief targets.  Unfortunately, our diets and lifestyles can do much to destroy our abilities to make as many enzymes as we need.  But first, let's learn how else enzymes heal.

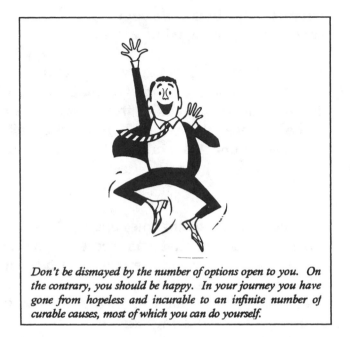

*Don't be dismayed by the number of options open to you. On the contrary, you should be happy. In your journey you have gone from hopeless and incurable to an infinite number of curable causes, most of which you can do yourself.*

Since enzymes "dissolve" antigen-antibody complexes, they are crucial for the person in pain with auto-immune disease (rheumatoid arthritis, ankylosing spondylitis, lupus arthritis, psoriatic arthritis, fibromyalgia, etc.) to turn down or turn off the inflammatory process in a natural and unharmful way. For these attached immune complexes or antigen-antibody complexes cause the release of harmful substances that eat away at bone, destroying cartilaginous surfaces of knees and hips and shrinking vertebral bones that are supposed to protect our discs. The antibodies, you recall, can be directed toward any food, chemical, or mold that we become allergic to. These antibodies are made by our immune system when it goes out of control. *Enzymes and fasting are the only safe ways to pull antigen-antibody complexes off from joints.* Less desirable ways are with prednisone whose damaging side effects include hemorrhaging to death from ulcers, death of the hip joints requiring bone grafts, mental breakdown, and more.

It turns out that most diseases eventually make auto-antibodies if ignored long enough. Even arteriosclerosis and Alzheimer's or presenile dementia are auto-immune phenomena (Fillit).

I know it's not easy learning immunology just so you can get out of pain. So let me make this as painless as possible. When an area first is damaged by an injury, chemical exposure, food allergy or toxin, the body sends in the troops to clean up the debris. It does not want old blood cells and poisons lying around. It wants everything neat and tidy.

But if you have not adequately nurtured the area, have covered up pain with drugs, continue to aggravate it, and have not found the underlying cause and corrected it, the process continues. It is labeled chronic. So now the special forces are called in: auto-antibodies. Auto-antibodies are the Pontius Pilate of the immune system, because they turn against the very body they have been designed to protect and then they destroy it, cell by cell.

Besides Alzheimer's, auto-antibodies have been identified for cancers, arthritis, Crohn's, ulcerative colitis, chronic pancreatitis, hepatitis, ankylosing spondylitis, vasculitis, neuropathy, high cholesterol, claudication, cardiomyopathy (a fatal heart disease), multiple sclerosis, glomerulonephritis, arteriosclerosis, etc. The cells that were designed to clean up and rescue eventually turn on us and start destroying if the process continues too long.

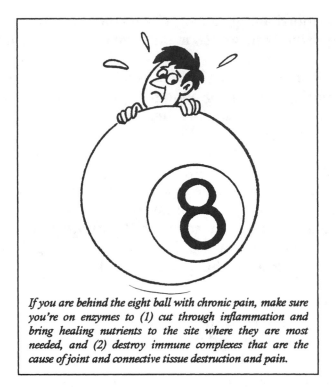

*If you are behind the eight ball with chronic pain, make sure you're on enzymes to (1) cut through inflammation and bring healing nutrients to the site where they are most needed, and (2) destroy immune complexes that are the cause of joint and connective tissue destruction and pain.*

To give you an idea on how well enzymes help penetration into inflamed areas, consider this. Oral enzymes have been used so successfully to improve blood flow, that they minimize antibiotic need in hard to reach areas of severely painful pelvic inflammatory disease, post-herpetic pain, prostatitis, and chronic cystitis. This enabled serious cases to be treated at home; not needing high doses of intravenous antibiotics once enzymes paved the way. Think of the money saved!

In addition, enzymes are able to minimize the harmful effects of radiation and speed healing as in thrombophlebitis (blood clots), as further examples, as well as lower lipid (cholesterol) levels. So from multiple levels of causation, and regardless of the label or concomitant diseases, enzymes are a must for at least the first 2-6 months (in concert with a total program) for persons in pain.

As a physician, I was taught very little about enzymes 35 years ago in medical school, aside from the use of a few to improve digestion and speed healing after surgery. Currently the biggest news in medicine about enzymes concerns the "clot busters" like streptokinase and urokinase for breaking up clots in coronary and brain arteries as an emergency intravenous procedure. As a specialist in environmental medicine, we have also used this knowledge about the power of enzymes to dissolve antigen-antibody complexes in many diseases, like arthritis, food allergies, and celiac disease, all of which can be potent causes of pain.

As we have described in our newsletter and other books, enzymes also dissolve the protective coating off from around cancer cells, leaving them vulnerable for attack by the immune system. There is a sialoglycoprotein, sort of a protein-mucous suit of armor that cloaks the cancer cell so that the immune system cannot recognize and destroy it. By using enzymes as we have described in *Wellness Against All Odds*, this protective coating can be removed without harm to the rest of the body, so that now the cancer cells are nakedly defenseless and can be much more readily captured and destroyed by the body's own immune system. However, if cancer is the source of your pain and you use enzymes, you must follow them with the detox protocol I'll describe later. Otherwise, the massive killing of many cancer cells can leave you lethally toxic.

To review this important modality, enzymes are triply useful in pain syndromes: (1) They dissociate antigen-antibody complexes, (2) penetrate the swelling and inflammation to bring more nutrients to the sick area, and (3) have an anti-inflammatory nature of their own, reducing the swelling and inflammation. In fact, they do such a good job that they have been used to improve the blood flow to areas that are difficult to reach like sinus, ovarian, bladder and prostate infections. Therefore they would be indispensable in conditions requiring long term antibiotics like some cases of Borrelia-caused Lyme arthritis.

Useful in breaking down antigen-antibody complexes not only in cancers but in other areas that are easy targets for auto-immune damage like the kidney, also means enzymes are useful in cases of lupus arthritis with auto-immune antigen-antibody complexes. As well, they have been used successfully for years to reduce the edema and swelling after surgery and accidents. For example women with lymph nodes removed from under the arm for breast cancer can get serious swelling and pain of that arm. Enzymes have paved the way for improved circulation and reduced swelling.

Never forget enzymes in cases of surgery or acute injury or trauma, as they speed up the dissolution and carrying away of the by-products of injury, thereby speeding up healing.

There are many good sources of enzymes. Organic pancreatic enzymes (available from lamb, pork or beef, from Nutricology/Allergy Research Group) are the most popular, being taken 1-4 with meals to improve digestion, but more importantly, 4-8 just before bed around 11 p.m. and another 4-8 in the middle of the night, say between 2 and 4 a.m. Since the body does most of its healing when you sleep, you want the enzymes working at those two precious times when the body does not have to use up its enzyme capacity for digesting food.

For these nighttime doses, measure out your enzymes and set them beside a large 8-ounce glass of water. In this way you won't have to turn on the lights and prematurely signal your brain's pineal gland to awaken your other glands for the day. Soon you'll learn the top dose you tolerate (start low) and the perfect dose of water so you'll awaken naturally between 2 and 4 a.m. for round two.

If you awaken in the morning more achy than usual, this is a good sign. Do the detox procedure described later on in this chapter. It is important to do in order to speed up getting rid of these toxic antigen-antibody breakdown by-products. Awakening even more achy after taking enzymes is a good sign that they are working and hoeing out old garbage.

Other great enzyme products if you do not tolerate animal-based glandulars, would include Total-Gest (Klabin Marketing or N.E.E.D.S.) which contains 14 enzymes and is a vegetarian source. Another excellent combination plant and yeast source would be Similase® (Tyler), 1-4 with meals, and 4-8 at 11 p.m. and 2 a.m. And don't forget Wobenzyme® (Pain & Stress Center), the classic upon which the majority of enzyme studies were done.

A pineapple source is Bromase (Bio-Tech) or Bromelain (Metabolic Maintenance, Pure Encapsulations, Jarrow), 500 mg capsules, taken as 1-4 with meals and 4-8 at 11 p.m. and 4-8 at 2 a.m. Always have a large 8-ounce glass of water with enzymes as it facilitates their action.

### Protect Yourself

This may sound off the wall to many, as it did to me when I was first exposed to the concept, but chemicals in the air have a predisposition to an area of previous weakness or damage, like an old back injury, as an example. Since we are the first generation of man ever to be exposed to such a high number of chemicals every day in our air, food and water, it is no easy matter to avoid them. Fortunately the old 80/20 rule has shown us over the decades that most people will improve with just a few of what we call **environmental controls.**

The first environmental control would be to reduce the amount of formaldehyde that outgasses from your mattress into your body as you snuggle a third of your life on it. For you get measurable blood levels of not only the foam stuffing's formaldehyde, but fire retardant that is in there by law. If formaldehyde and fire retardant were not enough, there are usually liberal amounts of pesticides as well. You are literally sleeping on a toxic heap.

Luckily, you can protect your system from becoming overloaded while it is attempting to heal at night (and in the daytime if you are bed-ridden with pain) by covering the mattress with several layers of heavy duty restaurant grade aluminum foil, shiny side up. Any restaurant supply store in the yellow pages of the phone book should carry it. Then you can put a couple of cotton blankets or sheets over it to minimize crinkling. Be sure they are natural organic cotton and not polyester permanent press, colorfast, or wrinkle-resistant, as these will defeat your efforts since they also outgas formaldehyde and other chemicals.

An alternative is barrier cloth covers for mattresses, sheets and pillows (Janice's, Nontoxic Environments and other sources in Resources). Also be sure to prop your back and neck with all cotton pillows.  My favorites are available from KB Cotton Pillows.

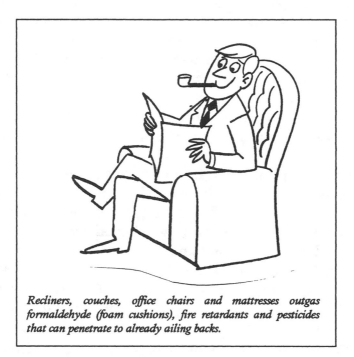

*Recliners, couches, office chairs and mattresses outgas formaldehyde (foam cushions), fire retardants and pesticides that can penetrate to already ailing backs.*

I recall one night I was suddenly nailed with the most excruciating flare-up of my back pain in a hotel room in London where I had been lecturing.  Fortunately at that time, we were at a different stage of knowledge, so I suspected right away that it must be a new mattress full of chemicals to be slowly released over the next 6 years.  I had precipitously awakened in such agony that my poor husband had to get dressed and begin a hunt after midnight on the streets of London for aluminum foil and a cotton blanket.  He is exceedingly resourceful and I slept like a baby the rest of the night.

When I was first exposed to this concept, I was accustomed to arriving from airplane flights with a severe flare-up of my back pain. It would also happen after much sitting in the office, at medical meetings, or anywhere for that matter. Being a dumb doctor, I blamed it on the seats, never dreaming it could be the chemicals outgassing from them. But you can diagnose and protect yourself as I did. I made a thick pad of several layers of aluminum foil and placed it in an attractive cotton flannel pillowcase that I could unobtrusively roll up and not be embarrassed carrying.

I soon found out (thanks to the enormous patience of Dr. Bill Rea, director of the Environmental Health Center in Dallas), that it was not the seats, but the chemicals outgassing from the seats that made a beeline to weakened areas of previous injury. All I can say is don't knock it until you have tried it. I get too much positive feedback from others that it has helped to ignore including it as part of the 80/20 rule. Chemical sensitivity may very well be a part of your total load of pain stressors. By remembering that an area of previous injury or weakness is the most common target organ for toxic chemicals, this may throw a different interpretation on your next "mysterious" flare-up of pain.

To recap a very inexpensive and important concept, many people, myself included, have derived tremendous benefit from going to a restaurant supply store to get a large roll of heavy-duty aluminum foil. Place 6 layers on your side of the bed, shiny side up. Then put one or two cotton blankets over it to keep it from crinkling and breaking up. Don't make your spouse sleep on foil, just put it on your side only. Many people have a dramatic reduction in back pain when they are not absorbing formaldehyde from a mattress or toxic phenols outgassing from a plastic waterbed all night long.

228

And if it helps you, don't forget to make a little aluminum foil pad to put inside of a cotton flannel pillow case to put on other places where you sit all day at the office, in the car, on a plane, bus, subway, or in a business meeting. And don't forget your favorite chair in the evening for watching television. I know it sounds ludicrous but if it hadn't helped me so dramatically and so many other people, we would not even bother mentioning it. It is encouraging how often some of the least expensive solutions are the best.

And the results may trigger you to dig deeper. You won't be the first person to be aghast at learning formaldehyde in kitchen cabinets or toluene from carpets added to their back pain. I recall one 35 old engineer who had a consulting job out of town a few days a week. As much as he disliked travelling, it was a blessing to learn that his total body pain which doctors had labeled as arthritis was gone when he was not at home. The cause we found and corrected? Very high levels of formaldehyde in his brand new home.

Other unexpected yet common chemical causes of chronic pain are natural gas. The kitchen and laundry rooms have more than their share, but many pain victims have had a bedroom over the basement gas water heater or a leaky gas heating system that provided a constant trigger for headaches or musculoskeletal pain.

Others had a bedroom located over the garage where cars were warmed up plus paints, weed whackers; kerosene, greases, pesticides and solvents were stored. Add to this concoction the motor oil spills and stored lawn mower gasoline, and it was enough to keep them chronically awakening in pain. Merely a little common sense clean-up with a large metal trash can holding many of the smellier products, baking soda to cover the leaked oil, and warming the car up outside of the garage can go a long way in relieving the situation. More details for diagnosing and fixing the problem in *The E.I. Syndrome, Revised,* then *Chemical Sensitivity* and *Tired or Toxic?*

I was extremely surprised to find that natural gas and other airborne chemicals that are in all of our homes and offices contributed to my back pain severely. In fact even after I learned about it from Dr. Rea, I staunchly resisted and denied the issue for years. I just could not fathom how everyday objects, appliances and furnishings could have any bearing on my severe back pain. Besides I was a physician and knew the pain could be explained by the damage on x-ray findings. After all hadn't I had enough accidents and x-ray findings to justify such pain? Fortunately, God does not give up on dumb doctors and several incidents made it so blatantly clear that even I could not deny it.

As one example, I had been lecturing in China for 3 weeks with a number of my colleagues, including Dr. William Rea and Dr. Theron Randolph, the "father of chemical sensitivity". As we entered a Chinese hospital kitchen on our tour, I smelled a tremendous amount of natural gas. I turned to leave when my back went into such violent spasm that it dropped me to the floor. Many other surprise attacks, directly related to the chemical environment, drove home the message. But it is only when you are particularly unloaded or cleaned out that these incidents can hit with such unmistakable clarity.

Clearly natural gas, propane, and furnaces with old tanks in the basement that often are over-filled and out-gas into the rest of the home air provide common chemicals that can provoke pain, weakness or muscle spasm (or all three), especially in a place of previous damage or injury. It is a pity to suffer when you have complete control over finding and getting rid of the source. If chemical sensitivity contributes to your pain, you merely need to follow the directions in *The E.I. Syndrome, Revised* to identify the causes and do the appropriate **environmental controls** to rev up your ability to detoxify. Review the preceding chapter for detoxification and see the resources for safer home products.

## Fortify Yourself:

Many nutrients other than boron, niacinamide, DLPA, or magnesium that you have learned about have worked wonders for pain. For example, tendon conditions like carpal tunnel syndrome, resulting in wrist pain from computer work, for example, have responded beautifully to high doses of pyridoxine or vitamin B6, negating the need for, the standard treatment recommended by conventional medicine, surgery.

The connective tissues that house the nerves and tendons in the wrist and hand can become inflamed from computer and other repetitive hand work, like painting, brushing, screwing, scrubbing, or sweeping. As the tissue inflames, it puts pressure on the hand and arm nerves giving pain with paresthesias (numbness and tingling). Often a mere 100-200 mg of vitamin B6, 2-3 times a day with various other nutrients as discussed here, has completely resolved the problem. Surgery was cancelled.

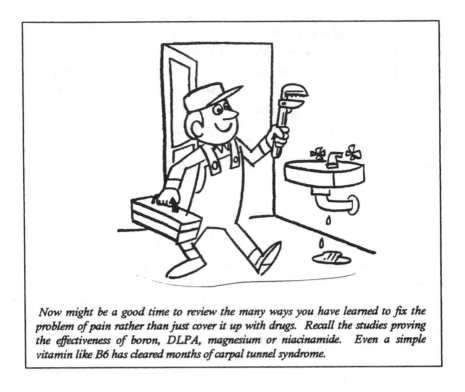

*Now might be a good time to review the many ways you have learned to fix the problem of pain rather than just cover it up with drugs. Recall the studies proving the effectiveness of boron, DLPA, magnesium or niacinamide. Even a simple vitamin like B6 has cleared months of carpal tunnel syndrome.*

## Lubricate Yourself

Those rickety old joints need a lube job, just as any moving part does. In fact, many pain victims are in need of a whole oil change. For we all have in our systems varying amounts of *trans fatty acids* or "bad" oils from our years of eating fast foods, French fries, commercial salad dressings, commercial breads, convenience foods, grocery store hydrogenated oils, restaurant foods, snack foods, margarines, and much more.

The high heat that is needed to hydrogenate an oil so that it survives in our pantries indefinitely without going rancid, changes the chemistry from what we call a cis (normal, healthy) form to a trans form. In this shape, the fat molecule

232

causes damage and disease (plus accelerates aging) once it gets incorporated into our cell membranes and arteries.

For recall that the cell membrane is the primary site of release of all those inflammatory mediators or messengers that turn on inflammation; and inflammation leads to leaky vessels resulting in swelling and pain. White blood cells come flocking in to dissolve and clean up the mess, destroying bone and cartilage in the process and more pain results. If the cell membrane is made of abnormal chemistry from years of ingesting these "plastic" fast foods like French fries, pretzels and chips and processed foods like commercial breads and salad dressings, then it does not function properly and lets loose with the inflammatory mediators much more readily. Fortunately, many medical studies show that by giving someone an oil change they can turn their thermostat for inflammation and pain way down.

The most commonly deficient category of essential fatty acids is the omega-3, obtainable from non-farm raised fish in the diet. Unfortunately most of the fish in supermarkets are farm-raised and fed omego-6 oil containing feed. This gives them the wrong chemistry to benefit you. Or if they are ocean or lake fish, high levels of mercury and other pollutants often contaminate them. Cod liver oil or flax oil are the best forms to restore omega-3 fatty acid deficiencies. I prefer Carlson's Cod Liver Oil® because you get both Omega-3's (EPA or eicosapentaenoic acid and DHA or docosahexaenoic acid) plus vitamins A and D, also needed for pain control. And I have seen the independent lab's assay substantiating no mercury.

The **first step for an oil change** is to stop eating any trans fatty acids. Eat nothing that has been fried or that contains vegetable oil, hydrogenated soybean oil, margarine, shortening, or cottonseed oil. **Next, cook with olive oil; use butter on toast and baking or organic cold-pressed corn oil or organic cold-pressed walnut oil.** Then take 1-3 tsp (3 tsp. = 1 tbs.) of flax oil a day. It can also be hidden on salad or whole grain, but do not cook with it. After a month, lower the dose to just one teaspoon. If you are worse, you may not have an omega-3 fatty acid deficiency or lack other nutrients.

Eventually make the switch from flax to even more nutritious cod liver oil. Carlson's Cod Liver Oil®, one teaspoon a day or 3 capsules a day is the best mercury-free form I have found. If the thought of cod liver oil each day still turns you off, you can take 1 tbs. twice a week, for the body stores this nutrient. Whichever you choose, you have 3 wonderful choices with which to correct an omega-3 fatty acid deficiency, the most common form to cause chronic pain.

If you are worse, you may not have an omega-3 deficiency but, an omega-6 deficiency, or more likely, the inability to convert omega-6 oils to their useful form, gamma linolenic acid. This presumed deficiency is corrected with Efamol Evening Primrose Oil® (Emerson Ecologics), 1-2 capsules, 2-3 times a day. Best, of course, is if you measure your membrane fatty acids and determine precisely which ones are low. Have your physician call MetaMetrix Laboratories, or Great Smokies Diagnostic Laboratory for instructions on assaying for fatty acid deficiencies. You should become well-versed on the importance of an oil change by reading *Depression Cured At Last!*

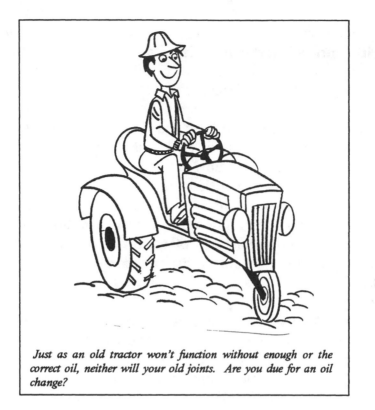

*Just as an old tractor won't function without enough or the correct oil, neither will your old joints. Are you due for an oil change?*

Recall that CM (Chapter 3) is also a fatty acid. And judging by the impressive results I have witnessed in all sorts of pain, it is definitely an unappreciated essential fatty acid for those who benefited from its remarkable relief. We know that in the grand scheme of things, we are in our infancy and have not begun to discover all the nutrients essential for health.

But by far, it just may be that the best way to lubricate those cell membranes (where the chemistry is released that turns on pain) is with Lyprinol® (Prevail, Tyler) that you learned about in chapter 4. For decades New Zealanders used extracts from the New Zealand green-lipped mussel (*Perna canaliculus*) to stop pain. In fact studies show that if you hang in there for 1-3 months, over 70% of rheumatoid arthritis and osteoarthritis sufferers get equal or more pain relief than they did with the nasty NSAIDs, but without the potentially fatal side effects.

And the relief is more potent than the results obtained by taking the well-researched essential fatty acids you just learned about. In addition, Lyprinol's anti-inflammatory advantages extend to other diseases like asthma and autoimmune diseases like inflammatory bowel. And Lyprinol® safely inhibits one of the inflammatory pathways that contribute to metastases of cancers, so it is a uniquely powerful anti-inflammatory without the gastrointestinal side effects.

Use Lyprinol® two capsules twice a day for 1-3 months, then see if you can reduce the dose to one twice a day after the therapeutic relief is obtained. So far the research and patient results make it a nutrient that should far outstrip Celebrex®, Vioxx® and the other COX-2 anti-inflammatories, which are infinitely more expensive, have had several deaths, and still have the potential of gastric hemorrhage.

Celebrex® may have the $800 million in sales per year and the *Wall Street Journal* coverage that goes with the money territory, but Lyprinol® has the safety, economy, infinitely longer history, more studies, and results that can't be duplicated. It has the unique and coveted capacity to repair the source of the problem, not just mask the symptom.

### Purge Yourself

"Ugh! How disgusting! I don't do enemas, so I'll skip this section."

Just hold on a moment. I've heard every negative there is regarding enemas. But even more frequently, I have heard folks chastise themselves for not doing the detox enema sooner. For to their surprise, they discovered that it caused instant pain reduction and accelerated healing. How they wished they had done it sooner.

Granted the word "enema" turns off many folks who say they could never even consider such a sordid procedure. But I can attest to thousands of folks, myself included, for whom it has been a lifesaver many times. If you are sick in any way, and especially if you know you have gotten into something that is flaring up your gut or other target organ, try it.

Whenever the body has an undesirable symptom, for sure the body's ability to detoxify its daily onslaught has been surpassed. In contrast, when our detoxification system is functioning on all cylinders, we can eat, drink, inhale, and be merry. The toxins and the total load of stressors to the body don't seem to phase us.

So the logical thing to do is speed up the body's ability to detoxify by decreasing the load of work it has to do before you can start feeling great again. Let me put it another way. If you had a howling night out with too much alcohol, you would feel lousy the next day. But you know that in another day or two, you can be your bright-eyed and bushy-tailed self again. This time lag is due to the fact that the body takes that much time to detoxify the excess alcohol.

Well why not speed up the detoxification work so you don't have to wait 2 days to feel great again? What's wrong with feeling great again in a few minutes or hours? That's what the detox enema does.

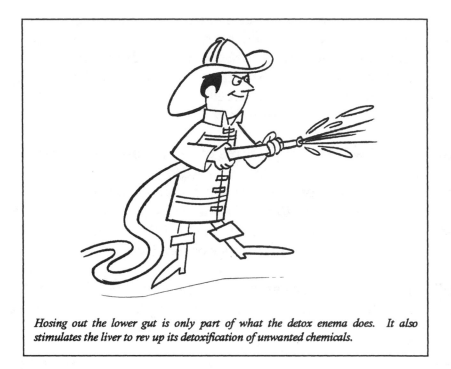

*Hosing out the lower gut is only part of what the detox enema does.  It also stimulates the liver to rev up its detoxification of unwanted chemicals.*

The last stage of detoxification in the body is when our chemicals from air, food, water, and uninvited germs march down the gut to be excreted.  Unfortunately as they hang around in the gut waiting to be eliminated, they can get reabsorbed, especially if the gut is leaky.  This is one reason why folks with constipation feel so crumby.  They get reabsorption of toxins and chemicals from the stool (that they have already wasted energy on detoxifying).

The reabsorption of these toxins further overburdens the detox system and with this double-whammy you get more symptoms on top of your usual ones. But if you can clean up the toxins a day or so earlier, you unload the detox system. This gives it a chance to catch up and clean out other toxins that are making you sick.  Now you can see why it *shortens the course of any illness,* and in many cases folks feel better within an hour or less.

The procedure is simple. Get one enema bag (N.E.E.D.S.) and Folgers® fully caffeinated coffee (red can). Put 4 cups of filtered water into a pan, add 4 tbs. of Folgers® and bring to a boil for 2 minutes and turn off. Let it cool to baby bottle temperature, gently warm. Pour liquid only (not the grounds) into the enema bag and hang it at waist level in the bathroom. It is easier if you make it the night before and merely warm it up in the morning.

Lie on the floor and insert lubricated (with water or saliva) tube into your rectum. Unclamp the hose and let half (2 cups) flow into the rectum. Rest and read something peaceful for 10 minutes. Get up and expel the enema into the toilet. Repeat once. What could be simpler? (More details in *Wellness Against All Odds* for those who need more direction or convincing, as it is a must for folks with cancer and other serious illnesses.)

Remember that you are going to be getting rid of a lot of toxins and inflammatory by-products in the work of getting well. For the basis of real healing is to first identify and stop the toxic overload causing inflammation and pain. Then the body has the monumental task of cleaning up all these toxic leftovers before it can begin the task of rebuilding the damaged bones and other tissues.

How does the body deal with these toxins? It has a whole specialized system designed to do just that: detoxify the body. It does so in two steps. In **Phase I** of detoxification, it switches the electrons around on the toxin so that it is prepared to enter Phase II.

In **Phase II,** a heavy molecule is attached to the toxin that can drag it out of the blood into the urine, sweat, and liver sinusoids. Once in the liver, where most of our toxins go, they dump into the bile ducts and their storage tank, the gall bladder. Here is it dumped into the gut and we eventually flush our toxins down the toilet.

When you are in pain, you want to accelerate the detoxification process so that you can be out of pain sooner. There are lots of ways to do this. One is to rev up Phase I and Phase II with your own DETOX COCKTAIL. The recipe is easy: a heaping teaspoon of Ultra Fine Pure Ascorbic Acid Powder (Klaire) and 400-800 mg of Recancostat Powder (Tyler) in a large 8 oz. glass of water. Have a second 8-oz glass of water with two 300 mg Lipoic Acid capsules (Metabolic Maintenance). You can do this 1-4 times a day as able.

Another way to rev up the detox procedure even quicker is to do a **detox enema.** If you still get all hot and bothered and say disgusting things you will regret, I need to remind you that this is one of the best, safest, quickest, cheapest, and easiest techniques to do in order to get relief from your pain. To pass this up is to put yourself through a lot of needless pain. Do you think I am any different from you, or got a medal for being perverse when graduating from medical school over 30 years ago? I had the same reaction of instant rejection when I first learned about detox enemas for accelerating detoxification. In fact I vowed I would never even divulge the subject to a patient, much less write about it for the public, much less do one myself. But people write in or tell me in the office every day how the detox enema saves the day for them, just as it has for me, many times over.

In fact, it is so beneficial that it is a must for any cancer patient as well. It can be done in less than 20 minutes, is simple after you have mastered your first one, and can be modified for the individual who is in such back pain, for example, that he cannot yet get down on the floor. In that instance, it is even more necessary to have one, but the irony is that you are in such pain that you cannot manipulate your body into the regular position to do it. So merely squat over the toilet, gently insert the tube 2" and do the enema in the seated (or even standing) position. For there is no way you would be able to move quickly enough off the floor when nature calls. In this case you will need to hang the bag a little higher; the shower head or door top is a perfect height.

Before you completely scratch the detox enema off your "to do list", recall that it was a normal part of medicine for over a century. It was in the *Merck Manual*, a standard medical text for decades, until the 1970's when it was displaced by more drugs which now make up the vast majority of medical cover-up (I can hardly call it treatment, for they do not cure, but merely mask).

### Brace Yourself

Once you are mobile, you will need to protect the hurting area while it is healing. There are countless thoughtless things we promote in medicine, but not much comes close to our encouraging people to abuse painful areas by wearing flimsy aces and braces and sucking down NSAIDs to mask their pain while they go out and run around on an inflamed body part. I shudder every time I'm biking down the road and see self-abusing joggers wearing knee braces. Pain is nature's message to stop beating up on a part. Areas of pain need rest, protection and immobilization for maximum

241

healing and to decrease the chance of arthritic deformities years later.

**Knee:**
First let's look at a common problem, the damaged knee. Knees are in the news as celebrities join the ranks of yuppies, or as *USA Today* calls them the "aging boomers", who have chronic knee problems. But age is irrelevant, as you will see in any weekend athletic event a plethora of braces and elastic bandages being sported by all ages. When *USA Today* did their 1997 pain survey they found that knee problems were one of the most common sources of pain for the aging baby boomers. And as a 41-year-old interviewee reported "Just about everyone we know in our age group who is into sports has some kind of knee problem."

So what is the cause of all this pain? *Weekend warriors* would be more appropriately called *weakened warriors,* for along with inadequate conditioning, nutrient depletion is at the core. First we are progressively more sedentary as a society. For many, their maximum daily exercise is walking to the water cooler. Being able to turn quickly as in soccer, basketball, racket ball, squash, lacrosse, tennis, rough terrain jogging, baseball, golf or volley ball requires balance among the supporting muscles of the knee joint. But many rarely stretch prior to play much less do daily knee bends and other stretching and strengthening exercises.

More importantly, as the mineral levels fall in our bodies, preferential areas become depleted. This causes a loss of tensile strength. You can actually see this mineral loss in other visible organs; look at the strength of the nails, hair, look at the skin for accelerated pouching, sagging and bogging, or just regard the overall level of vitality and enthusiasm.

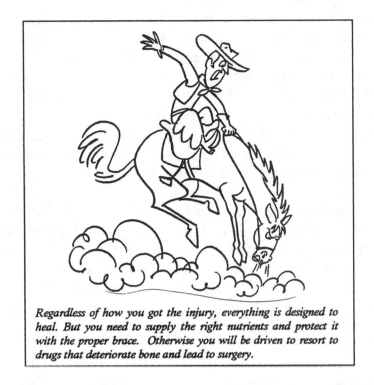

*Regardless of how you got the injury, everything is designed to heal. But you need to supply the right nutrients and protect it with the proper brace. Otherwise you will be driven to resort to drugs that deteriorate bone and lead to surgery.*

A quick test of the degree of aging is to pick up the skin on the back of your hand and see how long it stays tented versus that of a child which immediately resumes its shape. As we gradually lose our tissue elasticity and strength, the skin stays tented many seconds and sometimes minutes longer. When we assess the mineral status of people in the office, we rarely find anyone who is normal anymore, because mineral deficiencies have become the norm.

Why? The soils are more depleted by repeated growing, food is picked before ripening and maturation instead of waiting for full nutrient content to appear, and more foods are imported from foreign countries that do not have our pesticide guidelines, thereby adding to the toxic load. As well, more processed foods that are robbed of minerals make up a larger part of the diet, plus poorer choices of foods are being made by the consumer as he is manipulated by advertising. As an example, most of the "guilt-free" chips and other snacks contain Olestra or Olean. This turns off absorption of not only fat, but fat-soluble vitamins and causes diarrhea so minerals are lost as well! The body can rob Peter to pay Paul only so long before some area comes up deficient. Plus the work of having chronic inflammation itself uses up or depletes minerals.

But a worse problem looms in the horizon for the victim of knee injury. Whether it is a "torn cartilage" or torn ligament (anterior cruciate or posterior cruciate are the most common), or a "slipped patella" (kneecap) let's look at the standard treatment. If surgery is warranted immediately, there's no contest. But most have only partially damaged an area, in which case they are given the standard ice, elevation and stabilization with elastic bandage, brace or cast.

After a brief immobilization of weeks, physical therapy and exercise are encouraged and so are medications to help with the pain. This should be your first indication that you are on the wrong track. For pain is one of nature's warnings that you should not be doing what you are doing. It should not take a rocket scientist to figure that out. But instead we turn off this warning with any of a number of non-steroidal anti-inflammatory drugs (NSAIDs) to mask the pain.

As you learned, NSAIDs like Aleve®, Advil®, Motrin® (ibuprofen), etc., cause deterioration and eventual bone loss. They can go on to cause the leaky gut that can then proceed to cause food and chemical allergies, auto-immune diseases like thyroiditis, rheumatoid arthritis, MS, ulcers, and impaired nutrient deficiencies.

Worse, NSAIDs allow us to keep hammering away at the damaged area, almost guaranteeing that it will require eventual surgery. Each time you get one little twinge of pain in that knee cartilage means you have caused additional damage to provoke further inflammation which just may be the straw that breaks the camel's back. For you can function with just so much cartilaginous damage before you succumb to surgery.

Each seemingly harmless twinge of pain triggers further chemistry to protect the joint (to compensate for what you have failed to do). The result is arthritic spurs that eventually need surgery or loss of cartilage requiring total knee replacement. The work of healing is an inflammatory process where old damaged cells are gobbled up and replaced by healthy young ones. So why would anyone in their right mind want to suppress this natural protective and healing mechanism of the body by turning off inflammation with an anti-inflammatory drug?

The best treatment that I have observed (and first hand, as it happened to me as well) is to completely immobilize the knee for 6 months and allow it to permanently heal. Put it to rest. "Impossible!" you say, "I have to work." And so do we all.
If the brace is properly adjusted, there will be no pain, for the two inflamed joint surfaces never touch one another. A Joe Nameth type brace is the best. Your orthopedist makes a cast of your leg, saws off the cast and ships it to the brace manufacturer who uses this mold of your leg to create a brace that will optimally fit you. Still it is not perfect. You will need to anchor it around your waist with a couple of

thin cloth straps to keep it from slipping down around your ankle.

But with this, you can put it on when you awaken, do business as usual, even run through airports as I did; I even went horseback riding regularly with it. But it must be adjusted with the right amount of permanent flexion so that regardless of how much weight you put on it, you are never able to completely straighten the knee out and never able to produce pain.

I repeat: never once should you have a twinge of pain. If you do, it tells you the brace is not properly adjusted or you need evaluation for more of a problem. In the meantime, you should check your nutrient levels. I was astounded to find that the RBC zinc (red blood cell zinc is mandatory, because assays on the serum or plasma zinc are too insensitive), as an example, can drop 200 points during healing, even though folks are taking it. If you cannot get blood levels, the doses mentioned in the next chapter would be a good start. Take the brace off at night for passive stretches and any exercise as long as it does not produce even a twinge of pain. Exercising in a tub with 2 cups of Epson salts (magnesium sulfate) can help keep it from getting stiff and massage stimulates lymphatics.

The brace can be worn under trousers or skirts, and need not even be noticed. Sparing the knee completely of pain while it heals for 6 months, drastically reduces the likelihood of future surgery and problems.

I cannot over-emphasize: If it is properly adjusted there is never a need for any medication. For there should never be the opportunity for the two joint surfaces to touch one another to produce pain, while they enjoy complete healing

246

over at least 6 months. But as one orthopedic specialist told me when I explained my plan for my knee, "I consider that over-kill! We only use that brace if surgery has failed." and stomped out of the room. I venture to guess I'm the only ligament and cartilage injury to that extent that he did not get to operate on. And the next forty people I saw wearing the knee brace had, you guessed it, already had surgery!

Meanwhile, I and the people I have recommended this to have never had as much as a twinge of pain years after our knee injuries and are actively playing tennis, etc. And not one of us has had surgery, while over 40 people I talked with who used the conventional method, all had either arthroscopy, surgery, or had recurrent chronic pain and used frequent medications. Think about it. If you had a serious break of your leg, it would be about 6 months before the majority of healing had occurred. So why is the knee tissue any different? Just because it does not cover as large an area, it is the same physiology that is required to properly and totally heal.

The scariest people are the joggers I see along the road actually wearing knee bandages and braces while they jog, or the ones I hear bragging that they can jog as long as they take their medication. The NSAIDs cause bone to deteriorate. No wonder there are so many knee and hip replacements. One of the T.V. ads shows joggers bragging that they can perform as long as they premedicate themselves. I guess they will keep the orthopods in business a long time.

I have recently found a generic source for the knee brace. The source is *The Feel Good Catalogue*. Also try the Aircast Company, as they make an excellent ankle brace and most likely will eventually do the same for knees (see resources).

**Back:**

The same can be said for the back. After I had overpowered every corset and back brace prescribed for me, I was given a Raney jacket. Once again they make a cast of your body; several doctors wrapped my torso in plaster as I hung from monkey bars at the medical school. Once it dries, they saw it off and ship it to a brace manufacturer who customizes a fiberglass mold of it as a cast for your body. Mine had 6 one-inch thick straps to secure it, and in spite or the fact that it was terribly uncomfortable, it saved my sanity. For without it, I was in constant back pain and could not do any activity.

With it on, I was able to garden, ride my horse and water ski backwards and slalom. Of course it squeezes you so well that you'll end up with hemorrhoids, varicose veins and a hiatus hernia, but what price is sanity? I figured I would stop wearing it if my eyes began to bug out.

**Ankle:**

For ankle sprains nothing beats the Aircast Support Stirrup®, available in pharmacies across the U.S. and in sports stores, or direct from the manufacturers (Aircast, Summit New Jersey, 1-800-526-8785). For a reference junkie like myself it even comes complete with citations for the scientific studies to back up its therapeutic value and superiority over conventional prophylactic taping.

But nothing compares with the physical proof. Having sprained and chipped more ankles than I can keep track of, I was amazed at the mobility I suddenly had without the need for a cast. Within less than 24 hours of a "blowout" sprain where the ankle immediately tripled in size, it allowed me to comfortably navigate airports, thus not ruining a trip.

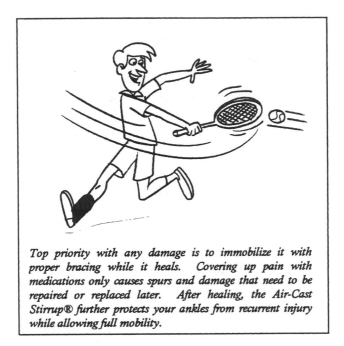

*Top priority with any damage is to immobilize it with proper bracing while it heals. Covering up pain with medications only causes spurs and damage that need to be repaired or replaced later. After healing, the Air-Cast Stirrup® further protects your ankles from recurrent injury while allowing full mobility.*

Being perfectly designed to support the commonly damaged areas enough to allow for comfortable navigation, it is superior to a cast (provided there are no broken bones or completely severed attachments). You can take it off nightly to passively exercise the area, thus saving you the time to rebuild the ankle that has atrophied or wasted away under a smelly cast for weeks. This speeds up recovery time.

If that were not enough of a gift, I was able to play doubles tennis within a month while wearing it, and singles in less than 2 months. Actually wearing bilateral stirrups makes it virtually impossible to sprain an ankle, but at the same time have complete mobility for vigorous tennis singles. It is smart to indefinitely wear bilateral ankle braces for weak-ankled folks prone to easy sprains, and they do not impair your game at all.

Meanwhile, if something is damaged, never take pain pills to mask the pain, except for the first 1-3 days of pain when you are completely immobilized. If there is chronic pain, it is nature's signal to immobilize and rest it. It needs support and complete protection from any weight bearing that could produce even a hint of pain. Fortunately with today's technology, we can immobilize and keep going as well. You may end up with a closet full of body parts like I have (braces for back, braces for knee, ankles, shoulders, fingers, etc.), but it is the best way to assure you will not end up with surgery.

Now you begin to appreciate how every injury is a warning sign. A ruptured Achilles tendon is often a result of three problems: (1) **mineral deficiencies**, from processed foods, that decrease tendon tensile strength, (2) **tight tendons**, from lack of proper stretching, and (3) **loss of bone at tendon attachments** from years of NSAIDs. Also recent reports show some popular antibiotics cause rupture of Achilles tendons. The same can be said for the epidemic of hip pain and often avoidable surgery. For bone and tissues can be regenerated once the cause has been stopped, corrected, and protected.

### Realign Yourself

Now that you are up and moving, you need to get put back in your best position. For when we have injuries or painful muscle spasms, or pain from inflammation and swelling, we get out of alignment. An excellent chiropractor can restore the correct positioning of bones, called their alignment. But many people in pain are leery of being damaged or hurt. So I recommend either of two much more gentle forms of chiropractic, either with the activator method or with what is called Network chiropractic.  Both are different but effective for many and do not entail the use of the classical more violent manipulations.

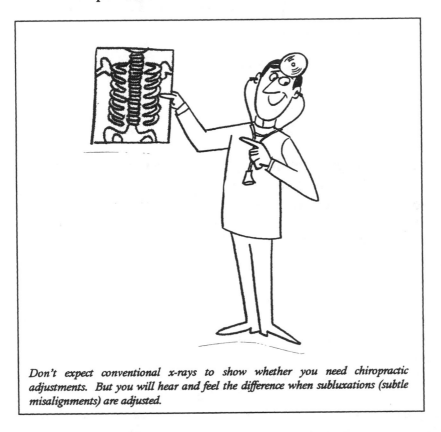

*Don't expect conventional x-rays to show whether you need chiropractic adjustments. But you will hear and feel the difference when subluxations (subtle misalignments) are adjusted.*

And once you are back in better alignment, you want to stay there.  In terms of office and computer work, if you have a bad back, definitely check out the more expensive versions of the kneeling chairs.  It throws your back in just the right position so that you do not miss a back support and you have no pain.  I find them so comfortable that I have used them in all my consultation and exam rooms for 20 years, even though I am healed.

And if you come out of alignment too soon after a chiropractic adjustment, remember the most likely cause is muscle spasm from magnesium deficiency or some hidden sensitivity to a food (like nightshades) or chemical (like formaldehyde or natural gas).

## Deep Heat Yourself

For areas of sprains, pulls and strains, you want to restore the circulation through the stagnation caused by swelling, spilled blood and abundant repair cells. The far infrared hair dryer (High Tech Health) does more than stimulate hair growth as it dries your hair. It also can be used to apply healing waves that penetrate into tissues as are found in the far infrared sauna. With the FIR hair dryer you can apply far infrared rays locally to any injury or painful area to accelerate healing.

Or for a larger area, a Thermotex® Pain Relief pad has the same infrared system with penetrating heat to bring increased circulation that brings nutrients to the area, fosters faster cellular debris cleanup, and encourages metabolism of lactic acid and speed healing in general (High Tech Health). It is especially good to use after the acute phase of the first 2 days of: muscle strain, tennis elbow, shoulder tendonitis, hip and back pain and sports injuries. Even a tense day at the office computer can be relieved by placing it over the upper back. Any place a heating pad would feel good, this does better, because of the penetrating and toxin-mobilizing effects of far infrared wavelengths. For recall these are the wavelengths that penetrate tissue to energize water and toxic molecules into harmonic resonance (a molecular dance if you will) to encourage the release of stored tissue toxins, a consistent companion to pain (Chapter 6).

## Sterilize Yourself

Wow! That sounds pretty serious. But actually, there is a whole wonderful world of unheard-of therapies that have bailed people out of incredible pain. There are mountains of evidence that many types of arthritis are due to infectious agents, from Lyme disease and Rocky Mountain Spotted Fever, to protozoa and bacteria, like mycoplasma. When I was lecturing at Oxford University a few of years ago, I heard Dr. Garth Nicholson who improved a significant number of Gulf War Syndrome victims with the generic antibiotic, tetracycline. This was very impressive and he has a wealth of data published on this phenomenon. However, for cases not responding to this therapy, it has been my experience that resistant Gulf War cases require a more comprehensive total body approach as described in *Depression Cured At Last!*

Antibiotics of the tetracycline class, particularly minocycline and doxycycline have produced such dramatic results in cases of very resistant arthritis that a whole foundation devoted to furthering the information has been formed. I have witnessed great results in people who were not my patients, but like anything else, there are those for whom it does not work.

In a study by O'Dell, who is chief of rheumatology at the University of Nebraska Medical Center, 46 patients with rheumatoid arthritis were treated with 100 mg minocycline or placebo twice a day for a year. Fifteen of the 23 in the minocycline group had 50% improvement. But minocycline is not acting merely as an antibiotic, for studies surprisingly demonstrate that it also has some anti-inflammatory, immuno-modulatory and chondro-protective effects in addition to its antibacterial activity. Dr. Passman at the department of molecular genetics at Albert Einstein College of Medicine has also demonstrated that minocycline definitely is able to exert control over gene expression as well. So there is a lot more going on here than just killing bugs.

Then there is a wealth of information by the Arthritis Trust (formerly the Rheumatoid Disease Foundation in Franklin, Tennessee, P.O. Box 8949, Topeka KS 66608-8949, or at *www.arthritistrust.org*). They have an extensive protocol on which I have seen many victims of recalcitrant arthritis and other painful conditions become pain-free. Even though the antibiotic protocol is demanding and can generate a painful healing crisis or Herxheimer reaction, plus invariably results in a leaky gut full of yeast, it is worth a try if you are at the end of your rope. I would suggest a thorough reading of the literature from the Arthritis Trust of America before embarking, because you want to be sure such a protocol is done properly.

For they do not advocate a solo antibiotic as some of the others do. Metronidazole (Flagyl®) is a top gun, with anti-fungals like Tinidazole and Clotrimazole being used as well. Other infrequently used antibiotics can be included in the protocol. The most interesting part is that most of the organisms that this protocol is geared to kill are not your average bacteria, but fungi, protozoa and other parasites that most likely made their way to joints from the gut. So even though these physicians made their discoveries years before leaky gut was recognized, their theories are backed up by modern discoveries. The foundation also has a list of physicians who use their protocols.

Since the protocol is lengthy and must be followed rigidly and the treatment itself can generate further problems, I would never suggest it to any one who had not done a 3 month's trial of the nightshade-free diet, CM, and checked for leaky gut and intestinal dysbiosis, first. For a year of minocycline is not without dangers. First it is in all likelihood going to create the leaky gut with Candida overgrowth, which will eventually have to be diagnosed and treated. Otherwise, these folks have a strong chance of going on to create the leaky gut tragedies you learned about in Chapter 4. Needless-to-say, you want to avoid that vicious cycle whenever possible.

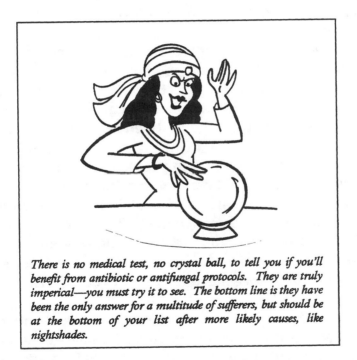

*There is no medical test, no crystal ball, to tell you if you'll benefit from antibiotic or antifungal protocols. They are truly imperical—you must try it to see. The bottom line is they have been the only answer for a multitude of sufferers, but should be at the bottom of your list after more likely causes, like nightshades.*

Harvard researcher, Dr. David Trentham looked at the effects of minocycline 100 mg twice daily in patients with scleroderma accompanied by painful Raynaud's phenomenon. Scleroderma is another auto-immune disease that medicine has no known cause or cure for and uses life-threatening medications like high doses of steroids and chemotherapy for. The skin gets so tight that it strangles the body and painful spasms occur in fingers, toes and other areas. Yet in this study 4 out of 11 people had total resolution of painful symptoms within a year.

Unfortunately as with any of these studies with great results, there is never an exhaustive search for other causes first. So we have no way of telling if many of these would have responded to the nightshade-free diet, CM, or a comprehensive environmental work-up.

On the flip side of this, there are multiple mechanisms why a long-standing trial of a broad spectrum antibiotic like minocycline would be so effective. For example, many people have hidden infection in root canals that unbalance meridians and over-stress the body enough to cause chronic pain and other symptoms in areas like joints that would never make you think of a tooth problem. In addition, there are numerous researchers who have demonstrated antibodies to these organisms in joint fluid (see references), substantiating their causative action. Cheaper, more efficacious and easier, if you are at the end of your rope, is a therapeutic trial, because science may not yet have the antibody test for the organism lurking in your joints.

In further defense of the antibiotic treatment, remember that one of the fastest ways researchers have of creating laboratory rats with arthritis for experiments is to inject them with a bacterium, Mycobacterium. And recall from the leaky gut section how bugs like Klebsiella and Streptococcus are already known for their ability to cause serious forms of arthritis. And we know how bugs from the gut can trek right into the blood stream and make a new home in any spot, including joints.

Clearly, infectious agents are the source of many types of arthritis, whether it involves one joint or many. All of these researchers have done a wonderful service for prisoners of pain in proving the bug connection to arthritis and other chronic pains and the need for antibiotics. However, it makes sense as part of the program to test for and clear up the leaky gut, not only because a leaky gut can allow bugs ready access to joints, but also because antibiotic therapy can then go on to cause a leaky gut! Definitely read DiFabio's book before embarking on long-standing antibiotic therapy.

The Nicholson's, the husband and wife Ph.D. research team from Houston have lectured widely and published much on the successful treatment of a significant number of folks (over 50%) with Gulf War Syndrome. Rheumatoid arthritis, fibromyalgia, and chronic fatigue syndrome have also benefited from this program. A major part of the program was the identification of mycoplasma infections in the blood, and patients were treated with several 6 week programs of antibiotics. Again, no one knows what percentage of sufferers a nightshade-free diet or a CM product, for example, might have been effective for.

In closing, because of the lengthy treatment and the chance of triggering Candida, leaky gut, auto-immune disease and many other problems, you want to be treated by someone who has studied all these papers and this book. A long-term antibiotic program of months is nothing you want to enter into lightly. Your physician should also contact Drs. Nicolson at the Institute for Molecular Medicine, 15162

Triton Lane, Huntington Beach, CA 92649, USA (714-903-2900) and read DiFabio's book.

I personally would do many of the other things in this book first to relieve my pain, like the nightshade-free diet, CM Plus®, heal the leaky gut, and the Far Infrared Sauna, which has such a great track record with fibromyalgia that they give a money-back guarantee. And don't forget that infection can't live long in a body that is hostile to it. This includes skin brushing and far infrared sauna to mobilize and get rid of toxins, an organic whole foods diet, anti-oxidants in high levels, the detox cocktail, detox enema, neutraceuticals like olive leaf that fight infection, and much more that you will learn to collate as you move through this program.

### Magnetize Yourself

If I did not have the greatest respect for Dr. William H. Philpott, M.D., and his pioneering publications that were literally decades ahead of their time (like *Brain Allergies*, Keats, New Canaan CT), I probably would never have explored the world of magnets. Although they are not the answer for everyone, folks with agonizing arthritis, degenerating back discs and other forms of chronic pain have been pleasurably improved, some totally. So it is worth learning about if you are at your wits end. They are so powerful that they have a beneficial effect even on healing of open ulcerous wounds, lessening scar, and even slowing the growth of cancer cells in experimental conditions.

And for non-union fractures that fail to heal, there is a wealth of data, researched and written about by Dr. Robert Becker. Properly applied electric currents which can amplify electromagnetic fields, can cause non-union fractures to finally knit, while magnetic fields have relieved pain in hips, backs, shoulders and literally every joint, as Newman's compilation of data will show.

Ceramic, high power gauss magnets do the best job. I suggest you write to Dr. Philpott for a catalog, for there is every type of magnet from penny-sized dots for tendon insertions to strips for scars and wraps for every organ; magnets of various sizes and shapes to strap on, shoe inserts, and seat cushions to entire mattresses which have cleared recalcitrant back problems with degenerating discs.

A great addition to your emergency non-drug box is to purchase what they call the **Soother-one**. It consists of two one and a half inch 3790 gauss ceramic magnets with velcro on the back plus an elastic band so they may be strapped onto any ailing joint or even on either temple for migraine relief. This pair of ceramic magnets is great for acute or chronic pain of the knee or ankle, Achilles tendonitis, tennis elbow, carpal tunnel syndrome, neck and shoulder aches and more. I especially like that the magnets are coated to protect them, stay charged for a lifetime, and that they have Velcro on the back side so you are sure to always put the negative (healing, south-seeking or north-compass needle-seeking) pole toward the body. Don't be scared by the ring of vasculitis you may see around the edges of the magnet contact point after prolonged use. Because the healing surface is the flat area, the sides have the non-healing polarity. So a vascular ring results where the sides have touched the skin. It is proof of the increased alkalinization, oxygenation and improved circulation to the central area and disappears within hours. But to avoid it, merely put a little cotton cloth pad between you and the magnet. This elevates it so the sides do not press in and create the vascular accumulation that occurs from being in contract with the wrong pole.

I recommend that for tough problems, like a bad tooth, to piggyback the two magnets and sleep with the pair over your bad tooth root. Within two months I have seen remarkable resolution of pain and sensitivity from cracked teeth roots after accidental biting on a nutshell. With colloidal silver, colostrum and other immune system boosters to keep infection at bay as well as lots of antioxidants plus nightly use of the magnets, the area became pain-free in two months without root canal or extraction, both of which can lead to lifelong problems in their own right.

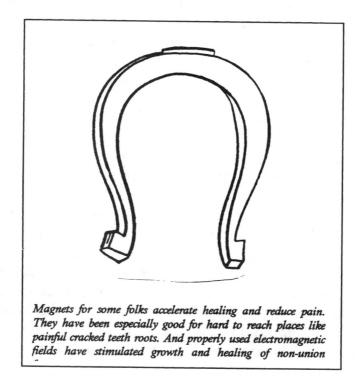

*Magnets for some folks accelerate healing and reduce pain. They have been especially good for hard to reach places like painful cracked teeth roots. And properly used electromagnetic fields have stimulated growth and healing of non-union*

Also the far infrared sauna should be remembered in these cases to improve circulation to the area. If you do not have one, the hair dryer or far infrared pad double as a local FIR source (High Tech Health), providing further deep heat and improved circulation to an area in trouble.

## Stretch Yourself

Yoga is indispensable for not only getting out of pain, but staying out of pain. Several poses can eliminate sciatica, for example, right while on the tennis court. Yoga is an effective substitute for chiropractic, for you will often hear your body correct its own subluxations as you hold a pose. It also stretches tight areas leading to greater mobility and resilience. This minimizes damage from falls. Furthermore, it opens blocked areas promoting circulation. Learning yoga is a priceless step toward a more pain-free life. There are many videos and books to assist you. Yoga literally saved my life.

### *Nightshade Nemesis Can Mimic Need for Emergency Decompression Surgery*

With all the calamities I had over 56 years, this one took the cake. I was tooling along in life, busy as ever, enjoying singles tennis for two hours at the start of each day. I had not a solitary ache or pain, no injuries; it was great. Then one day I awoke and realized that I had unmistakably had a nightshade ingestion. I searched my memory for the hidden source 36-48 hours prior and had my hostess check her trash. Sure enough the frozen lobster meat contained potato starch as a new ingredient, as this brand had not had it in the past and my hostess was fastidious about checking labels.

261

The next day I was measurably worse, much worse than I should have been with three bites of the lobster soufflé, so I searched again, only to find that I had had not one, not two, but four nightshade hits within the last few days. This was an unprecedented amount for me, so I had no idea what the consequences would be.

Within 2 more days, I was slammed with the worst pain I had ever endured in my entire life. It was a combination of every break (6 backs, 7 ankles, one shoulder and knee, 2 wrists, and many more minor catastrophes), for I was literally out of my mind with pain. The closest description of the pain I could give is that it was like having 4 men chain-sawing my leg off at once. The combination of emergency medications and the pain were so nauseating that I lost 20 pounds in 3 weeks. The first 3 days and nights I lay on the bathroom floor so that I could make it to the toilet with the least amount of effort. Unable to walk, I was lucky to be able to crawl on all fours, dragging my paralyzed leg.

The most interesting part of the whole ordeal was that the middle of the back (the lumbo-sacral area) which had always been the target in the past, was totally fine. Instead, the unbearable pain centered to the side of it in the S-I (sacro-iliac) joint, and extended throughout my entire right leg, right to the toes. In nearly every position I was literally screaming, out of my mind with chainsaw-type pain throughout the entire length of the leg.

It was obvious that I was wiping out my sciatic nerve. I had to somehow open up my S-I joint, which was so swollen that it was squeezing the life out of the biggest nerve in the body. And it had grabbed all five branches of it, L4, L5, S1, S2, and S3. Standing, sitting or lying on a bed was out of the question. But I soon found, writhing in extreme pain, that if I tried to open that joint as far as possible, and if I were maximally medicated, I could stand the pain. So I brought my right heel tightly into the crotch, then pushed my knee down and away from my body as far as possible, so that my thigh was on plane with the rest of my body. This effectively opened that S-I joint.

The problem was we could not maintain that position with any form of traction. So I had to actively hold myself in that extremely awkward position night and day for 7 grueling weeks. Each time I drifted off to sleep in exhaustion, I would lose the position and be explosively awakened with excruciating pain. As well, I had to keep a high dose of steroids and pain medications maxed out, or I was at my breaking point and literally out of my head with the pain. When any of the dexamethasone, aspirins, Darvon, codeine or Demerol would wear off, it felt like my leg was being chain-sawed off with a half dozen saws placed along the length of the leg. The paralysis of my lower right leg and complete loss of feeling in several areas paled in comparison to the pain. For the first 3 weeks I got no more than 20-minute snatches of sleep, because each time I would doze off I was jolted into reality by the pain. On top of that, with all those medications, I was doggy-style on the floor much of the first few days with projectile vomiting, until I figured out that chewing 4-6 soaked almonds just before the medications protected my stomach. Oh, it was a fun time.

At 7 weeks, the antigen-antibodies fell off the joint, and the pain left as precipitously as it had come. It took me 3 more weeks to rebuild the lost nerve and muscle function in my leg, as I couldn't even walk up stairs, but had to crawl. My muscles that would lift me up on a step (the hamstrings in the back of the thigh) were gone as well as the foot extensors (muscles that enable you to flex your foot and toes upward toward your body). In two months I was back to singles tennis as though none of this nightmare had ever happened.

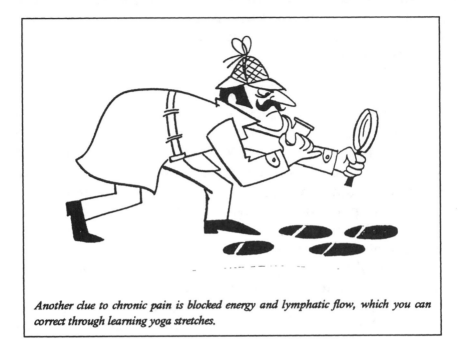

*Another clue to chronic pain is blocked energy and lymphatic flow, which you can correct through learning yoga stretches.*

What did I have to be grateful for from the experience? A ton.
(1) I am forever indebted to Janet Thompson for having taught me enough yoga theory in a few sessions so that I could figure out how to save myself. I never imagined that yoga could save my life. For if I could not have opened up that joint, I would have resorted to hospitalization and undoubtedly exploratory surgery to "save the day". Also I was grateful that she had taught me enough so that I could do the stretches sufficiently over the years to be limber enough to be able to even get into the position that saved me. The position was not one that most folks could get into, much less hold for several

minutes, much less hours, much less days, much less seven weeks.

(2) I was grateful to God for giving me another lesson. He never hesitates to use me as a guinea pig, and then provide me with all that I need to not only survive, but communicate the findings to others who may not have as many options available for a fortunate outcome. For I unquestionably had far more resources available to me with which to rescue myself from this harrowing experience than most.

(3) It made me realize that most folks would have succumbed to emergency decompression surgery, for not many could have tolerated that pain and paralysis for long. But knowing that God always puts me in pain for a good reason, I just looked up and asked if my lesson couldn't be speeded up a little this time (it wasn't). I know from 58 years that I always come out ahead after one of these experiences. It also helped me tremendously to understand and trust implicitly from past calamities that it was due to nightshades. For nothing slams as quickly as a food or chemical reaction. As horrible as the pain was, surgery was definitely not indicated and I had to trust that the reaction in time would turn off as precipitously as it had turned on, once the antigen-antibodies dropped off the joint. I had expected them to do so at their usual three to five weeks, for that was the time frame in the past. But due to the unprecedented number of exposures, it took longer than ever before.

(4) I was even more grateful than ever for my husband ("Luscious"), God's greatest gift to me, who took care of me night and day. No one could have done more for me, and I would not have survived without him. Unconditional love is an understatement and unfathomable.

No one will ever be able to comprehend the extent of the pain. As a physician who has broken and maimed more body parts than she has, and having been an emergency room physician as well, I know of very few people who would have endured this much pain and for this incredible length of time. I literally lost 2 months from my life, which I spent on the floor, day and night, medicated to the gills, and holding my leg in extreme extension.

But it made me reflect on all the elderly arthritics, many on fixed incomes who are living on French fries and Big Macs with ketchup daily. How many of these folks could end their suffering by just avoiding nightshades? How many eat highly spicy foods, loaded with nightshades, because their taste buds have dwindled from zinc and other mineral deficiencies? How many are sure to have tomatoes every day because they read how good lycopenes and other phytochemicals are for preventing prostate and other cancers as well as degenerative eye diseases?

This episode also reminded me that as much as I believe that natural medicines are superior for us, there is definitely a time and place (emergencies) for our wonderful medical armamentarium. I was in such unprecedented pain that I needed all the medications I could stomach. In fact it was the first emergency of my life where I did not use the detox enema. Why? Because it would have speeded up my body's metabolism of the drugs and I would have gotten rid of them sooner. Since the drugs (the most potent steroids and narcotic pain relievers) were barely enough to give me the slightest relief from pain, I needed all the drugs I could stomach. So the last thing I needed was to get rid of them quicker, as I dreaded when they wore off in stages at their appointed times, leading to more nausea and pain.

Likewise I did not do the enzymes to speed up the dissolution of antigen-antibody complexes from the joint, because I could not take any more in my stomach above and beyond the drugs. Between them and the pain (which never left one second in 7 weeks), the nausea was too great.

I think I was more nightshade sensitive also for a number of reasons. I had lost my cetyl myristoleate coverage after taking it a few months several years before. I think it got depleted again. In addition, because it had allowed me to be a lot more careless with nightshades, I think they bioaccumulated to a point where 4 miscalculations promptly nailed me as never before. In addition, seven months prior, I had a large dental project done which introduced a multitude of meridian-blocking chemicals. This reset my detoxification threshold.

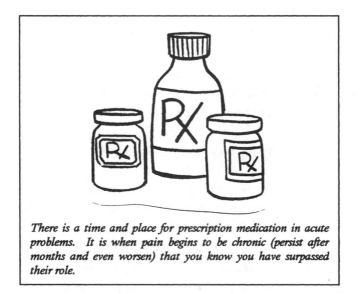

*There is a time and place for prescription medication in acute problems. It is when pain begins to be chronic (persist after months and even worsen) that you know you have surpassed their role.*

This episode also brought home more than ever how important a trust in God is and having a loving spouse. And it bore out how important it is to know your body and your sensitivities. If this had happened before I had known how nightshade sensitive I was, I would have been completely baffled and never have been able to endure such a protracted course of total disability with conviction. I would have had needless decompression surgery and who knows what complications.

Last, it showed me unmistakably that nightshades could mimic the most horrible pain. A pain that most surgeons would think must be operated immediately. And I cannot blame them, for who wouldn't try to put someone out of such emergent and protracted misery? And what about the prospect of permanent irrevocable nerve damage from such protracted paralysis? I was uniquely bestowed with the knowledge, conviction and resources to survive. That is why I believe it was not a mistake that it happened to me. It serves to make me incredibly cautious now, and spread the message to folks who would never even dream that mere food could cause such long-standing agony. And it brought to light once more the importance of the total load of factors, in this instance including knowledge of yoga. Don't miss the books and videos on self-instruction in chapter 10.

### Hyperoxygenate Yourself

High pressure oxygen, in the form of several sessions in a hyperbaric oxygen chamber, has brought remarkable relief to antibiotic-resistant Lyme arthritis, recalcitrant tooth pain, serious bone infection or osteomyelitis, non-union fractures that refuse to heal, strokes, aseptic bone necrosis (a serious side effect from steroids where the main vessel supplying a bone dies, bringing about a painful death of the bone), and more.

The high oxygen pressure in the chamber allows healing oxygen access to areas otherwise isolated by inflammation, swelling, infection, and/or scar tissue. This highly effective and unique therapy requires that you know more about it before you would embark on a course. Read the books in chapter 10 for more information.

## Experiment Yourself

Obviously a book this small cannot go into all the causes and cures of chronic pain, but it is an excellent start on the old 80/20 rule, and we will have lots more in future books and newsletters. In the meantime, if you are still a prisoner of pain, there are many more things you need to know.

If there is one thing that I have learned in over a quarter of a century in medicine, it is that each time I thought I had reached an impasse where everything was hopeless, the solution appeared. In case I may not have touched on all the aspects of your total load that are required for you to heal, do not ever give up. Arm yourself with a solid education in environmental medicine principles, and keep abreast of new findings via the newsletter, for it has eventually provided a solution for most.

I am constantly in awe of how often solutions to chronic pain turn out to be God-given natural techniques, foods or supplements that are readily available to most people. It reminds me of how ego-centric medicine can be in projecting the image that the answer to all disease must be found in expensive and dangerous drugs and high-tech surgery. For do not forget, as the *New England Journal of Medicine* (April 14, 1998) article taught us, the 4th leading cause of death in the U.S. is from a prescribed drug while in the hospital (and it ignores those deaths out of the hospital).  It further drives home the meaning of "Has God not made foolish the things of this world?" (1COR1)

There are all sorts of programs that have received very little recognition, but deserve mention because they have helped some very recalcitrant cases.  One such example is the program of Dr. Paul St. Amand, the chief of epidemiology at UCLA Medical School.  He discovered that a vast number of people with fibromyalgia no longer hurt if they take the prescription mucolytic drug Guaifenesin.  This is known as Robitussin, an expectorant that brings up mucous.  No one understands why it works in fibromyalgia.  Regular Robitussin would not be appropriate as it is only 100 mg per teaspoon and the dose that cleared most people in Dr. St Amand's experience was 600 mg 2-3 times a day, available from special pharmacies in the Resources (chapter 10).

The protocols here and in *Depression Cured At Last!*, *No More Heartburn*, and *Wellness Against All Odds* have been successful for most cases of fibromyalgia.  But because Dr. Amand has had such good results, it should be mentioned here for people who are resistant to all other treatments.  If you and your doctor are interested in the technique, which is lengthy, devour his book first.  There is a special diet that must also accompany the medication or it will not be successful.  The interesting thing is that the Guaifenesin has no recognized bad side effects although people can go through a severe worsening of their pain when they are on the program.  Another draw-back is that Guaifenesin and a very restrictive diet must be continued indefinitely.  But if you are at the end of your rope, this program can be a life-saver.  Read *What Your Doctor May Not Tell You About*

*Fibromyalgia* by Paul St. Amand, M.D. (Warner Books, NY, 1999).

### Elevate Yourself

In the meantime, there are many other things that contribute to the whole total package or total load of chronic pain as I have described in *Depression Cured At Last!*, as certain happy hormones in the brain, like endorphins, are also linked to reduction of pain. And since depression is a common partner to any medical problem, boosting more of your brain's happy hormones can also supply a missing piece of the pain puzzle. There is no problem in taking a safe, inexpensive, non-addicting, non-prescription, natural anti-depressant like 5-hydroxy-tryptophan. This amino acid is the precursor to serotonin, one of the brain's many happy hormones. The potentially addicting and suicide-inducing prescription anti-depressants like Prozac, Paxil, Luvox and Zoloft work on augmenting serotonin by slowing down its breakdown. But it makes more sense to boost its production naturally and without the dangerous side effects of drugs. You might as well make more of your own happy hormone and not take prescription anti-depressants with potentially dangerous side effects that include death from the serotonin syndrome or psychotic suicide.

A good start to put you on a brighter pathway of optimism and improved mood would be 5-Hydroxy-Tryptophan (Pure Encapsulations, Pain & Stress Center), one or two 50 mg capsules 2-3 times a day. You could add Hypericalm® (a reliable brand of St. John's Wort, an anti-depressant herb by Enzymatic Therapy/PhytoPharmica) that naturally slows the breakdown of serotonin without drug side effects. In fact, studies on St. John's Wort confirm it is as effective and yet safer than the prescription drugs. One or two capsules 2-3 times a day is the normal dose. Combine it with a multiple like one Multiplex-1 (Tyler), one MethylMax (Tyler), one tsp. of Phos Chol Concentrate (American Lecithin Co.) and 3 Magnesium Taurate (Ecological Formulas/Cardiovascular Research). The toll-free numbers for these companies are in the Resources chapter.

Studies clearly show that patients with fibromyalgia had less pain after revving up the happy hormones in the brain. In fact many pain clinics across the country rely on heavy doses of anti-depressants, because they fail to look for the total load of causes of the pain. So on a temporary basis, there is no problem with you feeling happier, as you look for the permanent cures of your pain. And you may even have a reduction in pain with these safe natural, non-prescription supplements.

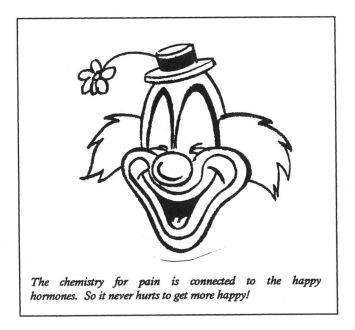

*The chemistry for pain is connected to the happy hormones. So it never hurts to get more happy!*

If you prefer a mood-boosting, relaxing supplement already made for you, try **Mood Sync** (Pain & Stress Center). It contains 175 mg of St. John's Wort, 125 mg of GABA, 110 mg Taurine, 75 mg of glutamine, 25 mg of 5-HTP, and 5 mg of pyridoxine (vitamin B6). It is a clever and effective combination of anti-depressants, calming amino acids and cofactors that jump-start and boost the system. Use 1-2 capsules, 1-4 times a day as needed.

## Connect Yourself

Connect with God. Is there a reason you have been forced into some down time? Have your priorities become unbalanced? Is He whispering to you that a reprioritization is long overdue? See starter books in chapter 10.

## Total Load

I have attempted in this book to make something concise and user friendly, and to capitalize on the old 80/20 rule. For after over 30 years in medicine, I know that 80% of the people will be better with only 20% of things that we have to offer. I offer those things in this book, knowing full well that a small portion of you will eventually need to cover the less common but often elusive and always important (especially if it is the trigger for your pain) causes.

There are numerous entities that I have omitted, some intentionally because of lack of efficacy, evidence, or ease of applicability. We do have scheduled (through the office) telephone consultations with myself to brain-storm about what would be your best options, tests you need, and the preferred course of action, or what might be missing from the total load, keeping you a prisoner of pain.

Other items were intentionally ignored because they allow the individual a "quick fix" without ever fixing what is really broken.  Yet some quick fix items have provided so much relief that they were mentioned.  Unfortunately, just like a drug, "quick fix" items allow the person in pain to carry on, not really making the responsible lifestyle changes, as in diet or environment, for example, to truly and permanently heal himself.

Acupuncture is an example.  Certainly it has volumes of evidence behind it, and it definitely works. But how? Science has proven that in addition to our arteries, veins, nerves and lymphatics we have yet another electrical system, the meridians. When there are blocked meridians in the body, energy is trapped and cannot flow normally.  This blocked or locked energy causes inflammation and pain. The acupuncture needle merely short-circuits the block and allows it to dissipate throughout the body, thus relieving the pain.  But did it force the individual to change his lifestyle, diet, or environment?  Did it give him any responsibility for and control over his pain?  There is no purpose in pain if somebody else has to patch us up; there is no purpose in pain if it does not teach us to fix what is broken.  There is no purpose in chronic pain if it does not force us to be increasingly responsible for our wellness.

As an example, I have a friend who excitedly told me how acupuncture had healed his severe asthma.  He could drink beer, sleep with his wife's cat on the bed, and do a myriad of things he could not do before and he needed no medications. That was fine, but it robbed him of the responsibility for and control over his health and in my view merely shifted

274

damaging energies to another spot. Indeed, the next year he had coronary bypass surgery, the next year disc surgery in his lower back, the next year neck surgery, the next year further medical problems. All a coincidence, maybe, but he still thinks that all the events, although in the same body, were unrelated and is happy to have doctors fix everything as it malfunctions.

There are copper bracelets but evidence is lacking (and I hardly think you will absorb enough copper into your super-oxide dismutase enzyme to rev up the anti-inflammatory detox capability). How does it work? We do not know. Then there are the bee stings, but how many people have access to these? I always believe that therapies or medical solutions should be accessible to everyone, as natural as possible, make sense in terms of fixing what is broken, and empower the person to maximize his terrestrial control over his body.

Additionally, there are many therapies about which I know little or nothing, and I welcome the opportunity to learn about them. And there are those that are very worthy, but I have no training in them. These include such things as electro-acupuncture by Voll with homeopathic remedies, via a machine like the Computron® or Interro®. In the hands of experienced physicians whom I have observed, they can locate harbored levels of some pesticide from 20 years ago or a latent viral infection from childhood that is interrupting the normal energy flow and creating this thing we call disease. They then use the same instrument to create a homeopathic treatment that will neutralize the effect. It definitely works, but is expensive and the operators are scattered over the country, not accessible to the masses and vary tremendously in skill. The same can be said for chelation therapy and prolotherapy and NAET.

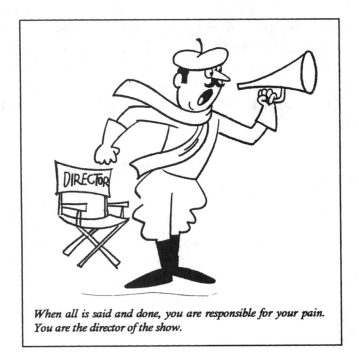

*When all is said and done, you are responsible for your pain.*
*You are the director of the show.*

For folks who know they need the total load and cannot possibly pull it off in their hometown, I recommend the Environmental Health Center in Dallas. Dr. William J. Rea, cardiovascular surgeon, author of the 4 volume textbook, *Chemical Sensitivity* (CRC Press, Boca Raton FL), and preeminent world renowned specialist in environmental medicine directs it. This is a place to get the all inclusive total load of tests mentioned here and more.

The program can include (but is not limited to) detoxification with intravenous supplementation, plus blood tests and fat biopsies to diagnose underlying nutrient deficiencies, hidden environmental poisonings and infections. Also special laser acupuncture to rescue autonomic nervous system imbalances are just a smattering of the modalities offered.  Autogenous transfer factor, and many advanced treatment modalities not available elsewhere all under one roof in one program with facilities for residing there a few weeks included.   No program is more complete for diagnosing and treating the underlying cause of pain and other conditions that have eluded medicine (see resources).

## The End or the Beginning?

After all is said and done, I believe as the natural hygienists of a century ago did, that pain is generally a toxicity of the body.  That is why fasting is so effective, diet changes, revving up the detox capability, improving the nutrient status, healing the leaky gut, purging stored toxins from the body, and reducing the environmental total load are so universally effective.  And the beauty of it all is, after you have learned to find the true underlying causes and to free yourself from pain, you have simultaneously opened yourself up to a world where you can keep yourself healthier than you ever dreamed.

## Message in a Nutshell

There is a seemingly endless array of causes and cures for pain. Knowledge is the key. *Seek and ye shall find (Matt 7).*

## Chapter 8

## The Daily Plan of Attack For
## Prisoners of Pain

### Are Your Priorities in Place?

Now that you know more about pain than you ever did before, I hope, how are you going to implement this into your already-stressed out life? You are already pressed for time for all the things you want to do, much less anything new. There is a wonderful little book on time management written years ago by Alan Lakein, *Getting Control Of Your Time And Your Life*, in which he recommended merely rating each item on a "to do list", A, B, C, or D.

If the item must be done or your life will be drastically changed for the worse (like neglecting to renew your license, forgetting your anniversary or procrastinating past the deadline for your income tax), that item is an "A". If the item is something that must be dealt with within the next week (like a business report or grocery shopping for food), this would be a "B". The "C" category was things that should be done but life will not come to a screeching halt if they are not done. Last, all the other items fall into "D" (for dreams?) and can be left undone, although you would prefer not to.

So life can be reduced to priorities. Where are yours? If you cannot promote your pain relief plan to an "A", maybe you don't hurt that much. In which case don't you dare grumble about the pain and make miserable the ones who worry about and love you. They don't deserve the added stress in their lives regarding something they have no control over (but you do!). They don't deserve this type of treatment. And if everything is an "A", you had better regroup in a hurry. Just imagine what the world would be like if you died tomorrow. Regardless of how important any one person is, sad to say the world doesn't even miss a heartbeat when they die. It keeps right on moving while a small few grieve with broken hearts. So just how important are all those A's again?

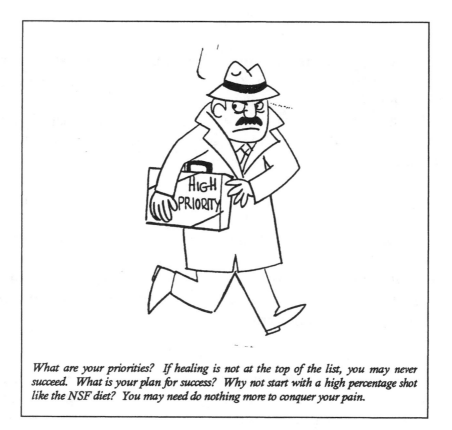

*What are your priorities? If healing is not at the top of the list, you may never succeed. What is your plan for success? Why not start with a high percentage shot like the NSF diet? You may need do nothing more to conquer your pain.*

The plethora of self-help books speaks to those hoping to find a secret, effortless, quick fix. Sadly, very few will succeed because it does take organization. But with a little concentrated effort, your years of pain can become ancient history within 3 months or less. Using our old friend the 80/20 rule, let's map out what you should do first, proceeding to the next most likely item to bring your pain under your control. Sure, you now have a lot of options, but you also have the 80/20 rule in your favor!

## Overall Plan
## Detox, Rebuild, and Protect

Before we lay out the various stages that you might need, let's look at an overall scheme. Then you can appreciate the big picture and how little of it you are going to have to do in order to become master of your pain. Fortunately most of you will not need all of the stages, and not even everything in a single stage. Basically, the approach is as easy as 1-2-3:

(1) **stop the toxicity**, and even get rid of it if you want to go one step further
(2) **rebuild the damage**, then institute an ongoing program to
(3) **protect the system** from here on to avoid future pain. This can include anti-oxidant nutrients, whole foods, and avoidance as well as continuing to detoxify future unwanted causative chemicals

**Detox:**
For some, in order to stop the toxicity that is triggering inflammation, it can be as easy as stage I, stopping the nightshades (Chapter 2); or diagnosing the cause and treating Candida and the leaky gut (Chapter 4). For others, they may need to identify one or more environmental (like natural gas or toluene or formaldehyde toxicity), nutritional and/or metabolic causes. They obviously have a much larger total

280

load triggering their symptoms. For some, avoidance is sufficient; for others, they must get rid of the underlying chemicals via the far infrared sauna (Chapter 6).

**Rebuild:**
Rebuilding can be as easy as taking 2-3 months of CM (cetyl myristoleate, Chapter 3) or Glucosamine Sulfate (or Mobil-Ease), or both (Chapter 5). Others need Lyprinol, Power Relief, and/or Rheumatol Forte (with its type II collagen and hyaluronic acid) or Arthropan; or restore cell membranes with pure phosphatidyl choline (Phos Chol), tocotrienols, EPA, IP6, TMG, MSM, and/or taurine and more; or heal the gut with UltraInflamX (Metagenics), or all of these and more.

But even before all that, be sure you have done a trial of 18% magnesium chloride solution (Pain & Stress Center), one teaspoon 4 times a day in water for 2-4 weeks. The reason? Over 50% of the population is magnesium deficient. And correcting it has totally terminated fibromyalgia, years of hip and knee pain, back pain from ruptured discs, and more. Don't overlook this simple, inexpensive and highly likely cause.

**Protect:**
Then the perennial protection involves maintaining an adequate level of protective anti-oxidants in the form of natural phytochemicals in the diet plus supplements to balance the destructive forces from the daily diet and environment that continually attempt to undermine health. Many need a steady flow of enzymes to promote digestion, dissolve sludge and keep antigen-antibody complexes at bay. This is another specific use for Wobenzyme (Pain & Stress Center), Total-Gest (Klabin, N.E.E.D.S.), Traumagesic (Tyler)

or Pancreatic Enzymes (Klaire or ARG). Or you may need to keep the gut tidy and bug-free with Kyo-Green, Kyo-Dophilus and Kyolic (Wakunaga) and Potent C (Seraphim).

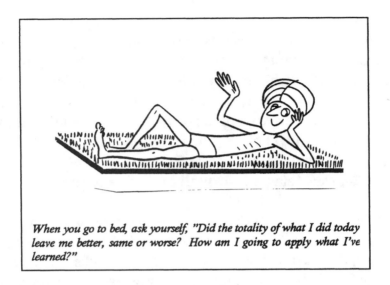

*When you go to bed, ask yourself, "Did the totality of what I did today leave me better, same or worse? How am I going to apply what I've learned?"*

For remember, the sum total of every day leaves us better, same, or worse. You want to stay ahead of the healing curve. When you finally nestle your head in your pillow you want to be able to say that the sum total for the day has left you further ahead than when you awoke. You need the positive factors to far outweigh the negative.

So with those parameters in mind, namely stopping the toxicity, rebuilding the damage, and perennially protecting, let's get under way to determine how much of this scheme you will need.

## Stage Ia
## Go Nightshade-Free

I have given you a lot of options here and some may look pretty tough. I know that you would like something very simple to get you out of pain. So let's start with Stage Ia. If you were going to do only one thing for your chronic pain, I would do the *nightshade free diet for 3 solid months*. It is the statistically most likely to provide life-long relief and the least expensive item to do. You have a good chance of having that be all that you need. Then I would go out and tie one on and have all the French fries, spaghetti sauce, green peppers, chili, cayenne, paprika, and crushed ground red peppers that you want and see what happens. But prepare yourself for 3 months of agony.

Start the nightshade-free diet. It is not easy. You must train your spouse in how to identify any nightshade sources, since it takes two to stay alert for the many ways the world has of trying to thwart your best efforts. Friends who invite you to dinner will appreciate a list to follow, and who knows, they may cure themselves of pain. Merely copy the list in the box and have a sheet ready for future hosts.

# Nightshades I Must Avoid

**Potatoes** the common potato sources include baked, mashed, scalloped, chips, fries, knishes, pierogies, plus potato water in breads, biscuits, matzo, soups and stews and vodka. Beware that potato is also included in these ingredients: hydrolyzed vegetable protein, modified vegetable protein (MVP), or modified food starch hidden in packaged meats, cold cuts and seafoods and other processed foods. Sweet potatoes are O.K. (a different family).

**Tomatoes** and their sauces (like barbecue and brown sauces), seasonings, condiments like ketchup and steak sauce, prepared meats (like meatloaf), baked beans, gravies, and salad dressings containing them.

**Peppers** include red, green, orange, yellow, jalapeno, chili, cayenne, curry, pimentos, and paprika. These are hidden in salads, cold cuts, pastas, sausage and deli meats, olives, tobasco, Worcestershire, steak sauce, coloring on nuts and fish, seasoning mixes, crackers, dips and spreads; black and white pepper are O.K.

**"Spices"** If the word "spices" or "natural flavorings" appear in the ingredients list, I cannot have it. These are hidden sources and nearly always in commercial salad dressings, mayonnaise, mustard, condiments, sauces, prepared (frozen) entrees, and soups; they could contain paprika, crushed red pepper, ground red pepper, cayenne, chili, or curry; all other specified spices are O.K.

Also avoid **eggplant** and **tobacco,** as well as soy products, since Monsanto is genetically modifying 80% of the soy with the petunia gene (a nightshade). That is no loss since the gene allows soy to be heavily sprayed with Monsanto's toxic pesticide, Round-up, and the most common form of soy is hydrogenated soybean oil which is full of damaging trans fatty acids that potentiate heart disease, cancer and more. I'm fine with olive oil, vegetables, fruits, meats, nuts, beans, wines, cheeses, grains and herbs. The purest or least adulterated form is safest.

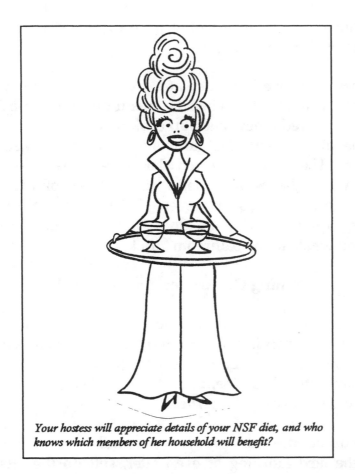

*Your hostess will appreciate details of your NSF diet, and who knows which members of her household will benefit?*

Just when you think you have it mastered, you will probably fall flat on your face as I did. Many times well-meaning friends would be especially careful to check every ingredient. Only when I felt the pain begin did we go back and double check to invariably find a hidden nightshade that they did not notice or realize was a nightshade. It is a tremendous burden for any cook. But with well over 30 million arthritics in the country, the odds are you will diagnose and cure someone else. Often you can spare them surgery for joint repair or replacement. This never would have happened if you hadn't been invited to dinner.

At other times, we had eaten at a favorite restaurant a couple of times a month, knowing the menu and recipes by heart. Then they hired a new back-up cook who was too innovative for me and spiked the garlic-olive oil with crushed red pepper. The microscopic red flakes were invisible without my reading glasses and after a glass or two of wine it just tasted more delicious than ever. But morning told the tale, unable to launch my loins alone, it was the old "carry the beached whale to the bathroom" trick.

### Turning Off An Accidental Ingestion

If you do realize you got hit with nightshades early enough, you can try to vomit it up, or if too late, start a heaping one or two teaspoons of vitamin C powder (Metabolic Maintenance or Klaire Labs Ultra Fine, Pure Ascorbic Acid Powder) every 1-3 hours until you get diarrhea.

If you do not discover your *faux pas* until the tell-tale signs of pain the next morning or even later, still do the vitamin C purge and then do the DETOX COCKTAIL (a huge 500-800 mg scoop of Recancostat powder (Tyler) or 1-2 of the 400 mg capsules and a heaping tsp. of vitamin C powder in an 8-16 oz. glass of good water) every 4 hours. Also do a detox enema every 8 hours and take 2 aspirins every four hours (to inhibit the domino effect of mediator release); do all for the first 24-36 hours. Lots of water is key, for **the solution to pollution is dilution.**

The detox cocktail accomplishes 4 goals at once. By turning off the prostaglandin cascade, revving up the detox pathway, alkalinizing the system, and speeding the gut transit time, you can often thwart the full force of the event. But I would definitely not recommend eating a nightshade intentionally while counting on this to save the day, as repeated ingestions can make future reactions stronger. Incidentally, taking aspirin for a couple of days is not going to cause leaky gut. It takes weeks or months of use to do that. And remember that detoxification includes getting other junk out of your diet; eat only healthful food while healing (*No More Heartburn* will guide you if you need further help).

### Stage Ib
### To Detox If Bed-Ridden or in Severe Pain

Begin the following regimen to start to tone down inflammation, speed up detox metabolism, turn off muscle spasm, break up antigen-antibody complexes, and improve circulation and blood supply. You can do any or all.

- If you are in severe pain and are bed-ridden, fast for 3-6 days. That means nothing but glass bottled spring water. If you need calories, use carrot, beet, celery, pear, or apple combination freshly prepared juices.
- After that go into the rare food diet described in *The E.I. Syndrome, Revised*, to identify your hidden food allergies.
- Foil your bed.
- Do the detox enema (in seated or squatting position over the toilet if pain inhibits getting on the floor).
- Begin carrot juicing every few hours as soon as you have terminated the fast. Clear vegetable broths are acceptable.

- Begin enzymes like Wobenzyme (Pain & Stress Center), Total-Gest (Klabin, N.E.E.D.S.), Bromelain 500 mg (Metabolic Maintenance) or Bromase (Bio-Tech) or Infla-Zyme (American Biologics), or Serraflazyme (Ecologic Formulas) or Pancreatic enzymes (Klaire or ARG) or Similase (Tyler) 4-8 before bed and at 2 a.m. to disassociate the immune complexes.
- Have one to two heaping teaspoons of Kyo-green (Wakunaga) in a large glass of good water, 2-8 times a day. Chlorophyll helps cleanse and heal the bowel. If the bowel is in more serious straits, use 1 scoop of UltraInflamX in water 2-3 times a day. This is also great to use if you are too weak or need to fast but need nutrients during it. If you have grain allergies you cannot use these.
- Do the DETOX COCKTAIL (400-800 mg Recancostat and a 1-2 heaping tsp. of vitamin C powder (Metabolic Maintenance, Klaire) in an 8-16 oz. Glass of water), 1-4 times a day.
- To turn off muscle spasm and down-regulate pain, start Magnesium Chloride Solution 18% (Pain & Stress Center, Ecologic Formulas or ARG; this is the best absorbed form, almost like an I.V.). Use 100 mg 4-6 times a day. Also include one 20 mg manganese picolinate (Thorne) a day, 1 Multi-plex-1 without iron (Tyler) a day, and Quercitin 500 mg (Jarrow) 1-2 capsules 2-3 times a day. Power Relief (Pain & Stress Center), 1-2 capsules 1-3 times a day kicks in the amino acids for control of the brain's pain center.

### Stage IIa
### Rebuild With CM and Magnesium

Start 2-3 CM (like CM Plus®) 2-3 times a day between meals with a digestant. For those who want a no brainer, what could be easier?  But to improve its effectiveness (and justify the cost!) it really should be combined with stages Ia and IIb; and stage IIc would give even more benefit.  Regardless, remember to strictly avoid nightshades (including tobacco), and in addition, avoid chocolate, coffee, citrus, sodas, and alcohol.  And mark your calendar for 4 months because you will probably have to remind yourself that you used to be a prisoner of pain.  Be sure to try 2-3 brands, for they all vary in formulation of this arthritis-zapping nutrient.

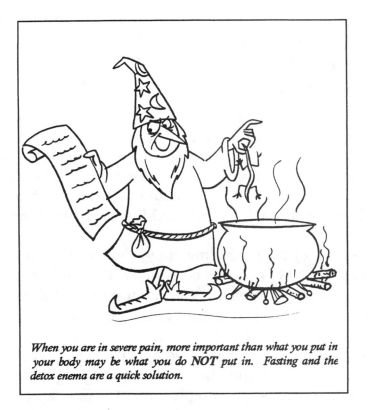

*When you are in severe pain, more important than what you put in your body may be what you do NOT put in.  Fasting and the detox enema are a quick solution.*

Clearly a vast majority will be free of pain in less than 4 months with a nightshade-free diet and CM.  But if you want an accelerated program or to increase your chances of success even more, you can look through the secondary phases (b and c) of stages I and II. Rebuilding may involve more than CM; you may need to rebuild the membrane, bone and cartilage (see II band Ic).

In the meantime time, start 1 teaspoon 4 times a day of Magnesium Chloride Solution 18% (Pain & Stress Center) for 2-4 weeks. Since over half the population is deficient (*Journal of the American Medical Association,* June 13, 1990) and its deficiency causes muscle spasm and pain, the odds are with you. I suggest you use the awful tasting liquid for 2-4 weeks. If you use better tasting capsules, it may not work. You'll think magnesium is not a factor. The solution is like an I.V. in making sure you get maximum gut absorption.

**Let me stop you right here. I know I've given you a lot of options, and that's because we are all biochemically unique. But if you want a quick fix for your pain, over 75% of folks will be out of pain with the combination of Stages Ia and IIa: Nightshade-free diet, CM and 18% magnesium. How simple could it be? If you do nothing else, do this trio.**

For phase II of the rebuilding stage, the addition of nutrients that support CM is best done along with it to improve your chances of being a success. You can use the formulations that accompany the CM products or create your own.

Because nutrients are expensive and there is a limit to what the stomach can handle, start any nutrient program in stages. Remember some people simply cannot take what others can take in a day. There is not another individual exactly like you. You may need to spread a day's worth of supplements out over two or three days. So be it. And if you come across a nutrient that you suspect does not agree with you, shelve it for a while and proceed to the next ones. You can always come back to it at a later date and retry it.

Unless otherwise stated, as in the case of CM, which should be taken between meals (or 1 hour before or after meals), most nutrients are best taken with meals when optimum digestive enzymes are at work to facilitate absorption. Examples of exceptions are nocturnal enzymes to break up antigen-antibody complexes, or Myristin® (a form of CM) taken 3 times a day 45 minutes before meals. Use your 18% Magnesium Chloride Solution any time you want, regardless of meals.

The brands are not limiting, but merely some of my trusted favorites for a variety of reasons. For example, many of the recommended companies I have known for 20 years and have come to trust their commitment to quality and respect their dedication to innovation. And they accomplished all this while maintaining an appreciation for our medical group (AAEM), which treats some of the most allergic folks from around the world. There are many look-alikes, imposters and knock-offs on the shelves, which are not worth the money and are even detrimental to health. Independent assays have even shown some do not contain what the label says, and toxic solvents are used in manufacturing. For others, like the majority of grocery-store vitamins, synthetic nutrients, like generic "vitamin E" are used which, for example, is actually detrimental and competes with natural vitamin E in foods for absorption. And in your body, synthetic vitamin E interferes with the action of real E.

The following protocols are examples of how you might group nutrients in regard to what you are trying to accomplish. They could eventually be additive, or you could have each group on a different day, or you could evaluate each group by itself for a few months. Obviously, any nutrient duplications from one group to another should not be done.

For example, if you are taking 400 mg a day of liquid magnesium for muscle spasm (from stage Ib), omit the magnesium taurate when you do glucosamine (in stage IIb), etc. You can also take select nutrients from several groups without doing the whole group. However, a multiple Multiplex-1 without iron (Tyler) to balance odd nutrients is advisable to cover the extra chemical work demanded of the body. As you see, there are more great nutrients available than a person could take. So you have to be selective after you get educated.

Stage IIb is geared toward enzyme-facilitated penetration of nutrients, reduction of muscle spasm and rebuilding bone. It would be a good accompaniment to Stage Ia (nightshade-free diet) or IIa (CM) or if osteoporosis is a problem. Stage IIc focuses on the cell membrane, energy, and liver. It would be a good accompaniment to any stage and is particularly good if chronic fatigue accompanies symptoms.

Then protective maintenance factors are relegated to stage IIIa. Some nutrients like Unique E (N.E.E.D.S.) or E-Gems Elite (Carlson), plus Tocotrienols (Carlson) and Methyl-Max (N.E.E.D.S., Tyler) should be taken everyday by everyone. But when you need to concentrate on the diet (Ia) and CM (IIa), you may not be able to handle these. Perhaps you could handle taking them once a week, however. Others like MSM or TMG depend on results of detoxification panel assays and how deficient the individual is, so they are in IIc. Once more, if you take nutrients from more than one stage, omit duplications and only take them once as indicated. Many stages over lap because the body chemistry is an orchestra that performs in concert.

## Stage IIb
### Enzyme-Facilitated Nutrient Penetration, Repair of Muscle Spasm and Bone Loss

For Stages IIa, b, and c, you could use any or all of the nutrients listed depending on the severity of your condition, stomach tolerance, and pocket book. Some need to spread out the nutrients for one day over 2 or 3 days or even over a whole week and that is fine. Anything is better than nothing and some bodies definitely heal better in a slow, gentle fashion. So don't feel anxious if you cannot do it all. You are not supposed to, but no one knows exactly what you do need. The doses given tend to be near the maximum so you have a general idea of what not to exceed.

The closest we can get to second-guess your system is what the vast majority of folks respond to. And even though measuring levels would improve precision, some of the most important nutrients do not have any levels yet. That is why a month-long trial is often the best guide.

The following stage uses enzymes, so you should do the detox enema each morning or the breakdown products can leave you unnecessarily achy.

- Glucosamine sulfate 500 mg (Enzymatic Therapy/ PhytoPharmica or Tyler), 1-2 capsules, 2-3 times a day or Mobil-Ease 1-2 capsules 2-3 times a day.
- Bovine cartilage 500 mg (Pure Encapsulations) or Mucopolysaccharide Concentrate (Cardiovascular Research), either 1-3 capsules, 2-3 times a day.

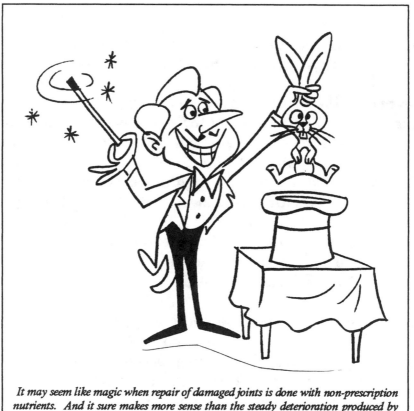

*It may seem like magic when repair of damaged joints is done with non-prescription nutrients. And it sure makes more sense than the steady deterioration produced by NSAIDs.*

- Magnesium Chloride 18% solution (Pain & Stress Center, Metabolic Maintenance, Ecologic Formulas or ARG/Nutricology), Magnesium Taurate (Ecologic

Formulas), Magnesium Glycinate (Tyler), or Magnesium Citrate 150 mg (Pure Encapsulations) at a total of 400-600 mg a day. Use any form, but remember the liquid absorbs the fastest, almost like an I.V. if you are in serious spasm.

- Wobenzyme (Pain & Stress Center), Organic Pancreatin (Klaire Labs or ARG/Nutricology), Bromelain 500 mg (Metabolic Maintenance, Jarrow or Pure Encapsulations), Bromase (Bio-Tech), Infla-Zyme (American Biologics), Serraflazyme (Ecologic Formulas), or Similase (Tyler): 4-8 before bed and at 2-4 a.m.
- MSM (Pain & Stress Center, Jarrow, Longevity Sciences, or Feidler) 500 mg, 1-4 capsules, 2-3 times a day, or Arthro Complex (Tyler).

You may need any solo nutrient from above or any combination. You can even add any of these below. For no one knows your chemistry, but these all have provided relief for many, depending on their individual needs.

- Rheumatol Forte (Ecologic Formulas) 2-6 capsules 2-4 times a day
- Lipoic acid 300 mg (Metabolic Maintenance, Ecologic Formulas, Carlson, Jarrow), 1-2 capsules 2-3 times a day.
- Osteo Complex (Tyler) or Bone-Up (Jarrow) 2-3 twice a day
- Manganese picolinate 20 mg (Thorne), 1 a day

So you have bone and cartilage builders (glucosamine, cartilage, Osteo Complex, and MSM), magnesium for muscle spasm and manganese to facilitate it, enzymes for penetration into inflamed tissues, the universal anti-oxidant lipoic acid, and collagen type II (Rheumatol Forte) to attenuate antigen-antibody complexes. But that's not all that may be needed to repair the damage. The good news is, when you repair bone, cartilage or membrane, you are repairing multiple unseen defects in blood vessels and elsewhere throughout the body. You are regenerating more than you realize.

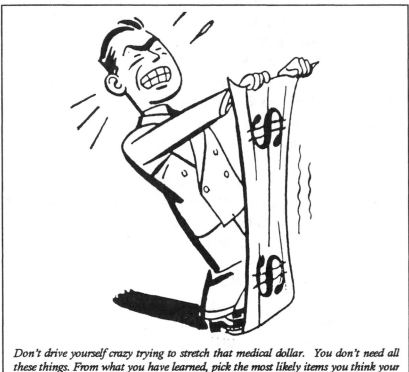

*Don't drive yourself crazy trying to stretch that medical dollar. You don't need all these things. From what you have learned, pick the most likely items you think your body needs. The rest may only apply to other folks or to you at another time.*

## Stage IIc
## Repair Cell Membranes

Don't be scared by how many nutrients it takes to repair the cell membrane for membrane repair is crucial for thorough healing and involves enormously interactive chemistry. Among the many important membranes, we'll concentrate on two: the mitochondrial membranes that direct energy syntheses, and the endoplasmic reticular membranes that direct detoxification. But what you see are some of the more important nutrients that are frequently the turning point. You can get a much more precise idea of what you need with a Detox Panel, RBC minerals and heavy metals and fatty acids analysis (MetaMetrix, Doctor's Data, Great Smokies Lab) with interpretation by a specialist in environmental medicine.

- Phos Chol Concentrate (American Lecithin), 1 tsp. a day
- Detoxification Factors (Tyler),1-2 capsules, 2-3 times a day
- Multiplex-1 without iron (Tyler), 1-2 capsules a day
- OptiQ-100 (Phillips Nutraceuticals), 1 tsp. 2-3 times a day, Q-Gel (Klabin, N.E.E.D.S.) 1-2, 2-3 times a day, or CoQ10 200 mg (Carlson) one twice a day
- Niacinol (Tyler), 1-2 capsules a day
- L-carnitine, 500 mg (Pure Encapsulations, Jarrow), 1 capsule twice a day
- Molybdenum picolinate 200 mcg (Thorne), 1-2 a day
- Selenomethionine 200 mcg (Solgar) 2 a day or Selenium Cruciferate (Ecologic Formulas) 4 a day
- Pure Cod Liver Oil (Carlson Labs) one tsp a day
- Water Oz Lithium (Water Oz) 150 mcg/tsp., 1-5 tsp. 1-6 times a day or Lithate (Bio-Tech) 5 mg one a day
- Thisilibin (BioTech) or ThistleRx (Enzymatic Therapy) 1-2 twice a day
- Calcium-D-Glucarate (Tyler) 2-4 twice a day
- IndolPlex (Tyler) 2 twice a day
- Biosil (Jarrow) 20 drops in water a day
- Coral Calcium (Premier Neutraceuticals), ¼ - ½ tsp. once or twice a day in water, or Calcium citrate/malate (Tyler) 3-6 capsules a day

- MSM 500 mg (Pain & Stress Center, Jarrrow, Klabin, Feidler)
- Ginkgo-Go (Wakunaga) one twice a day
- Lipoic acid 300 mg (Metabolic Maintenance, Ecologic Formulas, Carlson, Jarrow), 1-2 capsules 2-3 times a day.
- ThioNAC (Jarrow) 1-2 twice a day
- Cyto-Redoxin (Tyler) 1-2 twice a day
- Microhydrin 1-2 capsules 1-3 times a day (Fiedler)
- Boron (Bio-Tech) 1-2 capsules a day
- BioSil (Jarrow) 20 drops in water daily
- Sea Vive (Proper Nutrition) 2 capsules twice daily
- IP6 (Enzymatic Therapy) 2 caps 3 times a day between meals, as acid destroys it
- E-Gems Elite and Tocotrienols (Carlson), 1 or 2 a day of each

So you have, for example, pure phosphatidyl choline (Phos Chol), E, Ip6, Tocotrienols, MSM, Biosil (silicon), Cod Liver Oil, Coral Calcium and more to rebuild membranes including detox membranes. Also within this framework there are molybdenum (to boost aldehyde oxidase) and Lipoic acid, Niacinol and Microhydrin to facilitate phase I of detox, plus, silymarin and Calcium-D-Glucarate for glucuronidation of phase II of detox.

Lithium should not be underestimated, as it is a trace mineral necessary for stabilization of membranes and enhancing normal function. Yet with all these we haven't touched half of the beneficial nutrients like OPC or pycnogenol, a great anti-oxidant, or taurine (Ecologic Formulas, Pain & Stress Center) and germanium (Nutricology) two other great membrane stabilizers.

No, you cannot take them all, and certainly not in one day, nor do you need to. But these include some of the most usefully corrective nutrients which have enabled folks with diverse conditions to heal their pain.

## Stage IId
## Repair the Gut

Remember the gut houses over half the detoxification and immune systems, making it impossible to heal anything else if these are not healthy. In healing the gut, you may only need to kill the abnormal organisms, restore the good one, then repair, nourish and cleanse the gut. The following may be all; you need. If not, *No More Heartburn* will take you as far as you need to go.

- Kyolic, 2 twice a day (Wakunaga)
- Kyo-Dophilus, , 2 twice a day (Wakunaga)
- Kyo-green (Wakunaga), 1-2 tsp. in a large glass of good water 2-6 times a day
- UltraInflamX (Health Comm, Metagenics, N.E.E.D.S.) a large scoop with or in place of meals.
- Sea Vive (Proper Nutrition) 2 with meals, three times a day
- Permeability Factors (Tyler) 2 three times a day

## Stage III
## Protective Maintenance

Once you get well, you need to stay that way. Our air, food and water expose us minimum to over 500 chemicals daily, ready to thwart our health.

- Unique E (A. C. Grace or E-Gems Elite (Carlson), 1-2 capsules a day plus 2 Tocotriencols (Carlson) gives you all 8 forms of vitamin E
- Methyl-Max (Tyler), 1-2 a day or B-Compleet 100 (Carlson) one a day

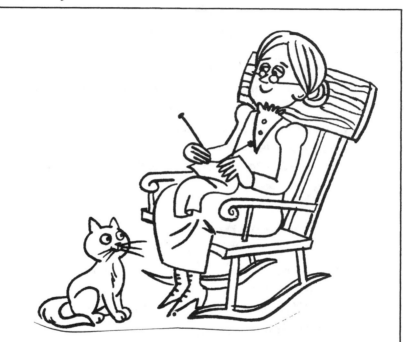

*Old Granny's adage, "A stitch in time saves nine", applies to health as well. And once you get well, it requires vigilance to stay that way. Never settle for even one symptom, for every one is an opportunity to fix what is broken before you get into worse trouble.*

- Phos Chol Concentrate (American Lecithin), 1 tsp. a day or every other day
- Multiplex-1 without iron (Tyler), 1-2 capsules a day
- Cod Liver Oil (Carlson) 1 tsp. a day or every other day or 1 tbs. twice a week
- Lipoic acid 300 mg (Metabolic Maintenance, Ecologic Formulas, Carlson, Jarrow), 1-2 capsules 2-3 times a day

- B Complete 100 (Carlson) 1 a day
- Detox cocktail 1-2 times a day (Recancostat (Tyler) 500 mg/scoop, 1 scoop, and Pure Ascorbic Acid Powder (Klaire, Metabolic Maintenance) 1 tsp in 1-2 large glasses of water
- Multiple Minerals Liquid or Chelated (Tyler, Carlson) one a day

And there are many other options that could be needed, depending on your individual chemistry, for example:

- L-carnitine, 500 mg (Pure Encapsulations, Jarrow), 1 capsule twice a day
- Quercitin 500 mg (Jarrow), or Tru-OPC 75 mg (Nature's Way) or Quercetone 200 mg (Thorne); all 1-2 capsules or tablets, 2-3 times a day
- Selenomethionine 200 mcg (Carlson) 1-2 a day
- TMG (Jarrow, Klabin/Longevity Science) 500 mg 1-2 capsules, 2-3 times a day or TMG powder (Longevity Science/Klabin)
- Silymarin as Thisilibin (BioTech) or ThistleRx (Enzymatic Therapy) 1-2 twice a day, etc.

Although this is a good maintenance, bear in mind:

- You can mix and match from other categories.
- You may not need everything each day; in fact, you may do quite well with nutrients only 2-3 times a week.
- There will be other things that you may need to add to it, for example, maybe you need 5-hydroxytryptophan, two twice a day for warding off depression, or Coenzyme Q10 for gum disease, or extra B6 for carpal tunnel, or extra

tocotrienols for high cholesterol, or hawthorn for congestive heart failure, or cesium for cancer pain.

- Be sure to give yourself a rest from nutrients every 3-6 weeks for a few days or a week, for every body is constantly changing; we are not stagnant.
- Options are to add a host of other nutrients, but they should be tailored to you. For example, you may have found that you don't have the stomach room or money to take many other nutrients because you still need glucosamine or Mobil-Ease or Lyprinol or Power Relief for a few more months until your body is more healed.
- Be sure to weed out duplications from other stages. For example, if you exceed around 600 mcg of selenium a day, it is possible for hair and nails to fall out.
- You will change with time and need rebalancing. The best is to find a physician who will measure levels. In the meantime, how you eat and how you feel are great guides. As well, too much stress or a too overloaded chemical environment will silently steal nutrients from you.

## Stage Ic
## Very Damaged or Overloaded, Needs Clean-Out

If you know you have "trashed" your body with high stress, bad diet, smoking, alcohol, and medications, you need a clean start.

1) Do the strict phase macrobiotic diet which entails following *You Are What You Ate* first, then *The Cure Is In the Kitchen*.
2) Sleep in a chemically less contaminated place. If you know someone who is chemically sensitive and has a "clean" house, you might ask if you can bring a sleeping bag over and sleep there for a couple of nights, or camp outdoors or by the

ocean. No place is perfect because air pollutants extend 30 miles out into the ocean and the woods contain molds and pollens. But being away from carpeting, natural gas, vinyl wall paper, and over-stuffed furnishings may be what your body needs in order to detox and heal. You wouldn't be the first person to discover they no longer hurt when they got out of a house with natural gas utilities. You need to find a way to discern this. Once you know you hurt less in a different environment, you have made a diagnosis that no doctor can and are on your way to healing. Read *The E.I. Syndrome* and *Tired or Toxic?* to learn more about chemical sensitivity, and how it can masquerade as chronic pain.

3) Time to get some tests if you are not better and find out what is missing. Get rbc (red blood cell) or erythrocyte minerals, heavy metals, fatty acids and vitamin panel (see MetaMetrix, Doctor's Data, Great Smokies Lab). Find out what is missing in your chemistry.

4) Do the leaky gut and CDSA tests (more described in *Depression Cured At Last!* and *No More Heartburn*), or merely begin to treat the presumed yeast and leaky gut as described in Chapter 4.

5) Get a Comprehensive Detox Panel (Great Smokies Lab) and learn why you cannot detox and heal. Go back to chapter 6 and take nutrients to repair the detox pathways. Reduce your total load to the detox system as described in *Depression Cured At Last!* and *The E.I. Syndrome, Revised.*

6) Check the status of your adrenal (stress) gland by getting an unconjugated DHEA drawn and do the magnesium loading test and the Cortrosyn stimulation test as described in *Tired or Toxic?* Salivary hormone tests are available through Great Smokies Lab.

7) Find a specialist in environmental medicine who is familiar with this total load approach who will do all of these

tests for you (Resources, next chapter). Find what heavy metal, pesticide, and chemical toxicities need to be cleared via the FIR sauna, for example.

8) Look at all of the other things in the total load that are missing as described in *Depression Cured At Last!*

9) See monthly newsletter for much more information and new findings and never give up hope.

## Stage Id
## Further Options

1) Heavy metal detox with the far infrared sauna. You may also want to add oral or intravenous chelators if heavy metals are elevated on blood tests. Mercury from dental fillings (even decades ago), paints, fish ingestion and industrial pollutants (downwind from incinerators) are common causes of chronic pain syndromes that elude all conventional diagnostic work-ups. Further diagnostic details are in *Wellness Against All Odds, Depression Cured At Last!*, and newsletters, *Total Wellness* 2000 and 2001, and *Detoxify or Die*. Remember, use the FIR sauna to get rid of pesticides, heavy metals and volatile organic hydrocarbons. For these combined with poor diet, ailing gut, and nutrient deficiencies are the backbone causes of pain.

2) Find a doctor willing to read the minocycline literature (see Resources: write the AAEM or the Arthritis Foundation for the names and addresses of physicians who already use the various antibiotic/anti-fungal/anti-protozoal medications with success).

3) Schedule a work-up with Dr. Wm. J. Rea, at the Environmental Health Center at 8345 Walnut Hill Lane, Ste. 205, Dallas TX 75231. Here people from all corners of the globe come as out-patients or in-patients for 3-6 weeks of

intensive biochemical and environmental work-ups. They are able to discern and detoxify the underlying causes, such as unsuspected levels of pesticides from decades prior or other xenobiotics (foreign chemicals) that have bioaccumulated over the years to disrupt their chemistry and promote pain.

4) Consider electro-diagnosis (Voll technique via computerized electro-dermal screening of meridians) with homeopathic and nutrient detox remedies.

5) Consider Dr. St Amand's Guaifenisen protocol.

6) Consider scheduling a phone consultation with myself to brainstorm on other diagnostic and therapeutic options.

---

### Some of the Key Features for the 3 Phases of Healing

| I – Detox | II – Rebuild | III - Protect |
|---|---|---|
| Nightshade-free diet | 18% Magnesium Chloride | Far infrared sauna |
| Treat Candida | CM | (For health maint.) |
| Treat Leaky Gut | Mobil-Ease | Phos Chol |
| Diagnosis heavy | Lyprinol | Lipoic Acid |
|   metals | Power Relief | Wobenzyme |
| Reduce exposure to | Arthropan | E-Gems Elite |
|   environmental | Boron | Tocotrienols |
|   chemicals | UltraInflamX | Multiplex-1 |
| Far infrared sauna | SeaVive |   without iron |
| Antibiotics | BioSil | Ascorbate |
| Detox Cocktail | Cod Liver Oil | Magnesium |
| Fasting or macro- | Permeability Factors | Cod Liver Oil |
|   biotic diet and | Measure RBC minerals, | Special tailored |
|   more |   fatty acids, detox |   nutrients |
| |   deficiencies, etc. | |

---

Then there are products like SeaVive (Proper Nutrition) that covers all 3 areas in the gut. It has B-glucan that helps detox by activating white blood cells (macrophages), hydrolyzed additional antibodies to protect the gut. You have many options. And there are enzymes that really function in all 3 phases to detox, rebuild and protect.

---

**Examples of Lab Tests for the Phases of Healing**

| I – Detox | II – Rebuild | III – Protect |
|---|---|---|
| • Comprehensive detox panel (GSDL) | • RBC minerals (MetaMetrix) | • ION panel (MetaMetrix) |
| • Environmental chemicals (Accu-Chem, Pacific Toxicology) | • Fatty acid (MetaMetrix) | • Cardiovascular panel (MetaMetrix) |
| • Heavy metals (MetaMetrix) | • Dysbiosis markers (MetaMetrix) | • Natural killers (Immuno-Sciences) |

---

## For the Acute or Emergent Problem

Over the years I have been forced to realize that when we hurt the most, we totally forget all we ever learned about how to get ourselves out of pain the quickest. Somehow pain seems to dull the mind. So at the risk of seeming repetitive, let's make this a section to which you and your family can refer when you most need it.

First, for days of serious sudden pain like the example of the acute attack of back pain, if it is very severe, one of the quickest ways to get out of it, if you are bed-ridden in absolute pain and no medications help, is to fast. Stop eating completely for a few days and drink only spring water in glass bottles. Do not buy water in carcinogenic, estrogen-mimicking plastic containers. Mountain Valley (1-800-643-1501) is an excellent one, and can usually be obtained at a health food store. You should add the detox cocktail to it.

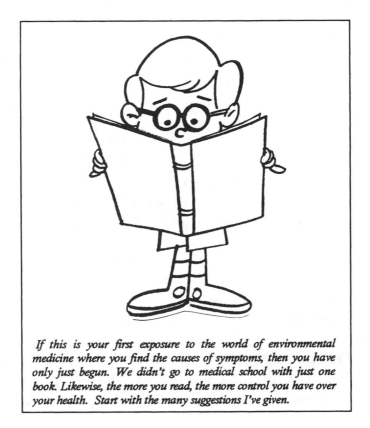

*If this is your first exposure to the world of environmental medicine where you find the causes of symptoms, then you have only just begun. We didn't go to medical school with just one book. Likewise, the more you read, the more control you have over your health. Start with the many suggestions I've given.*

Flood your system with water and drink at least 4 quarts a day, doubling that if you can. I know the big problem is getting out of bed to go to the bathroom and so for that reason you may want to cut the fluid volume down some. But the more you can drink, the faster you can flush your system out. **The solution to pollution is dilution** and the cells of inflammation escalate the pollutant load.

If you have an acute or sudden injury, you want to ice down the area and elevate it as soon and as high as possible. It should be packed in ice for 24 hours and make sure that you check periodically under the towels to see that you are not getting frostbite. Taking 2 aspirins every 4 hours during an acute injury will help to keep the amount of mediator release down so that you don't have as long a healing phase afterwards. Two days' worth is not going to cause leaky gut like chronic administration can.

During an acute pain attack, you can also do the detox enemas. Don't laugh, it may sound absolutely ludicrous, but it cuts your healing time in half, as it is a wonderfully safe and inexpensive way of detoxifying the body quicker. If you are in so much pain that you can't get down on the floor, just sit on the toilet and put the tube in the rectum and hang the bag up at ceiling level, on top of a door or on the shower head. Let 2 cups of the solution drip in, hold for the 10 minutes if you can according to the directions in the preceding chapter and then evacuate. In this way, you will not have to worry about getting down and up from the floor as is normally done with the enema. I cannot emphasize enough how much this accelerates healing and relief from pain.

I can hear in my mind's ear the thousand and one excuses for not doing it, for I have uttered them all myself and heard them from others for years. But if it had not been so highly successful, and if it did not still remain one of the mainstays for getting a pain victim out of misery quicker, I would not even mention it. It is best to start it now so that (1) you begin to lessen your pain, and (2) you are well-versed in it for emergencies.

Once you start to emerge from the severe pain, you may want to do the colon cleanse either with the Nature's Cleansing Program (Pure Body Institution, 1-800-952-PURE), or a more thorough cleanse as described in *Wellness Against All Odds*. The colon cleanse will also accelerate healing and rejuvenates the intestinal detoxification pathways. In addition, colon work is necessary not only to detoxify, but also because the effects of pain medicines, the actual pain itself, and the inactivity from being bedridden all contribute to severe constipation. This slows down healing, slows down detox and adds to your discomfort.

As you start to improve, make sure that you drink plenty of water before you go to bed so you will have to get up to go to the bathroom 2 or 3 times. Otherwise, when you awaken in the morning the lactic acid that has accumulated in the muscles that were not moving and pumping out the lactic acid waste build up will be extremely sore and stiff. This pain and stiffness upon arising in the morning can be worked out with gentle yoga stretches. Meanwhile if you are moving about several times in the night and stretching a little extra as you make your way to the bathroom, you will not only sleep better, but have less pain in the morning.

The addition of 10 minutes of gentle yoga stretches helps greatly. If your back is too sore, at least stretch your neck, arms, toes, and anything else you can or brush your body with a long-handled natural fiber body brush or loofa sponge; do anything you can do to stimulate lymphatic clean-up.

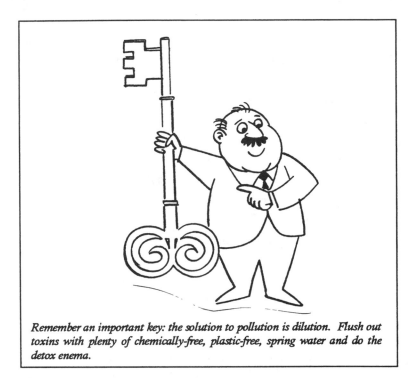

*Remember an important key: the solution to pollution is dilution. Flush out toxins with plenty of chemically-free, plastic-free, spring water and do the detox enema.*

As well, you might want to take a product that is easy to store for emergencies. Traumagesic (Tyler) contains plant enzymes to reduce inflammation and accelerate healing as well as multiple herbal components, like curcumin (more recognizable to you possibly as the Indian spice, tumeric or turmeric). The dose of Traumagesic for these items traditionally used for pain, inflammation and spasm due to traumatic injury, is 2-4 capsules every 3-5 hours on an empty stomach (Tyler). Have the capsules all counted out by the water bottle so you can take them in the dark when you awaken to urinate (turning on the light signals your pineal gland to start the day's hormone production that can cause insomnia). You could easily combine it with Power Relief (Pain & Stress), MSM, and others.

DMSO, dimethyl sulfoxide, is an old simple chemical that speeds up resolution of swelling and improves penetration of healing nutrients to the injured area. Although swelling physically protects an injury site, the swelling also physiologically isolates it. Yes, there is a place for such things as aspirin and DMSO when they are used for temporary periods of time and for acute (not chronic) relief from trauma. It is only inappropriate when they become chronically used and depended upon *in lieu* of taking responsibility for finding and rectifying the cause of chronic pain.

## A Quick Overview

**Detox**
- **Stage Ia**
  Nightshade-free diet (Chapter 2).
- **Stage Ib**
  If bedridden; water fasting or raw juicing, enzymes, Detox enema and detox cocktail, bowel cleansing, terminate spasm with magnesium, enzymes and other natural substances.
- **Stage Ic**
  Macrobiotic diet.
- **Stage Id**
  Get fatty acids, red blood cell minerals and heavy metals, and the detox pathways tested. If any bowel symptoms, test CDSA for Candida, etc. and leaky gut. Find missing parts of total load:

1. Chemical overload, like heavy metals, pesticides, volatile organic hydrocarbons, medications.
2. Food allergies, like nightshades.
3. Nutritional deficiencies, like magnesium or membrane repair.
4. Infection, either in joints like mycoplasma or in the gut as in Candida.
5. The rest of the total load, in books as described.

- **Stage Ie**
  Consider the far infrared sauna, the most logical and proven way to get rid of a lifetime of accumulated pain-producing poisons, as described in Chapter 6. Or you may need the specialty clinic, EHC of Dallas, a personalized phone consult, Minocycline or Guaifenisen protocols, etc. The sauna is the first choice as you will find a lifetime of use with it. The world will never run out of ways to poison us.

## Rebuild

- **Stage IIa**
  Cetyl myristoleate (Chapter 3) and 18% Magnesium Chloride Solution.
- **Stage IIb**
  Enzyme facilitated nutrient penetration, magnesium for reduction of muscle spasm, glucosamine, etc. for rebuilding bone (Chapter 5).
- **Stage IIc**
  Restore cell membrane: energy and detox functions.
- **Stage IId**
  Repairing the gut, kill unwanted buts (Chapter 4).

**Protect**

**Stage III**

Protective maintenance (keeping well once you get there is a delicate dance, since you are constantly exposed, reacting, repairing, eating, detoxifying, adapting and changing). A clean diet, environment and lifestyle are further protected by lifelong periodic use of the age-retarding far infrared sauna.

## Special Pain Situations:

### The Pain of Terminal Cancer

No pain is scarier than that of terminal cancer. And you will be as amazed as I was to discover that researchers have shown that it can be terminated in some cases in less than one day, in fact within a matter of hours with a simple over-the-counter mineral. This is in spite of these cases being resistant to morphine and other standard narcotic treatments. And even more excitingly, persistent use of this common mineral has been part of a program where inoperable or metastatic end-stage tumors have even shrunk and totally disappeared.

Cesium (pronounced seez' e um), is the non-toxic mineral, that in some folks has stopped cancer pain within 12-24 hours in many cases. And when combined with other minerals and vitamins, all non-prescription, it has caused complete disappearance of tumors within 3 months to two years in some cases (again, it depends on each person's total load and individual biochemistry).

Why haven't we heard of it? The same reason the media does not feature the stories of folks with end-stage cancer who have totally healed themselves of all cancer and metastases with diet and other non-prescription treatments. There is no money in it and more importantly it does not deify and empower those who want total control over your pain and health.

Normal cells get transformed into cancer cells via the combination of (1) environmental chemicals that generate free radicals and (2) nutrient deficiencies from a poor diet. Even government studies show that **95% of cancer is caused by diet and environment.** The free radicals in turn damage genetics and other regulatory mechanisms and membranes. With damaged cell membranes, as one example, oxygen can no longer readily enter the cancer cell, but glucose or sugar can. In fact, sugar is like fertilizer for cancer cells.

To better understand how cesium works, let's look briefly at the inside of a cancer cell and see what else makes it different from normal cells. Normal healthy cells live, breath and make energy via a process called aerobic (with oxygen) metabolism. They rely on oxygen. The cancer cell does not rely heavily on this process, having switched its chemistry to a fermentative process using much less oxygen, but lots of sugar (anaerobic). Now you can see why taking a box of candy to a cancer patient is like pouring gasoline on a fire. Sugar and alcohol are like fertilizer for cancer.

The cancer cell has literally become like a yeast cell. This adaptation to a metabolism of intracellular fermentation makes the internal cell very acidic (low pH). In turn, this acidity in the inside of the cancer cell further damages regulatory proteins. The loss of growth regulation results in unrestricted growth which is characteristic of metastatic tumors and pain. For an acidic internal cell environment

314

flames the fires of cancer, making it grow even more viciously.

This switch to anaerobic (without oxygen) yeast-like metabolism of cancer cells was discovered to predominate in cancer cells as early as 1925 by Nobel Prize laureate, Dr. Otto Warburg. The process snowballs as the pH drops and the cell gets even more acidic from poor diet, sugars, and environmental chemicals. As the pH goes lower (more acidic), more control mechanisms are damaged, and more metastases (spread) are triggered. If that were not enough, toxins from dead cancer cells not only poison the host, but also are powerful carcinogens by themselves and trigger further cell growth and spread.

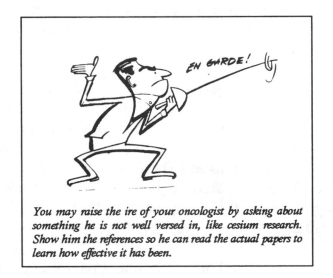

*You may raise the ire of your oncologist by asking about something he is not well versed in, like cesium research. Show him the references so he can read the actual papers to learn how effective it has been.*

There are many more differences in cancer cells versus normal. Cancer cells have only about one percent of the calcium in them as compared with normal cells. But it is calcium that helps transport oxygen into cells as well as alkalinize them or make them less acidic. The Coral Calcium in stage IIc is particularly suited to correcting this calcium deficiency.

The cancer cell (but not normal cells) easily and readily takes up cesium, a natural mineral, via potassium channels in cell membranes. It is attracted to very acidic cells but not normal, alkaline cells. Once cesium is inside the cancer cell, the pH rises from acid to alkaline, gradually killing off the cancer cell and shrinking the tumor mass. The normal pH of a cancer cell is 6.5, while a normal cell is 7.4. As soon as the pH of a cancer cell reaches 7.0, it stops growing; a little higher and it starts dying. For those doing this therapy, be absolutely sure to follow the precise detox enema protocol in *Wellness Against All Odds*, or the toxicity from dying cells can overwhelm the host and kill him, even though the tumor is shrinking.

In one study of 50 patients treated over a 3 year period with cesium chloride, the majority of patients were end-stage and unresponsive to all that medicine can offer. Regardless of cancer type (breast, colon, prostate, pancreas, lung, liver, lymphoma, sarcoma, unknown primary, etc.), there was over a 50% recovery. A constant finding was disappearance of pain within 3 days of starting cesium. Within days many tumors began visibly shrinking, ascites (fluid in the abdomen) and liver enlargements also improved.

In another study with 30 humans, cancer pain was gone in 12-36 hours, and tumor masses shrank. In most studies the effectiveness of cesium was improved by combining it with a macrobiotic diet (*The Cure Is In The Kitchen* gives the ultimate detailed directions, but start with *You Are What You Ate* for optimum orientation). Also important is to include nutrients that are also known to improve cancer survival, like at least 4-30 gm (one gm or gram of vitamin C equals 1,000 mg or milligrams) of vitamin C a day, plus high doses of vitamin A (use Cod Liver Oil, by Carlson, the only lab that could send me an independent laboratory assay to show their oil was not contaminated with mercury) and minerals like zinc, selenium, etc.

But the treatment of recalcitrant cancer is not the subject here and is covered progressively more in our other publications. For our purposes here, cancer pain can be improved dramatically. I would suggest anyone with terminal cancer pain should take this harmless and non-toxic dose (and if serious about trying to beat the cancer, have a phone consult to catch up with the current status of complementary therapies that have improved the survival odds. The aggressiveness, tenacity and resourcefulness of the individual appears to be a major determinant of the cancer patient's success over the disease. Clearly it is not for those who adopt a passive attitude toward their health, leaving it all up to the doctor.

The dose for cesium 500 mg (available from Bio-Tech or N.E.E.D.S.) is two grams (four 500 mg capsules) three times a day, however in the beginning start with 500-1000 mg every 3 hours to acclimate. The only side effects are nausea and diarrhea, or a transient tingling sensation, all dose related and unusual.

317

## Neuropathic Pain, Migraines, Tic Doloreux, Raynaud's, TMJ, Sympathetic Reflex Dystrophy, Trigeminal Neuralgia, Cluster Headaches, Shingles, Temporal Arteritis, Lupus, Gout, etc.

Aside from cancer, we have concentrated mainly on musculo-skeletal pains. But let's not neglect our friends with severe headaches, migraines, cluster headaches, vascular spasms masquerading as Raynaud's phenomenon, severe facial pain syndromes like tic doloreux, trigeminal neuralgia, temporal arteritis or sympathetic reflex dystrophy and jaw pain like TMJ (temporal-mandibular joint pain). And diabetes (diabetic neuropathy), amputations (including mastectomy) with phantom limb pain, even cancer drugs, and herpes zoster can cause excruciating torture, as well.

Those victims have **total load problems** and would be best advised to start with *The E.I. Syndrome, Revised,* then *Tired Or Toxic?,* then *Depression Cured At Last!.* For if I recall the last 100 people who presented with migraines, neuropathies, and vasculitis who got themselves well, no two people had the exact same set of causes for their pain. But their causes did fall into similar categories.

For example, most had hidden mold allergies, food intolerances and chemical sensitivities as well as undiagnosed nutrient deficiencies, magnesium and essential fatty acid deficiencies leading the list. Some also had leaky gut or Candida overgrowth in the gut, or hormone deficiencies. And all had harbored levels of pesticides, volatile organic hydrocarbons, and/or heavy metals. Fortunately most people only need to address a few of the causes to bring about relief. They don't have to get rid of all the causes. The work-up that

318

then takes you through all these is detailed in *Depression Cured At Last!* followed by *Detoxify or Die*.

As an example, I don't recall ever seeing a tough migraine patient who didn't have food and mold sensitivities as well as fatty acid and mineral deficiencies. Common accompaniments include harbored pesticides and other household chemicals like natural gas, cleansers, auto exhaust and other products of combustion, phthalates, toluene, and xylene from plastics and formaldehyde added to the total load. And don't forget stress!

One man's ten years of headaches cleared when we found and corrected mold allergies and a copper deficiency. Lots of migraine sufferers have found they can abort an attack with the detox cocktail, detox enema, and 2-4 teaspoons of 18% Magnesium Chloride Solution over an hour. Likewise, most folks with the painful blanched fingers of Raynaud's phenomenon have resistant magnesium deficiencies that require membrane repair with Phos Chol, EPA (cod liver oil), and other nutrients before magnesium repletion can take hold and turn off a lifetime of symptoms overnight.

"Why so many books to read?!?", you ask in exasperation. Because the world of conventional medicine uses mainly drugs and surgery. It does not stress finding the cause, nor does it stress empowering the patient with enough knowledge to diagnose the causes and heal himself. You can't learn a whole specialty or go to medical school in one book.

In actuality those who read the most and do the most on their own (after proper instruction) in conjunction with an environmentally and nutritionally-trained physician, often learn how to identify the causes and heal themselves. It is that simple. The answers are there for those willing to do their share. You cannot go to medical school in one book, much less learn a whole new 21st century mode of healing. And some people are just too plain sick to heal any other way. Yet it is the lack of understanding of all this that is the prime reason why many will never get better. They continually search for one simple quick fix, preferably in pill form, and it doesn't exist.

Sometimes those with migraine, tic doloreux or TMJ get lucky and with merely the environmental controls and diagnostic diet described in *The E.I. Syndrome, Revised* they get themselves significantly better. This energizes them to proceed to identify further causes. For example, some people have completely gotten rid of TMJ by identifying their hidden food allergies (*The E.I. Syndrome, Revised*) or by doing the magnesium loading test (*Tired or Toxic?*) or just correcting a magnesium deficiency. Suffice to say, if the musculo-skeletal suggestions in this book are not enough, do not give up, for you have barely begun to put yourself through medical school, enabling you to learn all the other possible causes.

And when all else fails, the macrobiotic diet (start with *You Are What You Ate* then proceed to *The Cure Is In The Kitchen*), the far infrared sauna program (Chapter 6), attention to environmental controls (*The E.I. Syndrome*) and correction of assayed nutrient deficiencies has been the key to healing the impossible.

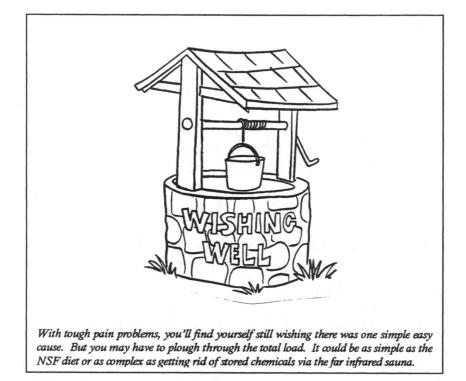

*With tough pain problems, you'll find yourself still wishing there was one simple easy cause. But you may have to plough through the total load. It could be as simple as the NSF diet or as complex as getting rid of stored chemicals via the far infrared sauna.*

For example, most diseases have an auto-immune component. Auto-immune type diseases or vasculitis-type diseases where the body painfully attacks its own tissues, including the blood vessels and joints themselves, are exemplified by lupus (systemic lupus erythematosis).  I have seen many end the misery of this "incurable" steroid-dependent disease with merely healing the leaky gut and doing the macrobiotic diet. Others needed to explore much more of the total load. For gout, sometimes a simple diet change can end the misery, whereas for others there are other biochemical glitches that need to be diagnosed and corrected, like a molybdenum deficiency since it runs the enzyme xanthine oxidase, important in purine metabolism.   Suffice to say, there is a cause and cure for everything. It is only drug-oriented medicine that treats all disease as a dead-end deficiency of pharmaceuticals.

But never neglect the basics. For any of these conditions, first do an 18% Magnesium Chloride Solution trial, one tsp 4 times a day in water for 2-4 weeks. Since the deficiency is extremely common and can mimic any pain, what do you have to lose with an inexpensive trial?

## Chest Pain

Medicine, true to form, even carves up hearts that do not respond to drugs. For years by-pass surgery has supplied new vessels, even when studies show that they will re-stenose (reclot or close up again) within 6 months to 5 years. Dr. Dean Ornish, however, has shown that the macrobiotic diet can not only terminate the pain of angina, not only leave the patient medication free, but also dissolve the clot! PET scans of the heart have proven that occlusion of the coronary arteries has been reversed on the diet. No drug can do that. The preferred (macrobiotic) diet is described in *You Are What You Ate*, then follow up with *The Cure Is In the Kitchen*.

Many people have cleared coronary artery pain, including the spasm of angina, or pain of arrhythmia, congestive heart failure or cardiomyopathy by merely healing the heart. A trial of 18% Magnesium Chloride Solution leads the success list. In addition, manganese, CoQ10, carnitine, taurine, DHA and EPA deficiencies are extremely commonly-missed 100%-correctable causes. For these cases it is preferred to have blood levels of nutrients done for better precision, as described in here. These same assays and nutritional recommendations are mandatory once someone has had a heart attack or bypass surgery, as studies confirm that a hefty level of anti-oxidants dramatically slows the progression toward re-stenosis or reclotting. Taking a handful of nutrients beats having part of your heart muscle permanently fried as is commonly done now. Ablation, used for "recalcitrant arrhythmias" and congestive heart failure, is criminal when these correctable nutrient deficiency causes have not been ruled out first. Unfortunately, these correctable causes are rarely looked for. Insist on RBC minerals, heavy metals and fatty acids and an interpretation by someone knowledgeable enough to insist on them, not the person you reluctantly had to persuade.

Unfortunately this life-saving information, straight from the most prestigious journals (*New England Journal of Medicine, Journal of the American Medical Association,* etc.) is ignored. Instead drugs which are powerless and actually speed aging and deterioration, remain the mainstay. Also if you have had chest pain, you need to get safe diagnostic tests to determine how extensive your disease is. The standard test, coronary angiography, includes the injection of a dye, from which you can die. But the **ultra fast heart scan** (you may have to drive to a bigger city) involves no injection. In fact the whole test is done within less than 10 minutes with all your clothes on. And since it can show if you have even the tiniest bit of calcification or clot forming in any of your coronary arteries, it is a wonderful crystal ball test for those who have not yet experienced any pain.

Once a person has chest pain, he can progress to congestive heart failure as more of the heart is damaged. But for the management of congestive heart failure that was resistant to drugs, medicine has mandated that up to a third of the heart be cut out and thrown away in order to reduce the load!  They are paring down what should have been repaired and built up.  Thousands have gotten out of CHF (congestive heart failure) and off drugs by remedying their deficiencies of nutrients, including carnitine, coenzyme Q10, taurine, magnesium, manganese, selenium, phosphatidyl choline, DHA, EPA, and much more.  In fact, many scientific studies show that carnitine, taurine, or coenzyme Q10 have reversed CHF in sufferers when physicians thought they were on their last legs, and when over a dozen medications had failed.  As well, in Mayo Clinic studies, the far infrared sauna has not only been well-tolerated by CHF patients (who could never tolerate regular saunas), but has enabled them to drop medicines and symptoms.

Ironically, the leading class of cholesterol-lowering drugs (called statins, like Mevocor® and Pravochol®) actually inhibits the body's ability to make life-sustaining and cardiac-sustaining coenzyme Q10.  Thus as with a cholesterol-lowering drug, you hurry the decline of the body and push it faster toward disease, pain and death.  And at the same time most cardiologists turn your care over to a hospital-based nutritionist who recommends plastic processed "low cholesterol" foods, like fake eggs, margarines, artificial creamers, grocery store corn oils and other "polyunsaturated" oils.  These are all high in hydrogenated soybean oil and other sources of trans fatty acids that actually promote arteriosclerosis and earlier heart death.  But due to the politics of medicine, the decades old and even current scientific findings are conveniently shelved.

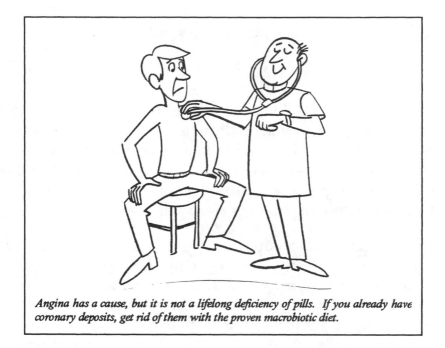

*Angina has a cause, but it is not a lifelong deficiency of pills. If you already have coronary deposits, get rid of them with the proven macrobiotic diet.*

Chest pain, one of the most serious of pains, is curable, if you have a doctor who knows how to look for the causes. Drugs are great for buying time, but nothing takes the place of detoxifying the cause and rebuilding the damage. As you can see from the very abbreviated presentation of evidence (see references), I would heartily suggest you quiz any prospective cardiologist on the use of the preceding cardiac nutrients. Ask him what their place is in cardiac disease and if he tests for them and prescribes them. For if the answers are wrong, you would be best advised to fire him on the spot. Medicine relies on drugs and attempts to bluff in order to cover up for ignorance of the scientific literature. It is one thing for a drug-oriented physician to be ignorant when it comes to your suffering from pain. It is even more inexcusable and mandatory that you take control when the source of pain is cardiac and has the potential to kill you.

## Acute Injuries

When you have a bad injury like road burns, lacerations, skin grafts, and loss of skin as through burns, there is a neat covering that accelerates healing, decreases the need for antibiotics and lowers pain. How does it work? Developed by orthopedic surgeon and trauma specialist, A. Bart Flick, M.D., it is a nylon dressing impregnated with silver.

Because silver is conductive, regenerative, analgesic and antimicrobial as well as hypoallergenic, it speeds healing while reducing scarring and need for antibiotics and pain medications. Silver has long been known to be one of nature's most universal antibiotics. As well, because of its conductive properties, it changes the electrical potential of injured tissue to a less negative surface potential, thereby allowing for less pain and faster repair of tissues. You might want to order some **Silverlon** (by Argentum, see Resources in chapter 9) to have on hand for emergencies.

## Gulf War Syndrome

By now you realize that anything as multi-factorial in symptomatology as gulf war syndrome is merely a total load problem. The key is to find as many causes as possible and then decide which ones are easier to correct. Each person carries an individual body burden of toxicities that must be dealt with and unloaded before healing of the body can take place. These folks with the wide variety of symptoms of gulf war syndrome have very damaged and overloaded detoxification pathways which is why they stump medicine, which is focused on finding a solo drug as an answer. Clearly the last thing you want to give someone with extensive damage to his or her detox pathways is another chemical to detoxify.

Although not the major symptom, joint, muscle, body pain, and headache are part of the gulf war syndrome for most victims. Often it is a bizarre total body burning or intense burning limited to one area like the face or an ear. Pain, wherever it is, is a major clue that toxic burdens of undetoxified pesticides and/or a myriad of hydrocarbon-based chemicals have been stored, and the body's ability to get rid of them has been exhausted. Long before the body can dump these, there has to be a concentrated and in-depth assay and correction of deficiencies in the detoxification pathways. A big mistake I see is when folks jump right in to detoxifying without first repairing the detox pathways. This makes them dangerously worse, for they are unprepared to handle the surge of chemicals that are pulled out of "safe" storage.

One of the aspects of this disease that is so frustrating is that it has horrendous political, social and legal ramifications that are paralyzing efforts to get on with its recognition and the medical cure. Suffice to say, with a total load this serious, you first need to find a physician who will measure all your detox capabilities and get them to maximum function before trying to unload your stored chemicals. Then assay what unwanted chemicals are on board and get rid of them. Otherwise, you can get much worse. And some may be lucky and not need a total environmental medicine work-up to get well. They may, for example, respond to the antibiotic treatment (described earlier) by Dr. Garth Nicholson.

## Colitis, Endometriosis, PMS,
## Cystitis, Prostatitis, etc.

In this era, we have more "-itises" and support groups for every one, than ever before. And they will keep growing as long as the focus is on naming or labeling the pain, and not on finding the cause. I have seen hundreds of these cases respond to total load reduction. Some people merely do the macrobiotic diet for a while in order to heal. It all depends on the individual. The bottom line is never give up.

If you truly want to get well, are willing to read and experiment, and do not expect someone else to do it all for you, chances are you will find the causes and the cures. For example, sometimes the cause of recurrent prostatitis or cystitis has been as simple as getting rid of a gut full of yeast, a few mold and food allergies and nutrient deficiencies. Unfortunately, medicine does not consider any of these but instead endless bouts of drugs and surgery on most patients.

For colitis, if you do not improve with the gut work outlined here, you need in depth work as described in *No More Heartburn*. And for endometriosis, try to avoid the drugs like Lupron, whose effect is really like a chemical castration. The strict macrobiotic diet (*The Cure Is In the Kitchen*) has totally healed many victims of this severely painful problem and they never needed to succumb to the threat of surgery. Many cases were triggered by food allergy combined with accumulated pesticides and other environmental chemicals like dioxins that were preferentially taken up in the uterus. That is why assay and correction of nutrient deficiencies, the far infrared sauna, and a macrobiotic diet, for example, have saved many from an unnecessary total hysterectomy.

The same goes for PMS, cystitis and prostatitis. So many, for example, have been affected in part, large or small, by Candida overload. Most have nutrient deficiencies, mold sensitivity and chemical overload as well. Often the chemical is the plasticizers or phthalates that cause the hormone receptors to malfunction.

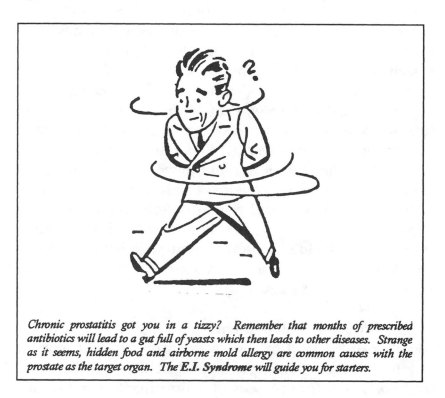

Chronic prostatitis got you in a tizzy? Remember that months of prescribed antibiotics will lead to a gut full of yeasts which then leads to other diseases. Strange as it seems, hidden food and airborne mold allergy are common causes with the prostate as the target organ. The E.I. Syndrome will guide you for starters.

## Diabetic Neuropathy

One of the nastiest forms of pain is from the dying-back of nerves in the extremities (fingers and especially toes) of diabetics. As nerve deterioration goes hand in hand with arterial deterioration, amputations have to be performed on infected gangrenous toes and even legs.

329

The diabetic needs a whole range of metabolic interventions such as special forms of vitamin E with all 4 tocopherols and tocotrienols (see Protective Stage III), phosphatidyl choline (Phos Chol), omega-3 fatty acids of EPA and DHA (cod liver oil), lipoic acid, IP6, and much more.

Since an entire book would need to be devoted to the diabetic's needs, let's look at one nutrient that has made a dramatic improvement in diabetics, hepatitis and other recalcitrant conditions, lipoic or thioctic acid. With Lipoic Acid 300 mg capsules (Metabolic Maintenance, Ecologic Formulas, Carlson, Jarrow, Pain & Stress Center) taken as 1-2 capsules 3 times a day, there has been reduction of pain within less than three weeks. Obviously, it should be taken for the life of the diabetic as it minimizes the adverse effects of sugar in a variety of ways. For example, it can also slow down cataract development and retinal deterioration that can lead to blindness. In fact because lipoic acid is one of the most universal anti-oxidants and a natural substance the body makes, it is one of those nutrients that should be taken by everyone daily and forever.

Another potent anti-oxidant that deserves mention is Microhydrin. I tend to shy away from pyramid marketing, mainly because in attempts to protect their patents they do not produce sufficient scientific documentation to support their claims. But the changes I have witnessed in folks, anecdotal as it may be, merit its mention here. A 1-3 month trial of 1-2 Microhydrin (Fiedler) taken 1-3 times a day is indicated if your condition needs more improvement.

Another nutrient, l-acetyl carnitine is made by the body just as is lipoic acid, and available also as a supplement. Some of its many functions include increasing acetylcholine, the nerve transmitter, as well as improving fatty acid metabolism, another defect especially prominent in diabetics. Consequently, it has been one of many nutrients that if used in concert, actually improves diabetic neuropathy. In my book, it is criminal not to prescribe these nutrients proven to help diabetics. As well, since diabetes is a perfect prototype of accelerated aging and arteriosclerosis, extra nutrients are needed, beyond prevention of its horrible consequences. Not only are additional nutrients needed for getting rid of stored toxins, but for correcting other nutrient deficiencies that are especially common in diabetes, like chromium, vanadium, and tocotrienols. These are all needed to down-regulate pain, especially once the disease has snowballed.

For folks with this type of serious pain, I would suggest a personalized phone consult and at least read *Depression Cured At Last!*, plus the newsletter, *Total Wellness*, which explores new issues continually.

### The Teleologic Reason for Pain

Last of all, I think God not only provides us with injury and illness so that we can learn how to heal ourselves, but He also gives injury at a time when we desperately need (and may be too stubborn to recognize it) a change of pace. Injury with immobilization is a perfect opportunity to slow down the pace, connect with God, and to assess whether our priorities are too entwined with the material world, and drifting away from our spiritual roots. Pain is a time to read, reflect, and appreciate how much our friends really care about us, and to be more sensitive to the pain of others, seen or not.

For everyone carries some unseen pain (physical or mental) which we all have a unique potential for lessening; if we choose to take the time to raise our sensitivity and caring level. Perhaps our pain is a message that we need to stop and pay more attention to a loved one, or to someone who is not loved enough. Or is it a signal that we are winding ourselves up faster every day with no end in sight? With the ever-escalating pace of the cyber-world, I wonder just how much faster we can all go. For some of us, I wonder if injury isn't a timely way for our minds and souls to say, "Stop the world, I need to appreciate", or "Stop the world, I need to reprioritize my life."

Whenever I have a medical problem including pain, I have learned now to look to God and ask, "What is the message this time? What am I supposed to learn?" (I also try to work in a prayer for making the message appear perhaps a little quicker this time.) For as a physician for 30 years, I have found that no illness, trauma, or pain was ever given to me without my benefiting from it. Sure I was on the pity-pot for years when I thought my life was over. I was racked in pain and drugged to the gills everyday. Now as I look back, it was one of the luckiest things that ever happened to me. It taught me how to get control over pain for myself and how to give that control to my patients and to you.

For example, I haven't mentioned half of my injuries. Just my neck alone has had untold trauma. I totaled 5 cars, rolled a truck upside down in a ditch (never had a seat belt on for any of these and walked away from them all), was flattened by a T-bar when it struck my head at a ski lodge, split my forehead open when I was distracted from a shallow dive that ended up being a deep dive into a shallow pool, fell onto my neck from a terrified run-away horse when the saddle cinch broke, landed on my neck again when a horse I was galloping down a hillside pavement tripped and threw us both on our necks. Yet with all this, I did not end up like Christopher Reeves.

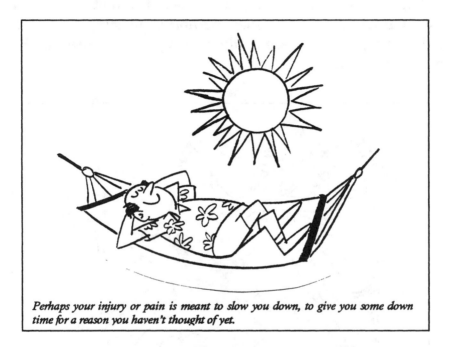

*Perhaps your injury or pain is meant to slow you down, to give you some down time for a reason you haven't thought of yet.*

That is what fuels me to share, as "Each one should use whatever gift he has received to serve others," (1PE4). And as I unearth these truths that empower people, as well as enabling them to obtain wellness, I am constantly reminded of how simple much of this is. "But God chose the foolish things of this world to shame the wise; God chose the weak things of this world to shame the strong. He chose the lowly things ..." (1COR1). I am convinced "that in all things God works for the good of those who love Him, who have been called according to His purpose." (RO8)

When we have pain, I often think that it is one of God's ways of slowing us down so that we will stop, smell the roses, perhaps reassess our journey and take a different path. It's a time that we can use for reflecting and connecting with God, and finding out if we are really serving the purpose that He intended us for.

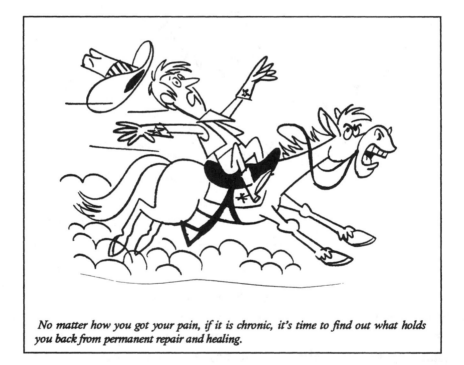

*No matter how you got your pain, if it is chronic, it's time to find out what holds you back from permanent repair and healing.*

Become a funnel or mirror of God's love. Set your goal to glorify his name in your small way. Bring as much love and comfort to others as possible and you will see it magnified many fold when you least expect it for yourself.

A major part of our toxic load is the mental toxic load, which can most effectively be corrected by connecting with God. Harbored anger, jealousy, guilt, fear, rage, hate, resentment and more all impede healing. Only forgiveness and love can put an end to them, most effectively when you surrender to your highest power and allow Him to make you a vehicle for his love. If you have no spirituality at all, perhaps your pain is meant or intended to keep you down until you take time to connect with God.

"Seek and ye shall find, knock and the door will be opened to you." For "Small is the gate and narrow the way that leads to life, and only a few find it." (MAT 7)

If you are down with pain and looking for a book to ease your boredom, perhaps this just might be the time for a major spiritual awakening. The books below reflect my personal bias, but don't let that dissuade you from exploring and following your own calling. Call a relative or friend whose spiritual convictions you admire to loan you some books or start with some that I have recommended below.

**Teleologic references:**
You may find it most helpful, regardless of your beliefs, to actually start to learn how to read and interpret *The Holy Bible*. For this I heartily recommend:

Stedman RC, *Adventuring Through the Bible. A Comprehensive Guide to the Entire Bible,* Discovery House Publishers, Box 3566, Grand Rapids MI 49501, 1997 (1-800-653-8333)

After that you may want to start with the simplest translation of the Bible, *The New Living Bible*, before you progress to understand the King James Version. Or better yet you could follow along with a side-by-side translation of several biblical forms in a concordance. For these I recommend *The Comparative Study Bible. A Parallel Bible presenting the New International Version, New American Standard Bible, Amplified Bible and King James Version,* Zondervan Publishing House, 1984, Grand Rapids MI 49506

If you just cannot get into this, you may enjoy a humorous, down-home and light-hearted approach of Bill Gillham in *What God Wishes Every Christian Knew About Christianity* (Harvest House Publ., Eugene Oregon 97402).

As well, a formerly agnostic scientist with a Christian wife had a miraculous healing of his cancer. After that he decided that as a scientist, he ought to be able to prove whether Jesus really existed as well as the many other miracles of the Bible. Robert W. Faid ended up writing, *The Scientific Approach to Christianity* (New leaf Press, PO Box 311, Green Forest AR 72638).

When he found folks who couldn't believe the miracles of the Bible, he explained how they occurred and documented their happening in *The Scientific Approach to Biblical Mysteries*, available through guideposts.com.

Another cancer-conqueror, Revered George Malkmus wrote *Why Christians Get Sick* to show folks how to heal with the live food diet (Destiny Image Publ., PO Box 310, Shippensburg PA 17257-0310, 1-800-722-6774).

## KISS Theory: Keep It Simple, Sherry

In keeping with my modus operandi, this to me houses a plethora of proven ways that have freed prisoners of pain. If it appears overwhelming to you, bear in mind that this is cause for rejoicing, for there are an infinite number of ways to get well.

The smart thing to do is explore what has helped the greatest number of people first. So you do the (1) nightshade-free diet, then (2) a trail of CM, next (3) check for Candida and the leaky gut, followed by (4) magnesium and other nutrient deficiencies, and (5) dental and other toxicities.

If clearing hidden infection doesn't bring relief, then you know you need a total load package.

## Just the Beginning

You now get the picture that chronic pain has many curable causes. I could have made this book 4 times its size if I had expanded on all the modalities. Many of you have already failed numerous pain and anti-inflammatory drugs, exercises, braces, manipulations, biofeedback, acupuncture, DMSO, anti-depressants, surgeries, and more in attempts to quell your pain. For in the end, a successful therapy should pinpoint the cause and be permanent.

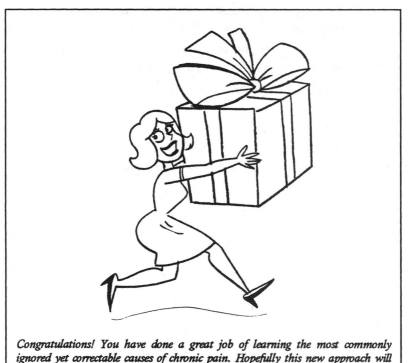

*Congratulations! You have done a great job of learning the most commonly ignored yet correctable causes of chronic pain. Hopefully this new approach will guide you in all your medical decisions.*

There are many other therapies, some of which have great merit, but I have tried to limit this to the entities that will help the greatest number of people and leave the more unique or complicated aspects for our subsequent books, consultations, and newsletters. For dramatic as their results can be, they are not in general the heavy hitters, meaning the therapies that help the greatest number of people. However, if they turn off your pain, they are 100% important to you.

Hopefully this book will keep you from exploring permanent nerve severance or nerve poisoning with toxic injections as performed in many medical school pain clinics as a spin-off of their anesthesia departments. And it goes without saying I would also hope you never experience the carcinogenic chemotherapy drugs increasingly prescribed for many auto-immune pain syndromes like rheumatoid arthritis.

Truly there never was a better time to be in pain. For there are more correctable causes than ever before to prove to you that you have absolute **power over your pain.**

# Chapter 9

# Resources

I'll just bet you were getting pretty worried in previous chapters about where on earth you were going to find some of the wonderfully healing remedies I've taught you about. Never fear, chapter 9 is here!  It has it all.

## Sources of Non-Prescription Supplements

N.E.E.D.S. has carried everything I prescribe for over two decades, even difficult to find items and items normally only available through nutritionally trained physicians or in bulk order.

>N.E.E.D.S.
>527 Charles Ave., 12-A
>Syracuse NY 13209
>1-800-634-1380
>www.needs.com

The following pharmacies and suppliers have unique products, hard to find products and the first four make custom compounded prescriptions for special needs:

| | |
|---|---|
| Wellness Pharmacy | 1-800-227-2627 |
| College Pharmacy | 1-800-888-9358 |
| Apothecure | 1-800-969-6601 |
| Abrams Royal Pharmacy | 1-800-458-0804 |
| American Environmental Health Foundation | 1-800-428-2343 |
| Emerson Ecologics | 1-800-240-9912 |
| NutriSupplies | 1-800-388-8808 |

Sources for prescription leaky gut test solution, Nystatin pure powder for Candida, some of the nutrients listed, guaifenesin, and more:

| | |
|---|---|
| Wellness Pharmacy | 1-800-227-2627 |
| College Pharmacy | 1-800-888-9358 |
| Apothecure | 1-800-969-6601 |
| Abrams Royal Pharmacy | 1-800-458-0804 |

Source of Nystatin pure powder (Bio-Statin) for Candida:

Bio-Tech    1-800-345-1199    www.bio-tech-pharm.com

## Whole Foods Catalogues

Even if you don't live near a big city or health food store, you can get tea tree oil, stevia, quality organic whole grains and beans, nuts and other foods from these sources by mail.

Natural Lifestyle
16 Outlook Dr
Asheville NC 28804-3330
1-800-752-277
www.natural-lifestyle.com

Kushi Institute Store
P.O.Box 500
Becket MA 01223-0500
800-645-8744

Goldmine Natural Foods
3419 Hancock St.
San Diego CA 92110-4307
1-800-475-3663
www.goldminenaturalfood.com

Garden Spot
438 White Oak Road
New Holland PA 17557
1-800-829-5100
www.gardenspotsfinest.com

Premier Neutraceuticals
(Formerly) Pacific Research Labs
2000 North Mays, Ste. 120
Round Rock, TX 78664
1-800-370-3447

# Tests
## (Need to Be Ordered By a Physician)

Note that these labs have many more tests than I have mentioned that would also be of interest.

## MetaMetrix Laboratory
4855 Peachtree Ind. Blvd
Ste 201
Norcross GA 30092
1-800-221-4640
fax: 770-446-6259
www.metametrix.com

This lab has important minerals and heavy metals in their panels that other labs do not offer.

**Tests Kits:**
RBC mineral panel or
Elemental analysis on erythrocytes
    (includes chromium, calcium and
    vanadium which other labs do not do)
Heavy metal panel (includes aluminum
    which other labs do not include)
Fatty acid panel
Candida antibodies
ION (Individualized Optimum Nutrition)
    Panel (a great bargain that includes
    many panels at a considerable savings)
Organic acids
IgG4 & IgE food antibody assays
Amino acids
SMAC, and much more
Candida antibodies
Dysbiosis markers (can determine if
    Candida and other gut pathogens are
    present even if they do not show on
    stool study)

**Great Smokies
Diagnostic Laboratory**
63 Zillcoa St.
Asheville NC 28801-1074
1-800-5224762
www.GSDL.com

**Test Kits:**
7 day Candida test
CDSA (comprehensive stool and digestive analysis)
Purged parasites
Leaky gut test (intestinal permeability)
Quantitative H. pylori antibodies
Vitamin panel
RBC mineral & heavy metal panels
Fatty acid analysis
Candida antibodies
Food allergy antibodies
Amino acids

Also have non-prescription-requiring hair analysis for minerals and toxic elements.

**Doctor's Data**
P.O.Box 111
West Chicago IL 60185
1-800-323-2784
www.doctorsdata.com

Whole blood elements (minerals and heavy metals)
Amino acids
Fecal toxic elements
Comprehensive stool
Intestinal Hyperpermeability (leaky gut) test

**ImmunoSciences Lab, Inc**.
8730 Wilshire Blvd, Ste 305
Beverly Hills CA 90211
1-800-950-4686
(310)-657-1053
www.immuno-sci-lab.com

Many other tests: Specialty tests
for H pylori antibodies, Candida
anti-bodies, sensitivity to
environmental chemicals,
cancer predisposition and
metastases and more.

> Natural killer activity
> Programmed cell death
> Chemical antibodies
> (formaldehyde, silicone, etc.)
> Food antibodies/human tissue
> Candida antibodies to human
> tissue
> Cancer antibodies
> Auto-immune antibodies
> 8-OHdG (metastases)
> Tumor necrosis factor
> Hs-CRP
> H. pylori by PCR

**American Environmental
Health Foundation**
8345 Walnut Hill Lane
Dallas TX, 75231
1-800-428-2343
www.AEHM.com

> Analysis of drinking water
> Tri-Salts (the preferred form
> for sauna detox)

**Pacific Toxicology Laboratories**
Los Angeles CA
1-800-32TOXIC
310-479-4911
www.pacifictox.com

> Chlorinated and other
> pesticide panels, heavy metals,
> volatile organic hydro-carbons
> and other harbored xenobiotics
> (foreign chemicals)

**Accu-Chem Labs**
990 N. Bowser Rd.
Richardson TX 75081
1-800-451-0016
972-234-5412
www: accuchemlabs.com

> Chlorinated and other pesticide
> panels, heavy metals, volatile
> organic hydrocarbons and other
> harbored xenobiotics

## "Where Can I Find a Doctor
## Who Does This Kind of Medicine?"

I am asked this question constantly. An organization comprised of physicians who are geared more toward cause and cure medicine versus drug-driven medicine is listed below. It does not mean that every physician in the organization does all of the things you have learned here; some do more, some do less.

> American Academy of Environmental Medicine
> 7701 E Kellogg ST.
> Wichita KS 67207
> Phone: 316-684-5500
> Fax: 316-684-5709
> www.AAEM@swbell.net

If you prefer a list of physicians in your area who have actually taken and passed the board examinations for environmental medicine, send a self-addressed, stamped envelope to:

> American Board of Environmental Medicine
> 65 Wehrle Dr.
> Buffalo NY 14225

# For Chelation Physicians

American College for Advancement in Medicine
23121 Verdugo Dr., Ste 204
Laguna Hills CA 92653
949-583-7666
fax: 949-455-9679
www.acam.org

## Environmental Units

Environmental Health Center –Dallas
8345 Walnut Hill Lane, Ste 220
Dallas TX 75231
214-373-5194
www.AEHM.com

Dr. Allan Lieberman
7510 North Forest Dr.
North Charleston, SC 29420
(843) 572-1600
www.COEM.com

## Manufacturers and/or Suppliers of
## Specific Nutrient Items Referred to Here.

Some do not sell small quantities or directly to the public, but all items are available at N.E.E.D.S. Also note that each of these companies offer many more great products than I have listed here that benefit health. And because most of them are on the cutting edge, they are continually developing more innovative products to add to their often one-of-a-kind lines. Send for their catalogues.

# Cetyl Myristoleate Products

**Longevity Science/**
**Klabin Marketing**
2067 Broadway,
Ste 700
NY, NY 10023
1-800-933-9440
(212)-877-3632

**CM-Plus®** (60 mg cetyl myristoleate and cetyl oleate 125 mg, plus cetyl myristate 75 mg in a base of mixed fatty acid esters and olive oil; vegetable source, no solvents

**CM-Plus Support Formula®**
ProBoost Thymic Protein A

**Knollwood, Inc.**
2250 E. Tropicana
Ste 19-321
Las Vegas NV 89119
1-800-829-1514

**CMO®** (100% cetyl myristoleate, but no precise number of mg specified)
**CMO Support Formula®**

**Jarrow Formulas, Inc.**
1824 S Robertson Blvd
Los Angeles Ca 90035-4317
1-800-726-0886
fax: 1-800-890-8955
www.jarrow.com

**True CMO®**
cetyl myristoleate extract (fatty acid complex) 760 mg

**EHP Products, Inc.**
P.O. Box 2027
Mt. Pleasant, SC 29465
1-888-EHP-0100
fax: 1-843-881-5789
www.cetylmyristoleate.com
email: myristin@logicsouth.com

**Myristin®**
260 mg cetyl myrstoleate, 260 mg cetyl oleate, 130 mg other oleates

**Myrist-Aid®** (support formula)

346

**Integris Corporation**
Irving TX 75063
1-888-737-7307
www.integriscorp.com

| |
|---|
| **Everlasting®**<br>275 mg cetyl myristoleate complex complex<br><br>**Everlasting Support®** |

**BioVita International**
**& Preventive Measures**
P.O.Box 768
Manson WA 98831
1-800-467-7810
also
**DNA Pacifica**
148-1 No. El Camino Real
Enchinitas CA 92024-2849

| |
|---|
| **Myristin®**<br>265 mg cetyl myristoleate, 265 mg cetyl oleate, 110 mg cetyl esters |

## Far Infrared Sauna and Products

**High Tech Health**
2695 Linden Dr.
Boulder CO 80304
1-800-794-5355
303-413-8500
fax: 303-449-9640
www.hightechhealth.com

| |
|---|
| **Far Infrared Saunas:**<br>Portable, many sizes and different materials such as poplar wood for the chemically sensitive, FIR hand-held hair dryer, FIR kitchen counter top oven/cooker, FIR Pain Relief Pad, Singer Spring Alkaline Water Machine |

## Orthotics (Braces)

### Aircast Air-Stirrup Ankle Brace
Excellent function and stability, especially for ankles, do not inhibit athletic activity at all, scientific back-up, many other braces.

Aircast
P.O. Box 709
92 River Road
Summit NJ 07902-0709
1-800-526-8785
908-273-6349
fax: 1-800-457-4221
www.aircast.com

## Important Nutrients

These fine companies have catalogues that do much more justice to their many products. I've merely listed here some of the key nutrients that have been recommended, difficult to find items, unique items, and/or items of exceptional quality.

(For companies that do not sell to the public or in small quantities, N.E.E.D.S., 1-800-634-1380, carries most items)

**Tyler Encapsulations**
2204-8 NW Birdsdale
Gresham OR 97030
1-800-869-9705
or (503)-666-4913
www.tyler-inc.com

Does not sell to public
(use N.E.E.D.S.)

Lyprinol
Mobil-Ease
Glucosamine sulfate
Osteo Complex
Multiplex-1 without iron
IndolPlex
Cal-Mag-K Chela-Max
Potassium Chela-Max
Mag-K Chela-Max
Arthro Complex
Detoxification Factors
OxyPerm
Recancostat
Mercury Detox
Alcohol Detox
Buffered C Powder

**Tyler Encapsulations**
(Products continued)

Cyto-Redoxin
Betaine HCl
Calcium-D-Glucarate
Traumagesic
Buffered C Powder
Bromelain
Multiple Minerals, chelated
Magnesium Glycinate Plus
Para-Gard
Eskimo-3
Fiber Formula
Candida Complex
Enterogenic Concentrate
Permeability Factors
Similase
MethylMax
Niacinol
Poly-C

**Pain & Stress Center**
5282 Medical Dr, #160
San Antonio TX 78229
1-800-669-2256
www.psctr@stic.net

Power Relief (DLPA and
    more)
Malic Acid Plus
Mag Link:
    Calcium (112 mg)
    Magnesium (65 mg)
5-HTP (tryptophan)
Magnesium Citrate 500 mg
Wobenzyme
Lipoic Acid 300 mg
MSM
MSM Cream or Lotion
18% Magnesium Chloride
    Solution
DLPA (for pain)
Potassium Citrate
Glucosamine Sulfate

## Pain & Stress Center
(Products continued)

Chromium
Vanadium
DHEA
Taurine
Arginine
Glycine
GABA
CoQ10
NAC
Manganese Picolinate
Melatonin
Carnitine
Liquid Serotonin
Alpha Keto-Glutaric Acid
Cal Mag Zinc Complex
Boswella Plus
P-5-P, B6
L-Glutamine
Super Glutamine 100 mg
St. John's Wort
Mood Sync
Mobigesic
Mobisyl
DMSO Cream
Cal:Mag 1:1
Selenium
Magnets, books and much
more

## Prevail
2204-8 NW Birdsdale
Gresham OR 97030
1-800-248-0885
email: info@prevail.com

Lyprinol
Mobil-Ease
Advance Multi-Vitamins
  with Minerals
Para-Gard
Eskimo-3

## Wakunaga of America
23501 Madero
Mission Viejo CA  92691
1-800-825-7888
1-800-421-2998
www.kyolic.com

| |
|---|
| Kyolic<br>Kyo-Dophilus<br>Kyo-Green<br>Ginkgo-Go |

You can get free samples of Kyo-Greens, Kyolic and Kyodophilus from the above number if you mention this book.

## Carlson Laboratories
15 College Dr.
Arlington Hts, IL 60004
1-800-323-4141
1-888-234-5656
www.carlsonlabs.com
email: carlson@carlsonlabs.com

| |
|---|
| Liquid Multiple Minerals<br>   (in capsules)<br>E-Gems Elite<br>Tocotrienols<br>Cod Liver Oil (purest, most<br>   mercury-free form I have<br>   found)<br>Mild-C Crystals<br>ACES Gold<br>E-Gems 800<br>Aloe Gold<br>B Compleet 100<br>Glutathione Boosters<br>Heartbeat Elite<br>Niacinamide<br>Niacin (B3)<br>CoQ10 200<br>Potassium<br>Liquid Magnesium 400 mg<br>   (in capsule)<br>Vitamin C Crystals<br>Individual chelated minerals |

## HealthComm/Metagenics International, Inc.
P.O. Box 1729
5800 Soundview Dr.
Gig Harbor WA 98335
1-800-843-9660
www.metagenics.com
Does not sell to the public (use N.E.E.D.S.)

UltraInflamX
UltraClear
Ultra Fiber

## Longevity Science/
## Klabin Marketing
2067 Broadway,
Ste 700
NY, NY 10023
1-800-933-9440
(212)-877-3632

**CM-Plus®** 60 mg cetyl
myristoleate and cetyl oleate
125 mg, plus cetyl myristate
75mg in a base of mixed fatty
acid esters and olive oil;
vegetable source, no solvents

**CM-Plus Support Formula®**
Pro-Boost Thymic Protein A
Total–Gest (enzymes)
TMG
MSM
ImmPower

## PhytoPharmica/
## Enzymatic Therapy
825 Challenger Dr
Green Bay WI 54311
1-800-553-2370/783-2286
1-800-376-7889
(920) 469-4418
www.phytopharmica.com
Does not sell to the public
(use N.E.E.D.S.)

Glucosamine Sulfate, GS 500
IP6
Garlinase
ZymeDophilus
Fiber Plus
Candimyacin
Rhizinate (DGL)
Gastro-Relief
GingerMax
Laxatol
Bromelain Complex
Bio-Zyme
Hypericalm
ThistleRx
PCO

## Metabolic Maintenance
68994 North Pine St.
Box 3600
Sister OR 97759
1-800-772-7873
(541) 549-3299
www.metablicmaintenance.com

This company puts high quality nutrients in dark glass bottles to protect you from phthalates and protect nutrients from light-induced deterioration.

Lipoic Acid 300 mg
Spaz Out
Magnesium Citrate 500 mg
Bromelain 750 mg
Vitamin C Powder
Calcium:Magnesium Citrate
    (100:100)
Potassium Citrate
SAMe
L-Carnitine
Glycine Powder and capsules
P-5-P
EPO 500 mg
Borage Oil 1000 mg
Silymarin (see Milk Thistle)
Magnesium
Rebuild Osteoporosis
    Formula
NAC (600 mg)
D, L-Phenylalanine (750 mg)
    with B6
Taurine (500 mg)
5-HTP
Buffered Vitamin C Powder
Milk Thistle (300 mg
    Silymarin) Extract
K/Mg Aspartate (99 mg)
K/Mg Citrate (99:125 mg)
Zinc Picolinate (30 mg)

## Pure Encapsulations

5490 Boston Post Rd.
Sudbury MA 01776
1-800-753-2277
888-783-2277
www.pureencapsulations.com

Bovine Cartilage  500 mg
L-Carnitine
Bromelain
Magnesium Citrate (150 mg)
CoQ10 500 mg
Silymarin 250 mg
Curcumin 250 mg
NAC 1000
L-Carnitine
Lactobacillus sporogenes
5-HTP
Lipoic Acid

## Thorne

25820 Highway 2 West
P.O. Box 25
Dover, ID 83864
1-800-228-1966
208-263-1337
fax: 208-265-2488
e-mail: info@thorne.com
www.thorne.com

Boron
Pure Ascorbic Acid Powder
Magnesium Aspartate
Magnesium Citrate
Molybdenum Picolinate
Manganese picolinate
L-Glutamine
Biogest
Citrocidal
Herbal Laxative
Betaine HCl
M.F. Bromelain
Basic Nutrients II
Super EPA
Undecyn
Quercenase, Quercetone
Folacal
Iodine
Potassium citrate
Potassium Aspartate
P-5-P

**Thorne**
(Products continued)

Copper Aspartate
Copper Citrate
Zinc Picolinate
CoQ10
Glucosamine Sulfate
Vanoxyl
5-HTP
Non-Hydrolyzed Whey
    (poor man's glutathione)

**Premier Neutraceuticals**
**(Formerly) Pacific Research Labs**
2000 North Mays, Ste. 120
Round Rock, TX 78664
1-800-370-3447

Coral Calcium Legend
PH paper
and much more

**American Lecithin Co.**
115 Hurley Rd., Unit 2B
Oxford CT 06478
1-800-364-4416
(203)-262-7100
www.americanlecithin.com

Phos Chol Concentrate
*(purest, most concentrated form*
*of phosphatidyl choline for*
*rebuilding membranes)*
Phos Chol 900 capsules

**ARG/Nutricology/**
**Allergy Research Group**
30806 Santana St
Hayward CA 94544
1-800-545-9960
800-782-4274
www.nutricology.com
Email: info@nutricology.com

Organic Pancreas
Magnesium 18% Solution
Magnesium Citrate 170 mg
L-Glutamine Powder
MSM
CoQ10 with Tocotrienols
Grape Pips
Proanthocyanidins
ParaMicrocidin
Germanium

355

**Water Oz**
Rt 1 Box 104B
Grangeville, ID 83530
1-800-547-2294
fax: 1-800-574-1897
www.wateroz.com

> Water Oz Lithium
> Water Oz Silver
> Water Oz Minerals

**Ecologic Formulas/**
**Cardiovascular Research**
1061-B Shary Circle
Concord, CA 94518
1-800-888-4585
Email: ecologicalformulas@yahoo.com

> Rheumatol Forte (collagen II)
> Fibromyalgin
> Tri-Salts
> Serraflazyme
> Allithiamine
> Laktoferrin
> Magnesium Solution 18%
> Lipoic Acid Crystals
> Magnesium Taurate
> Selenium Cruciferate
> Kyanthanol

**Jarrow**
1824 S. Robertson Blvd
Los Angeles CA 90035
1-800-726-0886
1-800-890-8955
www.jarrow.com

> BioSil (best form of silicon)
> TRUE CMO
> Bone Up (special
> osteoporosis formula)
> Thio NAC (for detox)
> L-Carnitine
> Jarrow-Dophilus
> Flax Fiber
> Yaemama Chlorella
> Whey
> L-Glutamine
> Bromelain
> L-Arginine
> Quercitin, and much more

## Jarrow
(Products continued)

Magnesium
    Citrate + K + Taurine
MSM
TMG
SAMe
Pycnogenol
Methylcobalamin 1 mg
    sublingual (best B12)


## American Biologics
1180 Walnut Ave
Chula Vista CA, 91911
800-227-4473
www.americanbiologics.com

Infla-Zyme
Dioxychlor
DC3


## BioTech
Box 1992
Fayetteville AR 72702
1-800-345-1199
fax: 501-443-5643
www.bio-tech-pharm.com
10% discount if you mention this book.

Cesium (for cancer pain)
Boron (for arthritis)
Bromase (dissolving enzyme)
Thisilyn (silymarin for detox)
PCN-200
DNZ


## Emerson Ecologics
18 Lomar Park
Pepperell, MA 01463
800-240-9912
800-654-4432
www.mmspro.com

Thisilyn Pro (140 mg)
Efamol's Evening Primrose
Oil
(carries many nutrient
    companies)

**Environmental Health Link**
301 N. High Street
Columbus grove, OH 45830
Email: smeeker@bright.net
419-659-5541

Stevia
(herbal sweetener for
cooking that does not trigger
Candida)

**Phillips Nutritionals**
26 Commerce Center Dr.
Henderson, NV 89014
800-514-5115
www.vitamins20.com

Bromelain
OptiQ-100
Evening Primrose Oil
Garlic Supreme
and much more

**Proper Nutrition**
PO Box 13905
Reading PA 19612
1-800-247-5656/1-800-555-8868
www.propernutrition.com

SeaVive
Sea Cure

**Carotec**
P.O. Box 9919
Naples FL34101
1-800-522-4279
www.carotecine.com
www.carotec.com

Wobenzyme
Ulva Rigida

**Klaire Laboratories**
1573 W. Seminole
San Marcos CA 92069-2589
1-800-859-8358
(760)-744-9364

Pancreas (beef, lamb, pork)
Ultra Fine Ascorbic Acid
    Powder
Taurine

**Kate Fiedler**
1-877-343-3537
(860 )434-9249
Email: katfiedler@aol.com

Microhydrin
MSM with Microhydrin

**Primary Services Int., Inc**
P.O.Box 812
Fairfield, CT 06430
1-888-666-1188
www.primarysourceopc.com

OPC-85
Pycnogenol

**Metagenics**
725 S Kirkman Rd.
Orlando FL 32811
1-800-843-9660
fax:407-445-0204
www.teamapn.com

Arthropan
UltraInflamX
Ultra Clear Sustain
Ultra Fiber
UltraGlycemX
Collagenics
Zinc Tally (taste test)
Zinc Drink
Magnesium Citrate
Pain & Inflammation
    Remedy (homeopathic)
Magnesium Glycinate

## Magnets

**Wm. Philpott, M.D.**
SE 29th St.
Choctaw OK 73020
405-390-1444
Fax 405-390-2968

Quality ceramic, all descriptions and indications for every body part from mattresses to wraps.

Send for descriptive catalogue.

**Argentum**
36 Lake Rabun Rd.
Lakemont GA 30552
706-782-6700
fax: 706-782-3903

## Products For a Cleaner Environment

## Air Purifiers For Home, Office, and Car

**E.L.Foust**
P.O. Box 105
Elmhurst IL 60126
1-800-EL-FOUST
1-800-353-6878

## Test Your Daily Drinking Water

Call for price and information about sending a sample of your water for analysis for undesirable contaminants that hold back health. Also water filters, air filters, safer paints and products for construction and furnishings, toiletries, supplements, health books, cotton products and many other catalog items for healthier home environment.

**American Environmental
Health Foundation**
8345 Walnut Hill Lane
Dallas TX, 75231
1-800-428-2343
www. ehcd.com

# Alkaline Water, Singer Spring

**High Tech Health**
2695 Linden Drive
Boulder CO 80304
1-800-794-5355
www.hightechhealth.com

## More Water Filters, Home Products, Foods, Etc.

**Nontoxic Environments, Inc**
P.O. Box 384
Newmarket NH 03867
1-800-789-4348
603-659-5933
www.nontoxicenvironments.com

## Mineral Waters

**Water Oz**
Rte 1
Box 104-B
Grangeville ID 83530
800-547-2294
www.wateroz.com

Special Magnesium
Lithium
Calcium
Platinum
Multiple Minerals
and other waters

**Mountain Valley**
Mountain Valley Spring Co.
PO Box 1610
Hot Spr. National Park, AR 71902
1-800-643-1501
www.mountainvalleyspring.com

Glass-bottled spring water

In general the purest, best
tolerated, readily available
glass-bottled water.

## Cotton Pillows

Avoid sleeping with your head nestled in foam pillows outgassing formaldehyde, fire retardants and pesticides all night.

**KB Cotton Pillows, Inc.**
1-800-544-3752
fax: (888)-829-5292
P.O. Box 57
DeSoto TX 75123
www.kbcottonpillows.com

## Cotton Bedding, Mattresses and Some Clothes

**Janice Corp.**
98 Rte 46
Budd Lake NJ 07828
1-800-JANICES
973-691-5459
www.janice.com

## Environmentally Safer Products, Cleansers, Clothing, Furnishings, bedding, Depollution Appliances

**American Environmental
Health Foundation**
8345 Walnut Hill Lane
Dallas TX 75231
1-800-428-2343
www.ehcd.com

**Natural Lifestyles**
16 Lookout Dr.
Asheville NC  28804-3330
800-752-2775
www.natural-lifestyle.com

**Nontoxic Environments, Inc**
P.O. Box 384
Newmarket NH 03867
1-800-789-4348
603-659-5933
www.nontoxicenvironments.com

**Harmony**
360 Interlocken BLVD, Ste 300
Broomfield CO 80021
1-800-869-3446
www.gaiam.com

## Yoga Videos

*Gentle Yoga, For the Physically Challenged*, Margot Kitchen, 4607 Coronation Dr. SW, Calgary, Albert Canada T2S 1M5,  1-403-243-1078. This would be a great start for anyone needing to learn safe yoga.

*Yoga Practice for Beginners* (by *Yoga Journal*), includes 52 page booklet, Natural Lifestyle 1-800-752-2775

*Total Yoga*, Natural Lifestyle 1-800-752-2775

*Yoga Practice Series* (6 hour or longer videos for different needs, Natural Lifestyle 1-800-752-2775

*A.M. and P.M. Yoga for Beginners* (for all ages and fitness levels, Natural Lifestyle 1-800-752-2775

*The Spirit of Yoga in Sedona*, World Research Foundation, 20501 Ventura Blvd, Ste 100, Woodland Hills CA, 91364, 1-818-999-5483. This is a more advanced video and definitely not for beginners nor even some intermediates.

## Other Resources

**R. Paul St. Amand, M.D.**
4560 Admiral Way
Marina Del Rey CA 90292
310-577-7510

**Apothecure**
Pharmacy for Guaifenesin
1-800-969-6601

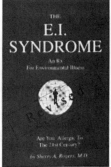

**The E.I. Syndrome, Revised** is a 635 page book that is necessary for people with **environmental illness**. It explains chemical, food, mold, and Candida sensitivities, nutritional deficiencies, testing methods and how to do the various environmental controls and diets in order to get well.

Many docs buy these by the hundreds and make them mandatory reading for patients, as it contains many pearls about getting well that are not found anywhere else. In this way it increases the fun of practicing medicine because patients are on a higher educational level and office time is more productive for more sophisticated levels of wellness. It covers hundreds of facts that make the difference between E.I. victims versus E.I. conquerors. It helps patients become active partners in their care while avoiding doctor burn-out. It covers the gamut of the diagnosis and treatment of environmentally induced symptoms.

Because the physician author was a severe universal reactor who has recovered, this book contains mountains of clues to wellness. As a result many have written that they healed themselves of resistant illnesses of all types by reading this book. This is in spite of the fact, that no consulted physicians were able to diagnose or effectively treat them. If you are not sure what causes your symptoms, this is a great start.

Many veteran sufferers have written that they had read many books on aspects of allergy, chronic Candidiasis and chemical sensitivity and thought that they knew it all. Yet they wrote that what they learned in *The E.I. Syndrome, Revised* enabled them to reach that last pinnacle of wellness.

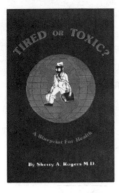

*Tired or Toxic?* is a 400 page book, and the first book that describes the mechanism, diagnosis and treatment of chemical sensitivity, complete with scientific references. It is written for the layman and physician alike and explains the many vitamin, mineral, essential fatty acid and amino acid analyses that help people detoxify everyday chemicals more efficiently and hence get rid of baffling symptoms, including chronic pain.

It is the first book written for laymen and physicians to describe xenobiotic detoxication, the process that allows all healing to occur. You have heard of the cardiovascular system, you have heard of the respiratory system, the gastrointestinal system, and the immune system. But most have never heard of the chemical detoxification system that is the determinant of whether we have chemical sensitivity, cancer, and in fact every disease.

This program shows how to diagnose and treat many resistant everyday symptoms and use molecular medicine techniques. It also gives the biochemical mechanisms in easily understood form, of how Candida creates such a diversity of symptoms and how the macrobiotic diet heals "incurable" end stage metastatic cancers. It is a great book for the physician you are trying to win over, and will show you how chemical sensitivity masquerades as common symptoms. It then explores the many causes and cures of chemical sensitivity, chronic Candidiasis, and other "impossible to heal" medical labels.

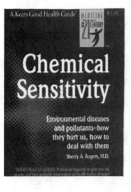

*Chemical Sensitivity.* This 48-page booklet is the most concise referenced booklet on chemical sensitivity. It is for the person wanting to learn about it but who is leery of tackling a big book. It is ideal for teaching your physician or convincing your insurance company, as it is fully referenced. And it is a good reference for the veteran who wants a quick concise review.

Most people have difficulty envisioning chemical sensitivity as a potential cause of everyday maladies. But the fact is that a lack of knowledge of the mechanism of chemical sensitivity can be the solo reason that holds many back from ever healing completely. Some will never get truly well simply because they do not comprehend the tremendous role chemical sensitivity plays. For failure to address the role that chemical sensitivity plays in every disease has been pivotal in failure to get well. The principles of environmental controls are of especially vital importance for cancer victims.

If you are not completely well, you need to read this book. If you have been sentenced to a life-time of drugs, whether it be for high blood pressure, high cholesterol, angina, arrhythmia, asthma, eczema, sinusitis, colitis, learning disabilities, chronic pain or cancer, you need this book. It matters not what your label is. What matters is whether chemical sensitivity is a factor that no one has explored that is keeping you from getting well. Most probably it is, and this is an inexpensive way to start you on the path toward drug-free wellness.

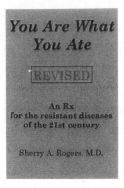

*You Are What You Ate.* This book is indispensable as a primer and introduction to the macrobiotic diet. The macrobiotic diet is the specialized diet with which many have healed the impossible, including end stage metastatic cancers. This is after medicine had given up on them and they had been given only months or weeks to live. Yes, they have rallied after surgery, chemotherapy and radiation had failed. Life was seemingly, hopelessly over.

Understandably, this diet has also enabled many chemically sensitive universal reactors, and highly allergic and even "undiagnosable people" to heal. It has also enabled those to heal that have "wastebasket" diagnostic labels such as chronic fatigue, fibromyalgia, MS, rheumatoid arthritis, depression, chronic infections, colitis, asthma, migraines, lupus, chronic Candidiasis, and much more.

Although there are many books on macrobiotics, this is one that takes the special needs of the allergic person and those with multiple food and chemical sensitivities as well as chronic Candidiasis into account. It provides details and case histories that the person new to macrobiotics needs before he embarks on the strict healing phase as described in *The Cure is in the Kitchen.*

Even people who have done the macrobiotic diet for a while will find reasons why they have failed and tips to improve their success. When a diet such as this has allowed many to heal their cancers, any other condition "should be a piece of cake".

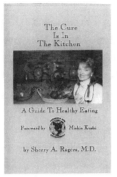

***The Cure is in the Kitchen*** is the next book you should read after ***You Are What You Ate*** to fully understand the healing macrobiotic diet. It is the first book to ever spell out in detail what all those people ate day to day who cleared their incurable diseases like MS, rheumatoid arthritis, fibromyalgia, lupus, chronic fatigue, colitis, asthma, migraines, depression, hypertension, heart disease, angina, undiagnosable symptoms, and relentless chemical, food, Candida, and electromagnetic sensitivities, as well as terminal cancers.

Dr. Rogers flew to Boston each month to work side by side with Mr. Michio Kushi, as he counseled people at the end of their medical ropes. As their remarkable case histories will show you, nothing is hopeless. Many of these people had failed to improve with surgery, chemotherapy and radiation. Instead their metastases continued to spread. It was only when they were sent home to die within a few weeks that they turned to the diet.

Medical studies confirmed that this diet has more than tripled the survival from cancers. And the beauty of this diet is that you use God-given whole foods to coax the body into the healing mode. It does not rely on prescription drugs, but allows the individual to heal himself at home.

If you cannot afford a $500 consultation, and you choose not to accept your death sentence or medication sentence, why not learn first hand what these people did and how you, too, may improve your health and heal the impossible.

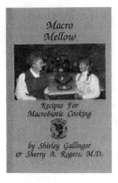

*Macro Mellow* is a book designed for 4 types of people: (1) For the person who doesn't know a thing about macrobiotics, but just plain wants to feel better, in spite of the 21st century. (2) It solves the high cholesterol/triglycerides problem without drugs and is the preferred diet for heart disease patients. In fact, it is the only proven diet to dissolve cholesterol deposits from arterial walls. (3) It is the perfect transition diet for those not ready for macro, but needing to get out of the chronic illness rut. (4) It spells out how to feed the rest of the family who hates macro, while another family member must eat it in order to clear their "incurable" symptoms.

It shows how to convert the "grains, greens, and beans" strict macro food into delicious "American-looking" food that the kids will eat. This saves the cook from making double meals while one person heals. The delicious low-fat whole food meals designed by Shirley Gallinger, a veteran nurse who has worked with Dr. Rogers for over two decades, use macro ingredients without the rest of the family even knowing. It is the first book to dovetail creative meal planning, menus, recipes and even gardening so the cook isn't driven crazy.

Most likely your kitchen contains a plethora of cookbooks. But you owe it to yourself and your family to learn how to incorporate healing whole foods, low in fat and high in phyto-nutrients into their diets. Who you have planning and cooking your meals has been proven to be as important if not more important than who you have chosen for your doctor. Medical research has proven the power of whole food diets to heal where high tech medicines and surgery have failed.

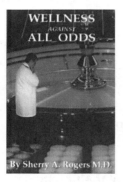

*Wellness Against All Odds* is the 6th and most revolutionary book by Sherry A. Rogers, M.D.   It contains the ultimate healing plan that people have successfully used to beat cancer when they were given 2 weeks, some even 2 days to live by some of the top medical centers.  These people had exhausted all that medicine has to offer, including surgery, chemotherapy, radiation and bone marrow transplants.   Some had even been macrobiotic failures. And one of the most unbelievable things is that the plan costs practically nothing to implement and most of it can be done at home with non-prescription items.

Of course, in keeping with the other works and going far beyond, this contains the mechanisms of how these principles heal and is complete with all the scientific references for physicians.   In fact, this program has been proven to more than quadruple cancer survival in the most hopeless forms of cancer (Gonzales, *Nutrition & Cancer*, 33(2): 117-124, 1999).

Did you know, for example, that there are vitamins that actually cure some cancers, and over 50 papers in the best medical journals to prove it? Likewise, did you know that there are non-prescription enzymes that dissolve cancer, arteriosclerotic plaque, and auto-antibodies like lupus and rheumatoid?  Did you know that there is a simple inexpensive, but highly effective way to detoxify the body at home to stop the toxic side effects of chemotherapy within minutes?  Did you know that this procedure can also reduce chemical sensitivity reactions (from accidental chemical exposures) from 4 days to 20 minutes?  Did you know that there are many hidden causes for "undiagnosable" symptoms that are never looked for, because it is easier and quicker to prescribe a pill than find (and fix) the causes?

The fact is that when you get the body healthy enough, it can heal anything.  You do not have to die from labelitis.  It no longer matters what your label is, from chronic Candida, fatigue, MS, or chronic pain to chemical sensitivity, an undiagnosable condition, or the worst cancer with only days to survive.  If you have been told there is nothing more that can be done for you, you have the option of kicking death in the teeth and healing the impossible.  Are you game?

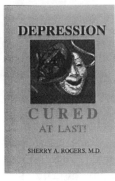

*Depression Cured at Last!* Just when you think all has been accomplished, along comes the most important book of all. Unique in many ways, (1) it is written for the lay person and the physician, and is appropriate as a medical school textbook. In fact, it should be required reading for all physicians regardless of specialty.

(2) It shows that it borders on malpractice to treat depression as a Prozac deficiency, to drug cardiology patients, or any other medical/psychiatric problem without first ruling out proven causes.

With over 700 pages and 1,000 complete references it covers the environmental, nutritional and metabolic causes of all disease. It covers leaky gut syndrome, intestinal dysbiosis, hormone deficiencies, hidden sensitivities to foods, molds, and chemicals, dysfunctional detoxication, heavy metal and pesticide poisonings, xenobiotic accumulations, and much, much more.

It is the best blue-print for figuring out what is wrong and how to fix it once and for all. If no one knows what is wrong with you, you need this book. If they know but say there is no cure, you need this book. If they say you need medications to control your symptoms indefinitely, you need this book. For it is the protocol for the environmental medicine work-up for all disease.

It is inconceivable that there is anyone who would not benefit from this book as it surely leaves drug-oriented medicine in the dust of the 20th century. And it does so by using the only disease that by definition sports a lack of hope. We chose this disease, depression, as a prototype to be sure to drive home the message that just when you least expect it, there is always **hope**. Every symptom has a cause and a cure.

The
Scientific Basis
for
Selected
Environmental
Medicine
Techniques

by

Sherry A. Rogers, M.D.

*Scientific Basis for Selected Environmental Medicine Techniques* contains the scientific evidence and references for the techniques of environmental medicine. It is designed with the patient in mind who is being denied medical payments by insurance companies that refuse to acknowledge environmental medicine.

With this guide a patient may choose to represent himself in small claims court and quote from the book showing, for example, that the *Journal of the American Medical Association* states that "titration provides a useful and effective measure of patient sensitivity". Or he may need to prove to his HMO that a U.S. Government agency states that "an exposure history should be taken for every patient". Failure to do so can lead to an inappropriate diagnosis and treatment.

It has sections showing medical references of how finding hidden vitamin deficiencies have, for example, enabled people to heal carpal tunnel syndrome without surgery, or heal life threatening steroid-resistant vasculitis, or stop seizures, or migraines, or learning disabilities.

This book is designed for patients who choose to find the causes of their illnesses rather than merely mask their symptoms with drugs for the rest of their lives. It is also for those who have been unfairly denied insurance coverage, or appropriate diagnosis by an HMO that is more concerned about profit than finding the cause of their patients' symptoms. And it is the ideal book with which to educate your PTA, attorney, insurance company, or physicians who still doubt your sanity.

In this era many HMO's tell people what diseases they can have, how long they can have them, and what treatments they can have. And all diseases seem to be deficiencies of drugs, for that is how they are all treated. It is as though arthritis were an Advil deficiency. This book arms you with the ammunition to defend your right to find the causes and get rid of symptoms and drugs

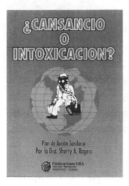

### *Cansancio o Intoxicacion?*

(*Tired or Toxic?* in Spanish) El lego informado reconoce que a medida que el mundo se vuelve más tecnológico, el hombre pierde proporcionalmente más control sobre su vida. Este libro le permitirá recuperar el control de su salud, ofreciéndole mayor capacidad para formar equipo con su medico para diagnosticar y tratar su condición.

Esta información es vitalmente importante ahora ya que a todos toca con cualquier síntoma tal como la sensibilidad química, alto colesterol, fatiga crónica, complejo relacionado a Cándida, depresion, Alzheimer, hipertensión, diabetes, enfermedad cardíaca, osteoporosis y más.

Dra. Rogers se encuentra en la avanazada de la educación pública sobre los efectos del medio ambiente en el individuo.

Otros libros escritos por Dra. Rogers que tienen que ver con prevenir enfermedades y restablecer la salud son **Eres lo que Has Comido, El Síndrome de E.A.,** y **La Cura Se Encuentra En La Cocina:** La Fase Curativa Estricta de la Dieta Macrobiotica.

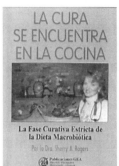

La Fase Curativa Estricta de
la Dieta Macrobiótica

Por la Dra. Sherry A. Rogers

Publicaciones GEA

### *La Cura Se Encuentra En La Cocina*
(*The Cure is in the Kitchen* in Spanish)
Este libro explora la relación entre dieta, medio ambiente, salud, y enfermedad y explica como la dieta macrobiótica, basada en cereales integrales, porotos y sus productos y otros alimentos naturales integrales puede prevenir enfermedades y restablecer la salud.

Nos explica cómo una dieta muy artificial contribuye a una variedad de problemas de salud y cómo ciertos aspectos de la vida moderna también nos pueden debilitar.

Un programa macrobiótico consiste de dos fases; pasar gradualmente a una dieta macrobótica o ponerse en una fase curativa estricta de carácter temporario. El objectivo de la fase curativa de esta dieta es aclarar una condición en particular. Es necesariamente, muy estricta e individualizada, y por eso razón, la persona debe consultar un doctor entrenado en la macrobiótica.

Otros libros escritos por Dra. Rogers que tienen que ver con prevenir enfermedades y restablecer la salud son **Cansancio o Intoxicación?, Eres lo que Has Comido,** y **El Síndrome de E.A.**

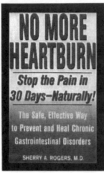

***No More Heartburn.*** The chance of healing any condition in the body is slim to none until the gut is healthy first. Heartburn, indigestion, irritable bowel, spastic colon, colitis, gall bladder disease, gas and bloating are far from benign, for they are all signs of an ailing gastro-intestinal tract.

Learn how the many prescription and over-the-counter drugs guarantee that you will not only have worse gut symptoms eventually, but that you can pile on new symptoms, seemingly unrelated to the gut, within the next few years like arthritis, heart problems or cancer.

Come learn how to find the many hidden causes of symptoms like food allergies, Candida overgrowth, Helicobacter, leaky gut, nutrient deficiencies, toxic environment and thoughts, and more. Then learn how to use non-prescription remedies to heal, not merely mask.

Since the gut houses over half the immune system and over hjalf the detoxification system, a silently ailing gut holds back healing any condition indefinitely. This book is also full of new non-prescription Candida and other yeast fighters and protocols, since this is a common unsuspected cause of many diseases.

Learn how heartburn masked with drugs is a fast road to a heart attack or cancer, chronic fatigue, chronic pain or fibromyalgia. Explicit clear directions are given for every symptom, their causes and cures. For an unhealthy gut is a primary reason for many folks to be stuck at a standstill, unable to heal any further. If your healing is stalled, chances are you need to start healing the gut first. You need to heal from the inside out, for **the road to health is paved with good intestines.** (Over 350 references)

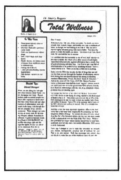

## Total Wellness Newsletter

For over a decade, this referenced monthly newsletter has kept folks and physicians up to date on new findings. Since Dr. Rogers is constantly researching, lecturing around the globe, maintaining a private practice, doing television and radio shows, writing for health magazines and physicians, and has published 18 scientific papers and over 12 books in 14 years, she is peddling as fast as she can.

There is literally an avalanche of new information, but we don't want you to have to wait for a new book on the subject to learn about it. We want that practical and useful instruction in your hands this month.

Furthermore, the field of environmental medicine, because it is so all encompassing, can be overwhelming at times. So in addition to bringing you the new, we also focus on the overall perspective and the practical solutions you can do today.

In this era, because we cannot get the information out to you fast enough, we use the newsletter as our communication link. By sending you to the medical school of the future each month, *Total Wellness* will teach you useful facts years before they will be presented elsewhere, and it is practical and action-oriented. For pennies a day or 75 cents a week, you really cannot afford to be without this life-altering unique information, in fact it more than pays for itself in saving you office visits galore. Cheaper than the newspaper by far, yet more crucial to your future, it is designed to get you independently healthy.

## Mold Plates

Since mold is unavoidably everywhere, and sensitivity to it can mimic nearly any symptom, you need to know what is in your environment. For as devastating and perplexing as mold symptoms can be, it is completely curable, but only if you have identified it as a possible cause. You need to know if you have too much and what types are present. By exposing special petri dishes (or mold plates) in your bedroom, family room, and office, you have effectively assessed your 24 hour mold environment.

Each plate comes with directions for exposure and a return mailer. In 6-9 weeks after the slow-growing fungi have appeared for identification, the report will be mailed to you detailing all of the specific molds and how many molds are present. We purposely take as long as we need, since we wait for the last molds to grow out before completing the report. We do not want to neglect the "slow growing" molds like other labs do, often sending reports back within days of receiving the plates. You will need to order one plate for each room you want to assess at home or work.

Mold allergy can mimic nearly any symptom. If you do not know how moldy your environment is, you may erroneously be attributing symptoms to chemical or food sensitivities or some "incurable" or mysterious problem with no known cause. It is always best to meet the enemy head on in order to identify the cause of the problem and solve it, once and for all.

Many people are stuck. They have an undiagnosable condition. Or they have a label but have been unable to get well. Or they have a "dead-end" label that means nothing more can be done. And many are not able to find a physician who is trained in what our books explore.

These people could benefit from a personal consultation with Dr. Sherry Rogers to explore what diagnostic and treatment options may exist that they or their physicians are not aware of. For this reason we offer prepaid, scheduled phone consultations with the doctor. These can be scheduled through the office by calling (315) 488-2856.

If you wish to send copies of your medical reports and/or also have your doctor on the line, this can be helpful as well. Reports must be received at least 3 weeks prior to the consult and not be on fax paper. They should be copies and not originals as they are not returnable. Do not send records without first having secured a scheduled appointment time, for records without an appointment are discarded.

Because you have not come to the office and been examined, you are not considered a patient (although you could elect to become one). In spite of that, you can learn what tests your physician could order and what plans you could follow. If he needs help in interpreting the tests, a scheduled follow-up consultation can allow you to explore treatment options with specific nutrient and other treatment suggestions. The point is, you do not have to be alone without guidance in your quest for wellness. And you owe it to yourself to explore the options that you might otherwise never even have heard of.

### PRESTIGE PUBLISHING
### P.O. BOX 3068
### Syracuse, NY 13220
### 1-800-846-6687 ◊ Fax 315-454-8119
### www.prestigepublishing.com

## Price List

| | |
|---|---|
| Depression Cured At Last! | $24.95 |
| The E.I. Syndrome Revised | $17.95 |
| Tired or Toxic? | $18.95 |
| Chemical Sensitivity (pamphlet) | $ 3.95 |
| You Are What You Ate | $12.95 |
| The Cure Is In The Kitchen | $14.95 |
| Macro Mellow | $12.95 |
| Wellness Against All Odds | $17.95 |
| The Scientific Basis of Environmental Medicine | $17.95 |
| No More Heartburn | $15.00 |
| Pain-Free In 6 Weeks | $19.95 |

*Spanish Translations*

| | |
|---|---|
| Cansancio o Intoxicacion? | $30.00 |
| La Cura Se Encuentra En La Cocina | $30.00 |

*Total Wellness Newsletter*

| | |
|---|---|
| Monthly referenced newsletter on current wellness and healing information/1 year (12 issues) | $39.95 |
| Back issues/1 year (12 issues) | $29.95 |
| Back issues/each | $ 4.00 |
| Mold Plates (one room) | $27.50 |
| Formaldehyde Spot Test Kit (test over 100 objects) | $45.00 |

Telephone consultations available with Dr. Rogers.
Contact Dr. Rogers' office (315) 488-2856 for scheduling information.

*Shipping/Handling:* $4.00 per single book/$1.00 each additional book. All other products $3.00 per single item/$1.00 each additional item.

***PRESTIGE PUBLISHING***
***P.O. BOX 3068***
***Syracuse, NY 13220***
***800-846-6687 ◊ 315-455-7862 ◊ Fax 315-454-8119***
***www.prestigepublishing.com***

## Order Form

- ❏ Depression Cured At Last!
- ❏ The E.I. Syndrome, Revised
- ❏ Tired or Toxic?
- ❏ Chemical Sensitivity
- ❏ You Are What You Ate
- ❏ The Cure is in the Kitchen
- ❏ Macro Mellow
- ❏ Wellness Against All Odds
- ❏ The Scientific Basis of Environmental Medicine Techniques
- ❏ No More Heartburn
- ❏ Pain-Free In 6 Weeks
- ❏ Cansancio o Intoxicacion?
- ❏ La Cura Se Encuentra En La Cocina
- ❏ Total Wellness Newsletter
- ❏ Total Wellness Back Issues per year, indicate year _____
- ❏ Total Wellness individual copies, indicate month _____
- ❏ Mold Plates
- ❏ Formaldehyde Spot Test Kit

Name: _____

Address: _____

City: _____ State: _____ Zip: _____

- ❏ Check - Amount Enclosed $_____ (NYS residents add 7% sales tax.)
- ❏ Money Order
- ❏ MasterCard/Visa

Card Number: _____ Exp. _____

Signature: _____

381

# Chapter 10

# References

## Chapter 1
• Lazarou J, Pomeranz BH, Corey PN, Incidence of adverse drug reactions in hospitalized patients, *J Amer Med Assoc*, 279; 15:1200-1205, Apr. 15, 1998
• Guttham SP, Rodriguez LAG, Raiford DS, et al, Nonsteroidal anti-inflammatory drugs and the risk of hospitalization for acute renal failure, *Arch Intern Med*, 156:2433-2439, Nov 25, 1996. (Taking NSAIDs raises the risk 4-fold of hospitalization)
• Page J, Henry d, Consumption of NSAIDs and the development of congestive heart failure in elderly patients, *Arch Intern Med*, 160:777-784, Mar 27, 2000
• Murray MD, et al, Adverse effects of nonsteroidal anti-inflammatory drugs on renal function, *Ann Intern Med* 112; 559, Apr 15, 1990
• Harris ED, Rheumatoid arthritis. Pathophysiology and implications for therapy. *N Engl J Med* 322; 1277-89, 1990
• Weinblatt ME, Methotrexate. In: Kelley W, Harris E, Ruddy S, Sledge C, Eds., *Textbook of Rheumatology. 4th ed*, WB Saunders, 1993; 767-778
• Langreth R, Burton TM, Merck's Vioxx gains on rival painkiller Celebrex, *Wall Street Journal*, B7, Nov. 24, 1999
• Solomon L, Drug-induced arthropathy and necrosis of the femoral head, 55B;246-51, 1973

**Note:** Many more references on the side effects of drugs in chapter 4

## Chapter 2
• Childers NF, *Arthritis – A Diet to Stop It*, Horticultural Publ., 3906 NW 31 Pl, Gainesville FL 32606, (5 editions 1977-1995), 1-888-501-8822
• Rogers SA, *The E.I. Syndrome Revised*, Prestige Publishing, Box 3068, Syracuse NY 13220, 1-800-846-6687
• Rogers SA, *You Are What You Ate*, Prestige Publishing, Box 3068, Syracuse NY 13220, 1-800-846-6687
• Rogers SA, *The Cure is in the Kitchen*, Prestige Publishing, Box 3068, Syracuse NY 13220, 1-800-846-6687
• Gallinger SM, Rogers SA, *Macro Mellow*, Prestige Publishing, Box 3068, Syracuse NY 13220, 1-800-846-6687
• Vogel J, Claudio M, *The Nightshade-Free Cookbook*, 1-888-501-8822 or 1-800-846-6687
• Childers NF, Margoles MS, An apparent relation of nightshades (Solanaceae) to arthritis, *J Neurol Orthop Med Surg*, 14:227-231, 1993

382

- Randolph T, *An Alternative Approach to Allergies*, 1-800-846-6687
- Nordlee J, et al, Identification of a Brazil nut allergen in transgenic soybeans, *New Engl J Med* 334; 11:688-92, 1996.
- Teitel M, Wilson KA, *Genetically Engineered Food: Changing the Nature of Nature*, Park Street Press, Rochester VT, 1999, available Natural Lifestyles 1-800-752-2775

## Mechanism for Physicians:

- Abbott DC, Field D, Johnson EL, Correlation of anti-cholinesterase effect with solanine content of potato, *Analyst* 85:375-376, 1960
- Alozie SO, Sharma RP, Salunkhe DK, Physiological disposition, subcellular distribution and tissue binding of a-chaconine (3H), *J Food Safety* 1:257-273, 1978
- Blankenmeyer JT, Atherton R, Friedman M, Effect of potato glycoalkaloids a-chaconine and a-solanine on sodium active transport in frog skin, *J Agric Food Chem* 43:636-639, 1995
- Childers NF, A relationship of arthritis to the Solonaceae (nightshades), *J Intern Acad Prev Med* 7:31-37, 1979
- Childers NF, *Arthritis – A Diet to Stop It*, Horticultural Publ, 3906 NW 31 Pl, Gainesville FL 32606, 904-372-5077 (5 editions 1977-1995), or phone 352-392-4711 ext 304 or 352-372-5077 or 1-800-501-8822
- Childers NF, Margoles MS, An apparent relation of nightshades (Solanaceae) to arthritis, *J Neurol Orthop Med Surg*, 14:227-231, 1993
- Childers NF, Russo GM, *The Nightshades and Health*, Horticultural Publications, Somerset Press Inc., Somerville NJ, 08876, 1977
- Claringbold WDB, Few JD, Renwick JH, Kinetics and retention of Solanidine in man, *Xenobiotica*, 12:293-302, 1982
- Corradino RA, Wasserman RH, 1,25-dihydroxycholecalciferol-like activity of Solanum malacoxylon extract on calcium transport, *Nature*, 252:716, 1974
- D'Arcy WG, *Solonaceae: Biology and Systematics*, NY, Columbia University Press, 1985
- Dawson RM, Reversibility of the inhibition of acetylcholinesterase by tacrine, *Neurosci Lett*, 118:85-87, 1990
- Durrell LW, Poisonous and injurious plants (potato included) in Colorado, *Colorado Agr Ext Sta Bull*, 412-A: 55, 1952
- Ewen SWB, Pusztai a, Effect of diets containing genetically modified potatoes expressing *Galanthus nivalis* lectin on rat small intestine, *Lancet* 354:1353-4, Oct 16, 1999
- Fenton B, Stanley K, Fenton S, Bolton-Smith C, Differential binding of the insecticidal lectin GNA to human blood cells, *Lancet* 354:1354-5, Oct 16, 1999Gibson GR, Whitacre EB, Ricotti CA, Colitis induced by nonsteroidal anti-inflammatory drugs, *Arch Intern Med* 152; 625-632, 1992
- Goodman LS, Gilman A, *The Pharmacological Basis of Therapeutics*, 5th Ed, MacMillan, NY, 1975
- Goodwin SD, Glenny RW, Nonsteroidal anti-inflammatory drug-associated pulmonary infiltrates with eosinophilia, *Arch Intern Med* 1`52:1521-1524, 1992

- Groen K, Pereoom DE, Fauw DPKH, Besamusca P, Beekhof PK, Speijers GJA, Derks HJGM, Bioavailability and disposition of 3H-Solanine in rat and hamster, *Xenobiotica* 23:995-1005, 1993
- Gutch CF, Nonsteroidal anti-inflammatory agents and acute renal failure, *Arch Intern Med*, 156:2414, Nov 25, 1996
- Guttham SP, Rodriguez LAG, Raiford DS, et al, Nonsteroidal anti-inflammatory drugs and the risk of hospitalization for acute renal failure, *Arch Intern Med* 156:2433-2439, Nov 25, 1996
- Harris H, Whittaker M, Differential response of human serum cholinesterase types to an inhibitor in potato, *Nature*, 183:1808-1809, 1959
- Hayes WJ, *Pesticide Studies in Man*, Baltimore MD, Williams and Williams, 1983
- Keeler RF, Comparison of the teratogenicity in rats of certain potato-type alkaloids and the veratrum teratogen cyclopamine, *Lancet*, 1187-1188, May 26, 1973
- Keeler RF, Young S, Douglas D, et al, Congenital deformities produced in hamsters by potato sprouts, *Teratology* 17:327-334, 1978
- Keeler RE, Baker DC, Gaffield W, Spirosolane-containing Solanum species and induction of congenital craniofacial malformations, *Toxicol* 28:873-884, 1990
- Krebs-Smith S, et al, Fruit and vegetable intakes of children and adolescents in the United States, *Arch Ped Adolescent Med* 150:81-86, 1996
- Kroker GP, Stroud RM, Marshall RT, et al, Fasting and rheumatoid arthritis: a multicentre study, *Clinical Ecology*, 2:137-144, 1984
- LaDu BN, Bartels CF, Lockridge O, et al, Phenotypic and molecular biological analysis of human butyrylcholinesterase variants, *Clin Biochem*, 23:423-431, 1990
- Layer PG, Cholinesterases during development of the Avian nervous system, *Cell Mol Neurobiol* 11:7-33, 1991
- Mammen L, Schmidt CP, Photosensitivity reactions: a case report involving NSAIDs, *Amer Fam Phys* 52:575-579, Aug 1995
- Michalska L, Nagel G, Swiniarski E, Zydowo MM, The effect of a-solanine on the active calcium transport in rat intestine, *Gen Pharmacol*, 16:69-70, 1985
- Morris SC, Lee TH, The toxicity and teratogenicity of Solonaceae glycoalkaloids, particularly those of the potato (Solonaum tuberosum): a review, *Food Technol. Australia*, 36:118-124, 1984
- Murphy PJ, Myers BL, Badia P, Nonsteroidal anti-inflammatory drugs alter body temperature and suppress melatonin in humans, *Physiol Behav* 59:133-139, 1996
- Nigg HN, Ramos LE, Graham EM, Sterling J, Brown S, Cornell JA, Inhibition of human plasma and serum butyrylcholinesterase (EC 3.1.1.8) by a-chaconine and a-solanine, *Fund Appl Toxicol*, 33:272-281, 1996
- Orgell WH, Vaidya KA, Dahm PA, Inhibition of human plasma cholinesterase in vitro by extracts of Solonaceae plants, *Science* 128:1136-1137, 1958

384

- Page J, Henry d, Consumption of NSAIDs and the development of congestive heart failure in elderly patients, an underrecognized public health problem, *Arch Intern Med*, 160:777-784, Mar 27, 2000

- Palmblad J A, Anti-rheumatic effects of fasting, *Nutrition and Rheumatic Disease/Rheumatic disease Clinics of North America,* 17; 2:351-362, May 1991

- Pierro LJ, Haines JS, Osman SF, Teratogenicity and toxicity of purified a-chaconine and a-solanine, *Teratology* 15:31A, 1977

- Quiralte J, Blanco C, Castillo R, Delgado J, Carrillo T, Intolerance to nonsteroidal anti-inflammatory drugs: Results of controlled drug challenges in 98 patients, *Ann Allergy* 98:3:678, Sept 1996

- Rea WJ, *Chemical Sensitivity, Vol II & III,* CRC Press, Boca Raton FL, 1993 and 1995)

- Renwick JH, Hypothesis: Anencephaly and spina bifida are usually preventable by avoidance of a specific but unidentified substance present in certain potato tubers, *Brit J Prev Soc Med*, 26:67-88 (and errrata 269)

- Renwick JH, Potato babies, *Lancet* 2:336, 1972

- Renwick JH, Diet and congenital defects, *Brit Med J*, 1:172, 1973

- Renwick JH, Claringbold WDB, McLean ACS, et al, Neural-tube defects produced in Syrian hamsters by potato glycoalkaloids, *Teratology* 30:371-381, 1984

- Roddick JG, Rijnenberg AL, Osman SF, Synergistic interaction between potato glycoalkyloids a-solanine and a-chaconine in relation to destabilization of cell membranes: ecological implications, *J Chem Ecol* 14:889-902, 1988

- Roddick JG, Rijnenberg AL, Weissenberg M, Membrane-disrupting properties of the steroidal glycoalkaloids solasonine and solamargine, *Phytochemicstry*, 29; 5: 1513-1518, 1990

- Roddick JG, The acetylcholinesterase-inhibitory activity of steroidal glycoalkaloids and their aglycones, *Phytochemistry,* 28:2631-2634, 1989

- Rogers SA, *No More Heartburn,* Kensington Publ;. NY 2000 (1-800-846-687)

- Seignalet J, Diet, fasting and rheumatoid arthritis, *Lancet,* 339:68-69, 1992

- Shankel SW, Johnson DC, Shankel TL, O'Neil WM, Acute renal failure and glomerulopathy caused by nonsteroidal anti-inflammatory drugs, *Arch Intern Med* 152:986-990, 1992

- Singh G, Ramey DR, Morfeld D, Shi H, Hatoum HT, Fries JF, Gastrointestinal tract complication of nonsteroidal anti-inflammatory drug treatment in rheumatoid arthritis, *Arch Intern Med*, 156:1530-1536, July 22, 1996

- Skoldstam L, Larsson L, Lindstrom FD, Effects of fasting and lactovegetarian diet on rheumatoid arthritis, *Scand J Rheumatol*, 18:83-123, 1984

- Smith DB, Roddick JG, Jones LJ, Potato glycoalkaloids: some unanswered questions. Review, *Trends In Food Science & Technology,* 7:126-131, Apr 1996

- Spoerke D, The mysterious potato, *Vet Hum Toxicol*, 36:324-326, 1994

- Sundquist T, et al, Influence of fasting on intestinal permeability and disease activity in patients with rheumatoid arthritis, *Scand J Rheumatol* 11;1:33-38, 1982

- Uden AM, et al, Neutrophil functions and clinical performance after total fasting in patients with rheumatoid arthritis, *Ann Rheum Dis*, 42; 1:45-51, 1983
- Ugent D, The potato: What is the botanical origin of this important crop plant, and how did it first become domesticated? *Science* 170:1161-1166, 1970
- Wasserman RH, Active vitamin D-like substances in Solanum malacoxylon and other calcinotic plants, *Nutrition Reviews* 33:1-5, 1975
- Wasserman RH, Henion JD, Haussler MR, Carcinogenic factor in Solanum malacoxylon, *Science,* 194:853-854, 1976
- West E, Emmel MW, Poisonous plants (to livestock) in Florida, *Florida Agr Ext Sta Bull*, 510:42-44, 1952

## Chapter 3
- Langreth R, Eminent journal urges moratorium on diet-drug use, *Wall Street Journal*, B1, B5, Aug 28, 1997
- Langreth R, Johannes L, Is marketing of diet pill to aggressive?, *Wall Street Journal*, B1, B5, Nov. 21, 1996
- Maremont M, Florida moves to restrict use of diet drugs, *Wall Street Journal*, B4, Sept 9, 1997
- Associated Press, Parents sue diet-drug makers, *Syracuse Herald Journal*, B1, May 6, 1997
- Langreth R, Glaxo Wellcome drug proves helpful in treating ailment linked to diet pill, *Wall Street Journal,* B4, Jan 29, 1998
- Losonczy KG, et al, Vitamin E and vitamin C supplement use and risk of all-cause and coronary heart disease mortality in older persons: The established populations for epidemiologic studies of the elderly, *Amer J Clin Nutr*, 64;2:190-6, Aug. 1996

## CM:
- Ashendel CL, Membrane lipids and signaling in cell growth regulation, pg 19, in Steele VE, Stoner GD, Boone CW, Kelloff GJ, eds. *Cellular and Molecular Targets for Chemoprevention*, CRC Press, Boca Raton FL, 1992
- Clegg CH, Ran W, et al, A mutation in the catalytic sub-unit of protein kinase A prevents myristylation but does not inhibit biological activity, *J Biolog Chem*, 264;33:20140-20146, 1989
- Cochran C, A little clarity on cetyl myristoleate, *Total Health* (1-888-316-6051) 22;2:34-35, April 2000
- Cochran C, *Arthritis and Cetyl Myristoleate*, Healing Wisdom Publ, 2067 Broadway, NY 10023, Feb 1998
- Cochran C, *CMO: Cetyl Myristoleate*, Healing Wisdom Publ, 2067 Broadway, NY 10023, 3rd ed., Mar 1997
- Cochran C, Dent R, Cetyl myristoleate—a unique natural compound valuable in arthritis conditions, *TLFD&P*, 70-74, July 1997

- Diehl H, May EI, Cetyl myristoleate isolated from Swiss Albino mice: an apparent protective agent against adjuvant arthritis in rats, *J Pharmaceut Sci*, 83;3:296-299, Mar. 1994
- Gordon JI, Duronio RJ, et al, Protein N-myristoylation, *J Biol Chem*, 266; 8647, 1991
- Griffin L, *CMO™ Information Packet*, G&S Marketing, 1-800-829-1514
- Hunt D, *Boom! You're Well With Cetyl Myristoleate*, Promotion Publishing, San Diego, CA, 1-800-231-1776
- Johnson DR, Cox AD, Solski PA, Gordon JI, et al, Functional analysis of protein N-myristoylation: Metabolic labeling studies using three oxygen-substituted analogs of myristic acid and cultured mammalian cells provide evidence for protein-sequence-specific incorporation and analog-specific redistribution, *Proc Natl Acad Sci USA*, 87:8511-8515, Nov 1990
- O'Brien C, Ward NE, Fan D, et al, A novel N-myristylated synthetic octapeptide inhibits protein kinase C activity and partially reverses murine fibrosarcoma cell resistance to Adriamycin, *Invest New Drugs*, 9:169-179, 1991
- Owen BL, *The Pure Cure for Arthritis*, Health Digest Books, Cannon Beach OR, 1-888-692-0800
- Resh MD, Membrane interactions of pp60 (v-src): a model for myristylated tyrosine protein kinases, *Oncogene* 5:1437-1444, 1990
- Sands L, *Arthritis Defeated At Last!*, Aquarius Holdings, 1998, available from G & S Marketing, 1442 E. Lincoln Ave, #247, Orange CA 92665, 1-800-829-1514
- Siemandi H, The effect of cis-9-cetyl myristoleate (CMO) and adjunctive therapy on arthritis and auto-immune disease, a randomized trial, *TLFD&P*, 58-63, Aug/Sep 1997

## Chapter 4
### Leaky gut, Candida, garlic, fibromyalgia references:
- Rogers SA, *No More Heartburn*, Kensington Publishing, NY 2000, 1-800-846-6687.
- Rogers SA, *Tired Or Toxic?*, Prestige Publishing, Syracuse, NY 1-800-846-6687
- Rogers SA, *The E.I. Syndrome, Revised*, Prestige Publishing, Syracuse, NY 1-800-846-6687
- Rogers SA, *Depression Cured At Last!*, Prestige Publishing, Syracuse, NY 1-800-846-6687
- Hunter JO, Food allergy—or enterometabolic disorder?, *Lancet*, 338:495-496, Aug 24, 1991.
- Bentley SJ, et al, Food hypersensitivity in irritable bowel syndrome, *Lancet*, 1983;II: 295-297, 1983.
- Barber AE, et al, Glutamine or fiber supplementation of a defined formula diet. Impact on bacterial translocation, tissue composition, and response to endotoxin, *JPEN*, 14:335-343, 1990.

- Gilliland SE, et al, Antagonistic action of lactobacillus acidophilus toward intestinal and food-borne pathogens in associative cultures, *J Food Prot* 40:820-823, 1977.
- Fernandes CF, Therapeutic role of dietary lactobacilli and lactobacillic fermented dairy products, *FEMS Microbiology Reviews* 46: 343-356, 1987.
- Page J, et al, Consumption of NSAIDs and the development of congestive heart failure in elderly patients, an underrecognized public health problem, *Arch Intern Med*, 160:777-784, Mar 27, 2000
- Jackson P, et al, Intestinal permeability in patients with eczema and food allergy, *Lancet* i: 1285-1286, 1981.
- Walker W, Transmucosal passage of antigens, Schmidt E (Ed.), *Food Allergy*, Vevey; Raven Press NY, 1988.
- Reinhardt M, Macromolecular absorption of food antigens in health and disease, *Ann Allergy*, 53:597, 1984.
- Editorial, Antigen absorption by the gut, *Lancet* ii:715-717, 1978.
- Stephansson K, Dieperink M, Richman DM et al, Sharing of antigenic determinants between the nicotinic acetylcholine receptor and proteins in Escherichia coli, Proteus vulgaris, and Klebsiella pneumoniae, *N Engl J Med*, 312:221-225, 1985.
- Paganelli R, Levinsky R, Atherton D, Detection of specific antigen within circulating immune complexes: validation of the assay and its application to food antigen-antibody complexes formed in healthy and food-allergic subjects. *Clin Exp Immunol*, 46:44-53, 1981.
- Berg R, Wommack E, Deitch EA, Imunosuppression and intestinal bacterial overgrowth synergistically promote bacterial translocation from the GI tract, *Arch Surg*, 123:1359-1364, 1988.
- Deitch EA, et al, Bacterial translocation from the gut impairs systemic immunity, *Surgery*, 109:269-276, 1991.
- Deitch EA, et al, The gut as portal of entry for bacteremia: the role of protein malnutrition. *Ann Surg*, 205,:681-692, 1987.
- Jenkins A, Trew DR, Crump BJ, et al, Do non-steroidal anti-inflammatory drugs increase colonic permeability? *Gut*, 32:66-69, 1991.
- Bjarnason I, Williams P, Smethurst P et al, Effect of non-steroidal anti-inflammatory drugs and prostaglandins on the permeability of the human small intestine, *Gut*, 27:1292-1297, 1986.
- Bjarnasson I, Williams P, Smethurst P, et al, Intestinal permeability and inflammation in rheumatoid arthritis: effects of non-steroidal anti-inflammatory drugs, *Lancet*, 2:1171-1174, 1984.
- Busch J, Hammer M, Brunkhorst R, Wagener P, Determination of endotoxin in inflammatory rheumatic diseases—the effect of nonsteroidal anti-inflammatory drugs on intestinal permeability, *J Rheumatol*, 47: 156-160, 1988.
- Berg RD, The translocation of normal flora bacteria from the gastrointestinal tract to the mesenteric lymph nodes and other organs review, *Microecology & Therapy*, 11:27-34, 1981.

- Galland L, Leaky gut syndromes: breaking the vicious cycle, *Townsend Letter for Doctors*, 145/146: 62-68, 1995.
- Hidaka H, et al, Effects of fructo-oligosaccharides on intestinal flora and human health. *Bifidobacteria Microflora*, 5(1):37-50, 1986.
- McKellar RC, et al, Metabolism of fructo-oligosaccharides by Bifidobacerium spp, *Appl Microbial Biotechnol*, 31:537-541, 1989.
- Fishbein L, et al, Fructo-oligosaccharides: A review. *Vet Hum Toxicol*, 30(2): 104-107, 1988.
- Schook LB, Lanskin DL, *Xenobiotics and Inflammation*, Academic Press NY, 1994.
- Well CL, Maddaus MA, Simmons RL, Proposed mechanism for the translocation of intestinal bacteria, *Rev Infect Dis*, 10:958- 968 (1988).
- Husby S, Jensenius JC, Svehag SE, Passage of undergraded antigen into the blood of healthy adults. Further characterization of the kinetics of uptake and the size distribution of antigen, *Scand J Immunol*, 24:447-455 (1986).
- Buist R, The malfunctional "mucosal barrier" and food allergies, *Internat Clin Nutr Rev*, 3:1-4, 1983
- Walker QA, Role of the mucosal barrier in antigen handling by the gut, in J Brostoff, SJ Challacombe, eds, Food *Allergy and Intolerance*, London, Bailliere Tindall, 209-222, 1987
- Inman R, Antigens, the gastrointestinal tract and arthritis, *Rheum Dis Clin North Amer (U.S.)*, 17; 2:309-321, 1991
- O'Farrelly C, Price R, Fernandes, L, et al, IgA rheumatoid factor and IgG dietary protein antibodies are associated in rheumatoid arthritis, *Immunol Invest*, 18; 6:753-764, 1989
- Spaeth G, Berg RD, Specian RD, Deitch EA. Food without fiber promotes bacterial translocation from the gut, *Surgery*, 108: 240-24, (1990).
- Souba WW, Klimberg VS, Hautamaki RD, et al, Oral glutamine reduces bacterial translocation following abdominal radiation, *J Surg Res*, 48:1-5, 1990.
- Hamilton IH, Cobden I, Rothwell J, Axon ATR, Intestinal permeability in celiac disease: The response to gluten withdrawal and single-dose gluten challenge, *Gut*, 23:202-210 1982.
- Ukabam SO, Cooper BT, Small intestinal permeability as an indicator of jejunal mucosal recovery in patients with celiac sprue on a gluten-free diet, *J Clin Gastro*, 7:232-236, 1985.
- Falth-Magnusson K, Kjellman N-Im, Odelram H, et al, Gastrointestinal permeability in children with cow's milk allergy: effect of milk challenge and sodium cromoglycate assessed with polyethyleneglycols (PEG 400 and PEG 1000). *Clin Allergy*, 14:277-286, 1984.
- Andre C, Objective diagnostic test of therapeutic efficacy by a measure of intestinal permeability, *La Presse Medicale (Paris)* 15:105-108, 1986.
- Leonard RE, Chicken feces fine to eat, says new USDA proposal, *Nutrition Week*, 24;27:4-5, July 22, 1994.

389

- Piccioni R, Analysis of data on the impact of food processing by ionizing radiation on health and the environment, *Int J Biosocial Res*, 9(2): 203-212, 198.
- Gledhill T, et al, Epidemic hypochlorhydria, *Br J Med*, 289: 383-386, 1985.
- Deitch, EA, Maejima K, Berg RD, Effect of oral antibiotics and bacterial overgrowth on the translocation of the gastrointestinal tract micro-flora in burned rats, *J Trauma*, 25: 385-392, 1985.
- Deitch EA, Berg RD, Specian RD, Endotoxin promotes the translocation of bacteria from the gut, *Arch Surg*, 22: 185- 190, 1987.
- Constantini AV, The fungal/mycotoxin connections: auto-immune diseases, malignancies, atherosclerosis, hyperlipidemias, and gout, Keynote speaker, American Academy of Environmental Medicine, Reno Nevada, 1993 (tapes available, Insta-Tape, Monrovia CA 1-800-NOW-TAPE)
- O'Dwyer ST, Michie HR, Ziegler TR., et al, A single dose of endotoxin increases intestinal permeability in healthy humans, *Arch Surg*, 123: 1459-1464, 1988.
- Caselli M, Trevisani L, Bighi S, et al, Dead fecal yeasts and chronic diarrhea, *Digestion*, 41: 142-148, 1988.
- Kane JG, Chretien JH, Garagusi V, Diarrhea caused by Candida, *Lancet*, 335-336, 1976.
- Gupta TP, Ehrenpreis MN, Candida-associated diarrhea in hospitalized patients, *Gastroenterol*, 98: 780-785, 1990.
- Alexander JG, Thrush bowel infection: existence, incidence, prevention and treatment, particularly by a lactobacillus acidophilus preparation, *Curr Med Drugs*, 8:3-11, 1967.
- Brabander JO, Blank F, Butas CA, Intestinal moniliasis in adults, *Can Med Assoc J*, 77: 478-482, 1957.
- Lau B, *Garlic and You: The Modern Medicine* (over 200 references) Apple Publ, 1997, Vancouver BC, Canada or Wakunaga)
- Pennsylvania State University and the National Cancer Institute, *Aged Garlic Extract, Current Research Papers from Peer Reviewed Scientific Journals and Scientific Meetings*, Wakunaga Co, Mission Viejo CA, 1-800-421-2998
- Piccioni R, Analysis of data on the impact of food processing by ionizing radiation on health and the environment, *Int J Biosocial Res*, 9(2): 203-212, 198.
- Gillette R, A practical approach to the patient with back pain, *Amer Fam Phys*, 53;2:670-676, Feb 1, 1996
- Reiffenberger DH, Amundson LH, Fibromyalgia syndrome: a review, *Amer Fam Phys*, 53;5:1698-1705, Apr 1996

## NSAID references:

- Murphy PJ, Myers BL, Badia P, Nonsteroidal anti-inflammatory drugs alter body temperature and suppress melatonin in humans, *Physiol Behav*, 59:133-139, 1996
- Gibson GR, Whitacre EB, Ricotti CA, Colitis induced by nonsteroidal anti-inflammatory drugs, *Arch Intern Med*, 152;625-632, 1992

- Mammen L, Schmidt CP, Photosensitivity reactions: a case report involving NSAIDs, *Amer Fam Phys* 52:575-579, Aug 1995
- Shankel SW, Johnson DC, Shankel TL, O'Neil WM, Acute renal failure and glomerulopathy caused by nonsteroidal anti-inflammatory drugs, *Arch Intern Med*, 152:986-990, 1992
- Gutch CF, Nonsteroidal anti-inflammatory agents and acute renal failure, *Arch Intern Med*, 156:2414, Nov 25, 1996
- Guttham SP, Rodriguez LAG, Raiford DS, et al, Nonsteroidal anti-inflammatory drugs and the risk of hospitalization for acute renal failure, *Arch Intern Med*, 156:2433-2439, Nov 25, 1996
- Goodwin SD, Glenny RW, Nonsteroidal anti-inflammatory drug-associated pulmonary infiltrates with eosinophilia, *Arch Intern Med*, 1;52:1521-1524, 1992
- Quiralte J, Blanco C, Castillo R, Delgado J, Carrillo T, Intolerance to nonsteroidal anti-inflammatory drugs: Results of controlled drug challenges in 98 patients, *Ann Aller* 98:3:678, Sept 1996 (periorbital angioedema was the most frequent symptom)
- Singh G, Ramey DR, Morfeld D, Shi H, Hatoum HT, Fries JF, Gastrointestinal tract complication of nonsteroidal anti-inflammatory drug treatment in rheumatoid arthritis, *Arch Intern Med*, 156:1530-1536, July 22, 1996
- Goldenberg DL, Fibromyalgia syndrome, *J Amer Med Assoc*, 257:20, 2782-2787, May 22/29, 1987; and editorial, Fibromyalgia, JAMA, ibid 2802-2803
- Newman N, et al, Acetabular bone destruction related to non-steroidal anti-inflammatory drugs, *Lancet 2*; 8445:11-14, 1985
- Woldes T, et al, Randomized placebo-controlled study of stopping second-line drugs in rheumatoid arthritis. *Lancet*, 347-352, 1996
- American College of Rheumatology, Issues and management guidelines for arthritis of the hip and knee, Amer Fam Phys, 53;3:985-986, Feb 15, 1996

## UltraInflamX references:

HealthComm will provide physicians with further references (see resources for number and address)

- Chan MM-Y, Inhibition of tumor necrosis factor by curcumin, a phytochemical, *Biochem Pharmacol*, 1995; 11:1151-6
- Huang M-T, Lysz T, Rerraro T, Conney AH, et al, Inhibitory effects of curcumin on in vitro lipoxygenase and cyclooxygenase activities in mouse epidermis, *Cancer Res*, 1991; 51:813-9
- Susan M, Rao MNA, Induction of glutathione S-transferase activity by curcumin in mice, *Drug Res* 1992; 42(7): 962-4
- Satoskar RR, Shah SJ, Shenoy SG, Evaluation of anti-inflammatory property of curcumin (diferuloyl methane) in patients with postoperative inflammation, *Intern J Clin Pharmaocol Toxicol*, 1986; 24:651-4
- Deodhar SD, Sethi R, Srimal RC, Preliminary study on anti-rheumatic activity of curcumin (diferuloyl methane), *Ind J Med Res*, 1980;71(12):632-4

- Skaper SD, Fabris M, Ferrari V, Leon A, et al, Quercetin protects cutaneous tissue-associated cell types including sensory neurons form oxidative stress induced by glutathione depletion: cooperative effects of ascorbic acid. *Free Rad Biol Med* 1997:22(4): 669-678

- Lichtman SN, Wang J, Sartor RB, et al, Reactivation of arthritis induced by small bowel bacterial overgrowth in rats: role of cytokines, bacteria, and bacterial polymers, *Infect Immunity,* 1995; 63:2295-2301

- Hazenberg MP, Intestinal flora bacteria and arthritis: why the joint? *Scand J Rheumatol,* 1995:24:207-11

- Srivastava KC, Mustafa T, Ginger (Zingiber officinale) in rheumatism ad musculoskeletal disorders, *Med Hypotheses* 1992; 39:342-8

- Ko TC, Beauchamp D, Thompson JC, et al, Glutamine is essential for epidermal growth factor-stimulated intestinal cell proliferation, *Surgery* 1993:114:147-154

### Kyo-Green references:

- Durham JJ, Ogata J, Nakajima s, et al, Degradation of organophosphorus pesticides in aqueous extracts of young green barley leaves (Hordeum vulgare), *J Sci Food Agric,* 1311-14, 1999

- Mitsuyama K, Saiki T, Kanauchi O, et al, Treatment of ulcerative colitis with germinated barley foodstuff feeding: A pilot study, *Alimentary Pharmacol Therapy,* 12:1225-30, 1998

- Cremer L, Herold A, Avram D, et al, Inhibitory capacity of some fractions isolated from a green barley extract upon TNF alpha production by cells of the THP-1 human monocytes line, *Roumanian Arch Miobiol Immunol,* 55:285-94, 1996

- Chemomorsky S, Segelman A, Poretz RD, Effect of dietary chlorophyll derivatives on mutagenesis and tumor cell growth, *Teratogenesis, Carcinogenesis and Mutagenesis,* 19:313-22, 1999

- Miyake T, Hagiwara H, et al, Possible inhibition of atherosclerosis by a flavonoid isolated from young green barley leaves, in *Functional Foods for Disease Prevention, Vol 2 : Medicinal Foods and Other Plants,* Shibamoto T, Terao J, Osawa T (eds.), American Chemical Society, 178-86, 1998

### SeaVive references (many more available from company):

- Playford RJ, Floyd DN, Marchbank T, et al, Bovine colostrum is a health food supplement which prevents NSAID induced gut damage, *Gut* 44(5): 653-8, May 1999

### Cox references:

- Langreth R, Drug makers zero in on new treatments that may slow the progress of arthritis, *Wall Street Journal,* b1, May 21, 1996

- Seibert K, Masferrer JL, Role of inducible cyclooxygenase (COX-2) in inflammation, *Receptor* 4:17-23, 1994

- Glaser K, Sung ML, O'Neill K, Belfast M, Hartman D, Carlson R, Kreft A, Kubrak d, et al, Etodolac selectively inhibits human prostaglandin G/H synthase 2 (PGHS-2) versus human PGHS-1, *Europ J Pharmacol*, 281:107-111, 1995

### Tylenol references:
- Easton T, et al, J&J's dirty little secret, *Forbes*, 42-44, Jan 12, 1998

### Lyprinol references:
- Gibson SLM, Gibson RG, The treatment of arthritis with a lipid extract of *Perna canaliculus*: a randomized trial. *Compl Ther Med*, 6:122-6, 1998
- Whitehouse MW, Macrides TA, et al, Anti-inflammatory activity of a lipid fraction (Lyprinol) from the NZ green-lipped mussel, *Inflammopharmacology*, 5; 237-246, 1997
- Rainsford KD, Whitehouse MW, Gastroprotective and anti-inflammatory properties of green-lipped mussel (*Perna canaliculus*) preparation, *Arzn Forsch*, 30-: 2128-32, 1980
- Gibson RG, Gibson S, Conway V, Chappel D, *Perna canaliculus* in the treatment of arthritis, *Practitioner*, 224:955-60, 1980
- Miller TE, Dodd J, Ormrod DJ, Geddes R, Anti-inflammatory activity of glycogen extracted from *Perna Canaliculus* (N.Z. green-lipped mussel), *Agents Actions* 38:C139-C142, 1993
- Kosugi T, Tsugi K, Ishida H, Yamaguchi T, Isolation of an anti-inflammatory substance from green-lipped mussel (*Perna canaliculus*), *Chem Pharm Bull* 34:4825-4828, 1986
- Macrides TA, et al, The anti-inflammatory effects of omega 3 tetraenoic fatty acids isolated form a lipid extract (Lyprinol) from the New Zealand green-lipped mussel. Abs, 88th American Oil Chemists Society Annual Meeting, Seattle WA, May 1997
- Whitehouse MW, Roberts MS, Brooks PM, Over the counter (OTC) oral remedies for arthritis and rheumatism: how effective are they? *Inflammopharmacology* 7; 2:89-105, 1999

### Power Relief and Malic Acid Plus/Boswellia references:
- Altura BM, Brodsky MA, Seelig MS, et al, Magnesium: Growing in clinical importance, *Patient Care*, 130-150, Jan 15, 1994
- Tso K, Barish RA, Magnesium: Clinical consideration, *J Emerg Med*, 10:735-45, 1992
- Abraham GE, Flechas JD, Management of fibromyalgia: rationale for the use of magnesium and malic acid, *J Nutr Med* 3:49-59, 1992
- Russell J, Michalek JE, Flechas JD, Abraham GE, Treatment of fibromyalgia syndrome with SuperMalic™: A randomized, double blind, placebo controlled, crossover pilot study, *J Rheumatol* 22:953-958, 1995

• Sahley BJ, *Malic Acid and Magnesium for Fibromyalgia and Chronic Pain Syndrome*, Pain & Stress Publ., San Antonio TX, 1996, 1-800-669-2256

• Fox A, fox B, Smith L, *DLPA To End Chronic Pain and Depression*, Pocket Books, NY, 1985

• Murray M, Pizzorno J, *Encylcopedia of Natural Medicine*, 2nd Ed., Prima Publishing, Rocklin CA, 1998

• Rogers SA, *Depression Cured At Last!*, Prestige Publ, Syracuse, NY, 1-800-846-6687, 1998

• Passwater RA, South J, *5-HTP: The Natural Serotonin Solution*, Keats Publ., 1998, New Canaan CT or 1-800-669-CALM

• Levine JD, Gordon NC, Fields HL, et al, The narcotic antagonist naloxone enhances clinical pain, *Nature* 272:826-7, 1978

• Budd K, Use of D-phenylalanine an enkephalinase inhibitor, in the treatment of intractable pain, *Advances in Pain Research and Therapy*, 5:3-5-8, JJ Bonica et al, Raven Press, NY, 1983

• Balagot TS, Ehrenpreis S, Greenberg J, et al, Analgesia in mice and humans by D-phenylalanine: Relation to inhibition of enkephalin degradation and enkephalin levels, *Advances in Pain Research and Therapy*, vol 5, 289-93, JJ Bonica et al, Raven Press, NY, 1983

• Hyodo M, Kitade T, Hosoka E, Study on the enhanced analgesic effect induced by phenylalanine during acupuncture analgesia in humans, *Advances in Pain Research and Therapy*, vol 5, 557-82, JJ Bonica et al, Raven Press, NY, 1983

• Ehrenpreis S, Balagot RC, Comaty JE, Myles SB, Naloxone reversible analgesia in mice produced by D-phenylalanine and hydrocinnamic acid inhibitors of carboxypeptidase A, *Advances in Pain Research and Therapy*, 3: 479-88, 1978

• Singh GB, Aral CK, Pharmacology of an extract of salai guggal ex-Boswellia serrata, a new non-steroidal anti-inflammatory agent, *Agents Actions*, 18:407-412, 1986

• Sharma ML, Bani S, Singh GB, Anti-arthritic activity of boswellic acids in bovine serum albumin (BSA)-induced arthritis, *Int J Immunopharm*, 11; 9:647-52, 1989

• Ammon HPT, Safayhi H, Mack T, Sabvieraj, Mechanism of antiinflammatory actions of curcumin and boswellic acids, *J Ethnopharmacol*, 38:113-19, 1993

• Safayhi H, Mack T, Sabieraj T, Anazodo MI, Subramanian LR, Ammon HPT, Boswellic acids: novel, specific, nonredox inhibotors of 5-lipoxygenase. *J Pharmacol Exp Thera* 261:1143-1146, 1992

• Etzel R, special extract of Boswellia serrata (H15) in the treatment of rheumatoid arthritis, *Phytomedicine*, 3; 1:91-94, 1996

• Sharma ML, Khajuria A, Atal CK, et al, Effect of Salai Guggal ex-Boswellia serrata on cellular and humoral immune responses and leucocyte migration, *Agents and Actions* 24; 1/2:161-3, 1988

## Chapter 5
## Glucosamine sulfate references:

- Lopes VA, Vaz AL, Double-blind clinical evaluation of the relative efficacy of ibuprofen and glucosamine sulphate in the management of osteoarthritis of the knee in out-patients, *Curr Med Res Opin,* 8:145-149, 1982

- Pujalte JM, Llavore EP, Ylescupidez FR, Double-blind clinical evaluation of oral glucosamine sulphate in the basic treatment of osteoarthrosis, *Curr Med Res Opin,* 7:110-114, 1980

- D'Ambrosio E, Casa B, Bompasi R, et al, Glucosamine sulphate: a controlled clinical investigation in arthrosis, *Pharmatherapeutica,* 2:504-508, 1981

- Tapadinhas MJ, Rivera IC, Bignamini AA, Oral glucosamine sulphate in the management of arthrosis: report on a multi-centre open investigation in Portugal. *Pharmatherapeutica,* 3:157-168, 1982

- Setnikar I, Antireactive properties of "chondroprotective" drugs, *Int J Tiss Reac* XIV (5) 253-261, 1992

- Muller-Fassbender H, et al, Glucosamine sulfate compared to ibuprofen in osteoarthritis of the knee, *Osteoarthritis Cartilage* 2:61-69, 1994

## Mobil-Ease references:

- Sreejayan RMN, Nitric oxide scavenging by curcuminoids, *J Pharm Pharmacol* 49; 1:105-7, Jan 1997

- Ammon HPT, Wahl MA, Pharmacology of Curcuma longa, *Planta Medica* 57:1-7, 1991

- Murray M, Pizzorno J, *Encylcopedia of Natural Medicine,* 2nd Ed., Prima Publishing, Rocklin CA, 1998

- Plummer SM, Holloway KA, Manson MM, Munks RJ, et al, Inhibition of cyclo-oxygenase 2 expression in colon cells by the chemopreventive agent curcumin involves inhibition of NF-kappaB activation via the NIK/1KK signaling complex, *Oncogene* 18; 44:6013-20, Oct 28, 1999

- Sidhu GS, Singh AK, Thaloor D, et al, Enhancement of wound healing by curcumin in animals, *Wound Repair Regen* 6; 2:167-77, Mar-Apr 1998

- Sidhu GS, Mani H, Gaddipati JP, Singh AK, et al, Curcumin enhances would healing in streptozotocin induced diabetic rats and genetically diabetic mice, *Wound Repair Regen* 7; 5:362-74, Sep-Oct 1999

- Kim SJ, Han D, Moon KD, Rhee JS, Measurement of superoxide dismutase-like activity of natural antioxidants, *Biosci Biotechnol Biochem* 59; 5:822-6, May 1995

- Safayhi H, Mack T, Sabieraj J, Anazodo MI, et al, Boswellic acids: novel, specific, nonredox inhibitors of 5-lipoxygenase, *J Pharmcaol Exp Ther* 261; 3:1143-6, Jun 1992

- Kapil A, Moza N, Anticomplementary activity of boswellic acids – and inhibitor of C3-convertase of the classical complement pathway, *Int J Immunopharmcol* 14; 7:1139-43, Oct 1992

- Wildfeuer A, Neu IS, Safayhi H, et al, Effects of boswellic acids extracted from a herbal medicine on the biosynthesis of leukotrienes and the course of experimental autoimmune encephalomyelitis, *Arzneimittelforschung* 48; 6:668-74, Jun 1998

• Srivastava KC, Extracts from two frequently consumed spices—cumin (Cuminum cyminum) and turmeric (Curcuma longa) — inhibit platelet aggregation and alter eicosanoid biosynthesis in human blood platelets, *Prostaglandins Leukot Essent Fatty Acids* 37; 1:57-64, Jul 1989

• Ammon HP, Safayhi H, Mack T, Sabieraj J, Mechanism of antiinflammatory actions of curcumine and boswellic acids, *J Ethnophamacol* 38; 2-3:113-9, Mar 1993

• Srivastava KC, Bordia A, Verma SK, Curcumin, a major component of food spice turmeric (Curcuma longa) inhibits aggregation and alters eicosanoid metabolism in human blood platelets, *Prostaglandins Leukot Essent Fatty Acids* 52; 4:223-7, Apr 1995

• Rohnert U, Schneider W, Elstner EF, Superoxide-dependent and –independent nitrite formation from hydroxylamine: inhibition by plant extracts, *Z Naturforsch* [C] 53; 3-4:241-9, Mar-Apr 1998

• Huang MT, Lysz T, Ferraro T, Conney AH, et al, Inhibitory effects of curcumin on in vitro lipoxygenase and cyclooxygenase activities in mouse epidermis, *Cancer Res* 51:813-19, 1991

• Mukhopadhyay A, Basu N, Gujral PK, et al, Anti-inflammatory and irritant activities of curcumin analogues in rats, *Agents Actions*, 12:508, 1982

• Bassleer C, et al, Stimulation of proteoglycan production by glucosamine sulfate in chondrocytes isolated form human osteoarthritic articular cartilage in vitro, *Osteoarhtritis Cartilage* 6; 6: 427-34, Nov 1998

• Qui GX, et al, Efficacy and safety of glucosamine sulfate versus ibuprofen in patients with knee osteoarthritis, *Arznitmettelforschung* 48; 5:469-74, May 1998

• Da Camara CC, Dowless GV, Glucosamine sulfate for osteoarthritis. *Ann Pharmacother* 32; 5:580-7, May 1998

• Deal CL, Moskowitz RW, Nutraceuticals as therapeutic agents in osteoarthritis. The role of glucosamine, chondriotin sulfate, and collagen hydrolysate, *Rheum Dis Clin North* Am 25; 2:379-95, May 1999

• Delafuente JC, Glucaosamine in the treatment of osteoarthritis, *Rheum Dis Clin North Am* 26; 1:1-11, vii, Feb 2000

## GAGs/ MSM/SAMe references:

• Leeb BF, et al, A meta-analysis of chondroitin sulfate in the treatment of osteoarthritis, *J Rheumatol* 27; 1:205-11, Jan 2000

• Ronca F, et al, Anti-inflammatory activity of chondroitin sulfate, *Osteoarthritis Cartilage*, 6 suppl A: 14-21, May 1998

• Murray M, The true arthritis cure; glucosamine sulfate vs. other forms of glucosamine and chondroitin sulfate, *Amer J Natural Med*, Arthritis Special Edition, 10-13, 1997

• Trentham DE, Dynesius-Trentham RA, et al, Effects of oral administration of type II collagen on rheumatoid arthritis, *Science* 261:1727-1730, 24 Sept 1993

• Prudden JF, Balassa LL, The biological activity of bovine cartilage preparations, *Semin Arthritis Rheum*, 3; 4:287-321, 1974

• Prudden JF, Allen J, The clinical acceleration of healing with a cartilage preparation; a controlled study, *J Amer Med Assoc*, 192:352-356, 1965

• Wolarsky E, Finke SR, Prudden JF, Acceleration of wound healing with cartilage; immunological considerations, *Proc Soc Exp Biol Med* 123:536, 1966

• Barnett ML, Conbitchi D, Trentham DE, A pilot trial of oral type II collagen in the treatment of juvenile rheumatoid arthritis, *Arthr & Rheumat*, 39; 4:623-628, Apr 1996

• Oberschelp U, Individual arthrosis therapy is possible, *Therapiewoche* 35:5094-5097, 1985

• Rosen J, Sherman WT, Prudden JF, Thorbecke GJ, Immunoregulatory effects of Catrix, *J Biol Response Modifiers*, 7:498-512, 1988

• Durie BG, Soehnlen B, Prudden JF, Antitumor activity of bovine cartilage extract (Catrix-S) in the human tumor stem cell assay, *J Biol Response Modifiers*, 4:590-595, 1985

• Jacob S, et al, *The Miracle of MSM: The Natural Solution for Pain*, Putnam, NY, 1999

• Lawrence R, Methylsulfonylmethane. A double-blind study of its use in degenerative arthritis, *Internat J Anti-Aging Med* 1; 1:50, 1998

• Mindell EL, *The MSM Miracle*, Keats Publ, New Canaan CT, 1997, or Pain & Stress Center, San Antonio, 1-800-669-CALM

• Ley BM, *The Forgottten Nutrient MSM: On Our Way Back To Health With Sulfur*, 1998, BL Publications, Temecula CA 92592, (909) 694-6283 or 1-800-669-CALM

• Walker M, *DMSO, Nature's Healer*, Avery Publ, Garden City NJ, 1993 or Pain & Stress Center, 1-800-669-CALM

• Gutierrez S, et al, SAMe restores the changes in the proliferation and in the synthesis of fibronectin and proteoglycans induced by tumor necrosis factor alpha on cultured rabbit synovial cells, *Brit J Rheumatol*, 37:27-31, 1997

• Gloriosos S, et al, Double-blind multicenter study of the activitry of S-adenosylmethionine in hip and knee osteoarthritis, *Int J Clin Pharmacol Res*, 5:39-49, 1985

• Osteoarthritis: the clinical picture, pathogenesis and management with studies on a new therapeutic agent, S-adenosylmethionine, *Amer J Med*, 83 (Suppl 5A), 1987 (includes numerous studies)

• Domljan Z, et al, A double-blind multicentre study of the activity of ademethionine vs naproxen in activated gonarthosis, *Int J Pharmacol Ther Toxicol*, 27,:329-333, 1989

• Marcolongo R, et al, Double-blind multicentre study of the activity of S-adenosylmethionine in hip and knee osteoarthritis, *Curr Ther Res* 5:39-49, 1985

• Tavoni A, Vitali C, Bombardieri S, Paero G, Evaluation of S-adenosylmethionine in primary fibromyalgia: a double-blind crossover study, *Amer J Med*, 83 (Suppl 5A): 107-110, 1987

• Jacobsen S, et al, Oral S-adenosylmethionine in primary fibromyalgia. Double blind clinical evaluation, *Scand J Rheumatol*, 20:294-302, 1991
• SAMe Part 4: Treatment for arthritis, *Life Extension*, 7-8, 57-59, Sept 1997 (1 800-544-4440)

## Boron references:

• Newnham RE, *Away With Arthritis*, Vantage Press, NY, 1994, or The Arthritis Trust of America, 5106 Old Harding Road, Franklin TN
• Newnham RE, Essentiality of boron for healthy bones and joints, *Environ Health Perspect*, 102 (Suppl 7): 83-85, Nov 1994
• Travers RL, Rennie GC, Newnham RE, Boron and arthritis: The results of a double-blind pilot study, *J Nutrit Med*, 1:127-132, 1990
• Nielsen FH, Gallagher SK, Johnson LK, Nielsen EJ, Boron enhances and mimics some of the effects of estrogen therapy in postmenopausal women, *J Trace Elem, Exp Med* 5:237-46, 1992
• Meacham SL, et al, Effect of boron supplementation blood and urinary calcium, magnesium, and phosphorus, urinary boron in athletic and sedentary women, *Am J Clin Nutr* 61:341-5, 1995

## Silicon/Biosil references:

• Carlisle EM, In vivo requirement for silicon in articular cartilage and connective tissue formation in the chick, *J Nutr* 106:478-484, 1970
• Carlisle EM, Silicon as an essential trace element in animal nutrition, *Silicon Biochemistry*, CIBA Foundation, 1986
• Carlisle EM, Silicon: A possible growth factor in bone calcification, *Sci* 167:279-80, 1970
• Carlisle EM, Curran MJ, Effect of dietary silicon and aluminum on silicon and aluminum levels in rat brain, *Alzhemier Disases and Associated Disorders*, 1:83-9, 1987
• Eisinger J, Clairet D, Effects of silicon, fluoride, etidronate and magnesium on bone mineral density: a retrospective study, *Magnesium Research*, 6:247-9, 1993
• Calomme MR, Cos P, Vanden Berge DA, et al, Comparative bioavailability study of silicon supplements in healthy subjects, *J Parental Enteral Nutr* 22:228-233, 1998
• Hott M, de Pollak C, short-term effects of organic silicon on trabecular bone in mature ovariectomized rats, *Calcified Tissue International*, 53:174-9, 1993
• Loeper J, Goy-Loeper J, et al, The antiatheromatous action of silicon, *Atherosclerosis*, 33:397-408, 1979
• Schwarz K, A bound form of silicon in glycosaminoglycans and polyuronides, *Proc Natl Acad Sci* 70:1608-1612, 1973
• Williams RJ, Introduction to silicon chemistry and biochemistry, in *Silicon Biochemistry, CIBA Foundation Symposium 121*, 24-39, John Wiley & Sons, NY

398

## Arthrogen/Niacinamide references:

• Jonas WB, Rapoza CP, Blair WF, The effect of niacinamide on osteoarthritis: a pilot study, *Inflamm Res* 1996; 45(7): 330-4
• Kroger H, Hauschild A, Ohde M, et al, Enhancing the inhibitory effect of nicotinamide upon collagen II induced arthritis in mice using N-acetylcysteine, *Inflamm* 1999; 23(2): 111-5
• Pero RW, Axelsson B, Siemann D, et al, Newly discovered anti-inflammatory properties of the benzamides and nicotinamides, *Mol Cell Biochem* 1999; 193(1-2):119-24
• Morin I, Li WQ, Su M, et al, Induction of stromelysin gene expression by tumor necrosis factor-a is inhibited by dexamethasone, salicylate, and N-acetylcysteine in synovial fibroblasts, *J Pharmacol Exp Ther*, 289; 3:1634-49, 1999

## Rebuilding membrane references:

• Kremer JM, N-3 fatty acid supplements in rheumatoid arthritis, *Am J Clin Nutr*, 71 (supple): 349s-351s, 2000
• Belch JJ, Hill A, Evening primrose oil and borage oil in rheumatologic conditions, *Am J Clin Nutr*, 71 (supple): 352s-356s, 2000
• Blok WL, Katan MB, Meer JWM, Modulation of inflammation and cytokine production by dietary (n-3) fatty acids, *J Nutr* 126:1515-33, 1996
• Clandinin MT, Jumpsen J, Relationship between fatty acid acretion, membrane composition and biological functions, *J Ped* 125; 5:S25-S32, 1994
• Shamsuddin AKM, IP6: An anti—cancer agent and more, *Natural Medicine* 1; 5:9-15, 1998

## Chapter 6

• U.S. Department of Health & Human Services, Agency for Toxic Substances and Disease Registry, *Case studies in environmental medicine*, Vol. 10, *Cadmium Toxicity*, 1-19, June 1990
• Sullivan JB, Kreiger GR, eds., *Hazardous Materials Toxicology: Clinical Principles of Environmental Health*, Williams & Wilkins, Baltimore, 1992
• Waalkes MP, Rehm S, Cherian MG, Repeated cadmium exposures enhance the malignant progression of ensuing tumors in rats, *Toxicolog Sci* 54:110-120, 2000
• Bernard A, Roels HA, Lauwerys R, et al, Characterization of the proteinuria in cadmium exposed workers, *Int Arch Occup Environ Health*, 38:19, 1976
• Kazantzis G, The mutagenic and carcinogenic effects of cadmium: an update, *Toxicol Environ Chem*, 15:83-100, 1987
• Nogawa K, Tsurintani I, Ishizaki M, et al, Mechanism for bone disease found in inhabitants environmentally exposed to cadmium: decreased serum 1a, 25-dihydroxyvitamin D level, *Int Arch Occup Environ Health*, 59:21-30, 1987
• Hallenbeck WH, Human health effects of exposure to cadmium, *Experientia*, 40:136-42, 1984

- Kido T, Honda R, Tsuritani, et al, Progress of renal dysfunction in inhabitants environmentally exposed to cadmium, *Arch Environ Health,* 43:213-17, 1988
- Sherlock JC, Cadmium in foods and the diet, *Experientia,* 40:152-6, 1984
- Yost KJ, Cadmium, the environment and human health: an overview, *Experientia,* 40:157-64, 1984
- Pelletier L, et al, Autoreactive T cells in mercury–induced autoimmunity, *J Immunol* 1988; 140: 750-4
- Brown EH, Hansen RT, *The Key To Ultimate Health,* 1998, Advanced Health Research Publ, Fullerton CA, 1-800-846-6687 or 1-888-792-1102
- Gregus A, Stein AF, Varga R, Klaasen CD, Effect of lipoic acid in biliary excretion of glutathione and metals, *Toxicol Appl Pharmacol,* 114;1:88-96, 1992
- Pelletier L, et al, Autoreactive T cells in mercury-induced autoimmunity, *J Immunol,* 140:750-754, 1988
- Summers AO, et al, Genetic linkage of mercury and antibiotic resistance in intestinal bacteria, *Antimicrobial Agents Chemother,* 37:825-834,1993
- Kolata G, New suspect in bacterial resistance: amalgam, *New York Times,* C1, Apr 27, 1993
- Sood PP, et al, Cholesterol and triglyceride fluctuations in mice tissues during methylmercury intoxication and monothiols and vitamin therapy, *J Nutrit Environ Med,* 1997, 7:155-162
- Salonen JT, et al, Intake of mercury from fish, lipid peroxidation, and the risk of myocardial infarction and coronary, cardiovascular, and early death in eastern Finnish men, *Circulation,* 91:645-655, 1995
- Vimy M, et al, Mercury released from dental "silver" fillings provokes an increase in mercury and antibiotic-resistant bacteria in oral and intestinal flora of primates, *Antimicrob Agents Chemother* 37:825-34, 1993
- Phillips H, Cole PV, Lettin AW, Cardiovascular effects of implanted acrylic bone cement, *Br Med J,* 3:460, 1971
- Gresham GA, Kuczmski A, Cardiac arrest and bone cement, Br Med J, 3:465, 1980
- Kepes ER, Underwood PS, Becsey L, Intraoperative death associated with acrylic bone cement, *J Amer Med Assoc,* 222:576, 1972
- Hyland J, Robbins RHC, Cardiac arrest and bone cement, *Br Med J,* 4:176, 1970
- Oppenheimer BS, Oppenheimer ET, Danishefsky I, Malignant tumors resulting from embedding plastics in rodents, *Sci,* 118:305, 1953
- Andrews LS, Clary JJ, Review of toxicity of multifunctional acrylates, *J Toxicol Environ Health,* 19:149-64, 1986

**FIR and sauna detoxification references:**
- Inoue S, Kabaya M, Biological activities caused by far-infrared radiation, A review, *Int J Biometerol,* 33:145-150, 1989
- Perera FP, Environment and cancer: Who are susceptible?, *Science* 278:1068-73, Nov 7, 1997 (95% ca is environ and diet)

- U.S. Environmental Protection Agency, *National Human Adipose Agency, Vols I-V*, EPA-560/5-86-039, Dec. 1986
- Coburn T, Vom Saal FS, Soto AM, Developmental effects of endocrine-disrupting chemicals in wildlife and humans, *Environ Health Perspect* 101:378-84, 1993
- Rea, WJ, Thermal chamber depuration and physical therapy in: *Chemical Sensitivity, Volume 4*, chapter 35, pp 2433-2479, CRC Press, Boca Raton, 1997
- Heuser C, Vojdani A, Enhancement of natural killer cell activity and T and B cell function by buffered vitamin C (ultra potent-C), in patients exposed to toxic chemicals: the role of protein kinase-C, *Immunopharmacol Immunotoxicol* 19:291, 1997
- Randolph TG, *Human Ecology and Susceptibility to the Chemical Environment*, Thomas Co, 1962, Springfield IL
- U.S. Environmental Protection Agency, *Broad Scan Analysis of the FY82 National Human Adipose Tissue Survey Specimens*, EPA-560/5-86-035, Dec 1986;
- *EPA Characterization of HRGC/MS unidentified peaks from the analysis of human adipose tissue*, EPA-560/5-87-002A, May 1987
- U.S. Environmental Protection Agency, *Chemicals identified in human biological media, a data base.* EPA-560/5-84-003, 1984.
- Kraul I, Karlong P, Persistent organochlorinated compounds in human organs collected in Denmark 1972-1973, *Acta Pharmacol Toxicol*, 38:38-48, 1976
- Morgan D, Roan CC, The metabolism of DDT in man, *Essays in Toxicol*, 5:39-97, 1974
- Findlay GM, deFreitas ASW, DDT movement from adipocyte to muscle cells during lipid utilization, *Nature* 229:63-65, 1971
- McVicker M, *Sauna Detoxification Therapy*, 1997, McFarland & Co, Box 611, Jefferson NC 28640
- James R, Cohn MS, Emmett EA, The excretion of trace metals in human sweat, *Ann Clin Lab Sci*, 8; 4:270-74, 1978
- Colucci AV, et al, Pollutant burdens and biological response, *Arch Environ Health*, 27:151-4, 1973
- Wolff MS, Anderson HA, Rosenman KD, Selikoff IJ, Equilibrium of polybrominated biphenyl (PPB) residues in serum and fat of Michigan residents, *Bull Environ Contam Toxicol*, 21; 6:775-81, 1979
- Schnare DW, Denk G, Shields M, Brunton S, Evaluation of a detoxification regimen for fat stored xenobiotics, *Med Hypoth*, 9:265-82, 1982
- Schnare DW, Ben M, Shields MG, Body burden reductions of PCBs, PBBs and cholorinated pesticides in human subjects *Ambio*, 13; 5-6:378-80, 1984
- Kilburn KH, Warsaw RH, Shields MG, Neurobehavioral dysfunction in firemen exposed to polychlorinated biphenyls (PCBs): Possible improvement after detoxification, *Arch Environ Health*, 44; 6:345-350, 1989b
- Wolff MS, Anderson HA, Selikoff IJ, Human tissue burdens of halogneated aromatic chemicals in Michigan, *J Amer Med Assoc*, 247:2112-2116, 1982

- Root DE, Reducing toxic body burdens advancing in innovative technique, *Occup Health Safety News Dig* 2;4, Apr 1986
- Root D, Lionelli GT, Excretion of a lipophilic toxicant through the sebaceous glands: a case report, *J Toxicol* 6; 1:13-17, 1987
- Cunliff WJ, et al, The effect of local temperature variations on the sebum excretion rate, *Brit J Derm* 83:650-4, 1970
- Vree TB, et al, Excretion of amphetamines in human sweat, *Arch Int Pharmacodyn*, 199:311-7, 1972
- Roehm DC, Effects of a program of sauna baths and megavitamins on adipose DDE and PCBs and on clearing of symptoms of agent orange (Dioxin) toxicity, *Clin Res* 31; 2:243A, 1983
- Williams M, et al, The effect of local temperature changes on sebum excretion rate of forehead surface lipid composition, *Brit J Dermatol*, 88:257-62, 1973
- Brain JD, Beck BD, Warren AJ (eds), *Variation In Susceptibility To Inhaled Pollutants*, Johns Hopkins University Press, 1988
- Metcalf RL, Sanborn J, LuP, Nye D, Laboratory model ecosystem studies of the degradation of fate of radiolabeled tri-, tetra-, and pentachlorobiphenyl compared with DDE, *Arch Environ Contam*, 3:151-63, 1971
- Schnare DW, Robinson PC, Reduction of hexacholorobenzens and polychlorinated bipheny human body burdens, International Agency for Research on Cancer, *Scientific Publication Series* (Oxford University Press), 77:597-603, 1986
- Rinsky RA, Smith AB, Hornung R, et al, Benzene and leukemia: an epidemiologic risk assessment, *N Engl J Med* 316:1044-50, 1987
- Oosterveld FGJ, Rasker JJ, van de Laar MAF, Koel GJ, Clinical effects of infrared whole-body hyperthermia in patients with rheumatic diseases, Departments of Rheumatology and Physiotherapy, Medisch Spectrum Twente and University Twente Enschede, P.O.Box 50 000, 7500 KA Enschede, The Netherlands
- Bellinger D, Levitron A, Waternaux C, Needleman H, Rabinowitz M, Longitudinal analyses of prenatal and postnatal lead exposure and early cognitive development, *N Engl J Med* 316:1037-43, 1987
- Lieberman AD, Craven MR, Reactive intestinal dysfunction syndrome (RIDS) caused by chemical exposures, *Arch Environ Health*, 53; 5:354-8, 1998
- Heckbert SR, Longstreth WT, Furberg CD, et al, The association of antihypertensive agents with MRI white matter findings and with modified min-mental state examination in older adults, *J Amer Geriatric Soc*, 1997; 45:1423-1433
- Stortbecker P, *Dental Caries As A Cause Of Nervous Disorders*, Bio-Probe, Inc., POB 58010, Orlando FL 32858-0160
- Hubbard LR, *Clear Body Clear Mind*, Bridge Publications, Los Angeles, 1-888-465-3396 (The originator to whom all the credit goes for sauna detox.)

## Chapter 7
## Fasting references:
- Kroker GP, Stroud RM, Marshall RT, et al, Fasting and rheumatoid arthritis: a multicentre study, *Clin Ecol*, 2:137-144, 1984

- Skoldstam L, Larsson L, Lindstrom FD, Effects of fasting and lactovegetarian diet on rheumatoid arthritis, *Scand J Rheumatol*, 18:83-123, 1984
- Palmblad J A, Antirheumatic effects of fasting, *Nutrition and Rheumatic Disease/Rheumatic Disease Clinics of North America*, 17; 2:351-362, May 1991
- Uden AM, et al, Neutrophil functions and clinical performance after total fasting in patients with rheumatoid arthritis, *Ann Rheum Dis*, 42; 1:45-51, 1983
- Sundquist T, et al, Influence of fasting on intestinal permeability and disease activity in patients with rheumatoid arthritis, *Scand J Rheumatol*, 11; 1:33-38, 1982
- Seignalet J, Diet, Fasting and rheumatoid arthritis, *Lancet*, 339:68-69, 1992

## Diet/Feeding references:

- Nussbaum E, *Recovery From Cancer*, Prestige Publ, Syracuse, NY, 1-800-846-6687
- Laughton MJ, Evans PJ, Halliwell B, Inhibition of mammalian 5-lipoxygenase and cyclo-oxygenase by flavonoids and phenolic dietary additives, *Biochem Pharmacol*, 42; 9:1673-1681, 1991
- Havsteen B, Flavonoids, a class of natural products of high pharmacological potency, *Biochem Pharmacol* 32; 7:1141-1148, 1983
- Nakagami T, Nanaumi-Tamura N, Shigehisa T, et al, Dietary flavonoids as potential natural biological response modifiers affecting the autoimmune system, *J Food Sci*, 60; 4:653-656, 1995
- Kjekdsen-Kragh J, Haugen M, Borchgrevink CF, Laerum E, Eek M, Mowinkel P, Hovi K, Forre O, Controlled trial of fasting and one-year vegetarian diet in rheumatoid arthritis, *Lancet* 338; 8772:899-902, 1991
- Panush RS, Food-induced ("allergic") arthritis: clinical and serologic studies, *J Rheumatol* 17:291-294, 1990
- Rogers SA, *You Are What You Ate*, Prestige Publishing, Box 3068, 3500 Brewerton Rd., Syracuse NY 13220, ph 1-800-846-6687
- Rogers SA, *The Cure Is In the Kitchen*, Prestige Publishing, Box 3068, 3500 Brewerton Rd., Syracuse NY 13220, ph 1-800-846-6687
- Rogers SA, *Tired Or Toxic?*, Prestige Publishing, Box 3068, 3500 Brewerton Rd., Syracuse NY 13220, ph 1-800-846-6687
- Rogers SA, *Wellness Against Odds*, Prestige Publishing, Box 3068, 3500 Brewerton Rd., Syracuse NY 13220, ph 1-800-846-6687
- Rogers SA, *The E.I. Syndrome, Revised*, Prestige Publishing, Box 3068, Syracuse NY 13220, phone 1-800-846-6687
- Jones V, Jacoby R, Cowley P, et al, Immune complexes in early arthritis, II. Immune complex constituents are synthesized in the synovium before rheumatoid factors, *Clin Exp Immunol* 49:31-40, 1982
- Paganelli R,Levinsky R, Brostoff J, et al, Immune complexes containing food proteins in normal and atopic subjects after oral challenge and effect of sodium cromoglycate on antigen absorption, *Lancet*, 1 1270-1272, 1979

- Paganelli R, Levinsky R, Atherton D, Detection of specific antigen within circulating immune complexes; validation of the assay and its application to food antigen-antibody subjects, *Clin Exp Immunol*, 46:44-53, 1981
- Darlington LG, Ramsey NW, Mansfield JR, Placebo-controlled blind study of dietary manipulation therapy in rheumatoid arthritis, *Lancet* 1:236-238, 1986
- O'Farrelly C, et al, IgA rheumatoid factor and IgG dietary protein antibodies are associated with rheumatoid arthritis, *Immunol Invest* 18:753-754, 1989
- Picq M, et al, Effect of two flavonoid compounds on central nervous system analgesic activity, *Life Sciences* 49:1979-1988, 1991
- Carter JP, Saxe GP, Newbold V, Peres CE, Campeau RJ, Bernal-Green L, Hypothesis: Dietary management may improve survival from nutritionally linked cancers based on analysis of representative cases, *J Amer Coll Nutr* 12; 3:209-226, 1993
- Neonan M, Helve T, Hanninen O, Effects of uncooked vegan food — "living food" on rheumatoid arthritis, a 3-month controlled randomized study, *Amer J Clin Nutr*, 56:762, 1992
- Darlington LG, Ramsey NW, Mansfield JR, Placebo-controlled, blind study of dietary manipulation therapy in rheumatoid arthritis, *Lancet*, 236-238, Feb. 1, 1986
- Adam O, Anti-inflammatory diet in rheumatic diseases, *Europ J Clin Nutr*, 49:703-717, 1995

**Water references:**
- Shirahata S, Kabayama S, Katakura Y, et al, Electrolyzed reduced water scavenges active oxygen species and protects DNA from oxidative damage, *Bioch Biophys Res Comm* 234:269-74, 1997
- Batmanghelidj F, *Your Body's Many Cries For Water*, Global Health Solutions, Inc., P.O. Box 3189, Falls Church VA 22043, 1995
- Bartmanhelidj F, Pain: a need for paradigm change, *Anticancer Res* 7; 5B: 971-990, 1987

**Alkalinizing references:**
- Shirahata S, Kabayama S, Katakura Y, et al, electrolyzed reduced water scavenges active oxygen species and protects DNA from oxidative damage, *Bioch Biophys Res Comm* 234:269-74, 1997
- Barefoot, R, *The Calcium Factor*, 1-800-THE-DIET
- Baroody TA, *Alkalinize or Die*, 1-800-794-5355 or 1-800-566-1522
- Anghileri LJ, Tuffet-Anghileri AM, eds, *The Role of Calcium in Biological Systems, Vol I*, CRC Press, Boca Raton FL, 1982
- Jarvis DC, *Folk Medicine*, Fawcett Publ, Greenwich CT, 1958

**Enzyme references:**
- Marsh, et al, Acute pancreatitis following cutaneous exposure to an organophosphate insecticide, *Amer J Gastroenterology*, 83:1158-1160, 1988

- Fillit, HM, et al, Antivascular antibodies in the sera of patients with senile dementia of the Alzheimer's type, *J Gerontol* 42(2): 180-184, 1987).

- Uffelmann K, Vogler W, Fruth C, The use of proteolytic enzymes in extra-articulator rheumatism, *General Medicine (Allgemein-Medizin)*, 19:4;151, 1990.

- Werk W, Horger I, The immune profile of rheumatoid arthritis patients before and after enzyme therapy (including a discussion of the mechanism of effectiveness), *Lab J Res Lab Med*, 7:273, 1980.

- Klein G, Pollmann G, Kullich W, Clinical experience with enzyme therapy in patients with rheumatoid arthritis in comparison with gold, *General Medicine (Allgemein-Medizin)*, 9:4:144-147, 1990

- Klein MW, Schwannn H, Kullich W, Enzyme therapy in chronic polyarthritis, *Natural and Holistic Medicine, Natur-Und Ganzheitsmedizin)* 1:112-116, 1988

- Miehlke K, Enzyme therapy in rheumatoid arthritis, *Natural and Holistic Medicine (Natur-Und Ganzheitsmedizin)* 1:108, 1988

- Netti C, Bandi GL, Pecile A, Anti-inflammatory action of proteolytic enzymes of animal, vegetable or bacterial origin administered orally compared with that of known antiphlogistic compounds, *Il Farmaco Ed P*, 27:453, 1972

- Rahn HD, Kilic M, The action of hydrolytic enzymes in traumatology. Results after two prospective randomized double blind studies, *General Physician (Allgemeinarzt)* 19; 4:183-187, 1990

- Reinbold H, Maehder K, The biological alternative in the treatment of inflammatory rheumatic disease, *J Gen Med (Zeitschr F Allgemeinmedizin)* 57:2397-2402, 1981

- Steffan C, Menzel J, Enzyme consumption from immune complexes, *J Rheumatology (Zeitschrift F Rheumatologie)* 42:249-255, 1989

- Vogler W, Enzyme therapy of soft tissue rheumatism. *Natural and Holistic Medicine, Natur-Und Ganzheitsmedizin)* 1:123-125, 1988

- Worschhauser S, Conservative therapy in sports injuries. Enzyme preparations for treatment and prophylaxis, *Gen Med (Allgemeinmedizin)* 19; 4:173, 1990

- Laffaioli RV, et al, Prognostic significance of circulating immune complexes in a long-term follow up of breast cancer patients, *Oncology*, 45:337-343, 1988.

- Ransberer K, Enzyme therapy of cancer, *Therapeutics (Dis Heilkunst)* 102:22-34, 1989.

- Seifert J, et al, Quantitative analysis about the absorption of trypsin, chymotrypsin, amylase, papain, and pancreatin in the G.I. tract after oral administration. *General Physician (Allgemeinarzt)*, 19:4, 132-137, 1990.

- Dittmar FW, Luh W, Treatment of fibrocystic mastopathy with hydrolytic enzymes, *Internat J Exp Clin Chemother*, 6:1, 9-20, 1993.

- Pastorino U, Hong WK, Eds, *Chemoimmuno Prevention of Cancer, 1st International Conference*, Vienna, Austria, 1990, Thieme Med Publ, 381 Park Ave S, NY, NY 10016, 1991.

- Dittmar FW, Weissenbacher ER, Therapy of adnexitis – enhancement of the basic antibiotic therapy with hydrolytic enzymes, *Internat J Feto-Maternal Med*, 2:3, 15-24, 1993.

- Wolf M, Ransberger K, *Enzyme Therapy*, 1972, Vantage Press, NY.
- Dasgupta MK, et al, Circulating immune complexes in multiple sclerosis: relation with disease activity, *Neurol* 32: 1000- 1004, 1982.
- Phelan JJ, et al, Celiac disease: the abolition of gliadin toxicity by enzymes from Aspergillus niger, *Clin Sci Molec Med* 53:35-43, 1977

## Chemical sensitivity references:
- Rogers SA, *The E.I. Syndrome, Revised*, Prestige Publishing, Box 3068, Syracuse, NY, 13220, prestigepublishing.com or 1-800-846-6687
- Rogers SA, *Chemical Sensitivity*, Prestige Publishing, Box 3068, Syracuse, NY, 13220, prestigpublishing.com or 1-800-846-6687
- Rogers SA, *The Scientific Basis of Selected Environmental Medicine Techniques*, Prestige Publishing, Box 3068, Syracuse, NY, 13220, prestigepublishing.com or 1-800-846-6687
- Rogers SA, *Tired or Toxic?*, Prestige Publishing, Box 3068, Syracuse, NY, 13220, prestigepublishing.com or 1-800-846-6687
- Rea WJ, *Chemical Sensitivity, Vol. 1-4*, CRC Press, Boca Raton FL, 1992-98
- Randolph TJ, *An Alternative Approach to Allergies*, 1-800-846-6687

## Nutritional references:
- Folkers K, Ellis JM, Watanabe T, Saji S, Kali M, Biochemical evidence for a deficiency of vitamin B6 in the carpal tunnel syndrome based on a cross-over clinical study. *Proc Natl Acad Sci USA*, 75:3410-3412, 1978
- Ellis JM, Folkers K, Levy, Shizukuishi S, Lewandowski J, et al, Response of vitamin B6 deficiency and carpal tunnel syndrome to pyridoxine, *Proc Natl Acad Sci USA*, 79:7494-7498, 1982
- Ellis JM, Folkers K, Clinical aspects of treatment of carpal tunnel syndrome with vitamin B6, *Ann New York Acad Sci* 585:302-320, 1990
- Shapiro JA, Koepsell TD, Voigt LF, Dugowson CE, Kestin M, Nelson JL, Diet and rheumatoid arthritis in women: a possible protective effect of fish consumption, *Epidemiology* 7:256-263, 1996
- Leventhal LJ, et al, Treatment of rheumatoid arthritis with gammalinolenic acid, *Ann Intern Med* 119:867-873, 1993 (dose used was 1.4 gm/d)
- Adam O, Review; Anti-inflammatory diet in rheumatic diseases, *Europ J Clin Nutr* 49:703-717, 1995
- McCarthy GM, Kenny D, Dietary fish oil and rheumatic diseases, *Seminars Arthr & Rheuma* 21; 6:368-375, June 1992
- Sperling RI, Dietary omega-3 fatty acids: the effects of lipid mediators of inflammation and rheumatoid arthritis, *Nutrition in Rheumatic Disease/Rheumatic Disease Clinics of North America*, 17; 2:373-389, May 1991
- Krewmer JM, Bigauoette J, Mickalek A, et al, Effect of manipulation of dietary fatty acids on clinical manifestation of rheumatoid arthritis, *Lancet* 1, 184-187, 1985

- Nielsen GI, et al, The effects of dietary supplementation with N-3 polysaturated fatty acids in patients with rheumatoid arthritis: A randomized, double-blind trial, *European J Clin Invest* 22:687-691, 1992
- Volker D, Garag, Dietary N-3 fatty acid supplementation in rheumatoid arthritis——mechanisms, clinical outcomes, controversies, and future directions, *J Clin Biochem Nutr*, 20:83-97, 1996
- Kremer JM, Jubiz, W, Lininger L, et al, Fish-oil fatty acid supplementation in active rheumatoid arthritis, *Ann Int Med*, 106; 4:497-502, 1987
- Tate G, Mandell BF, Zurier RB, et al, Suppression of acute and chronic inflammation by dietary gamma linolenic acid, *J Rheumatol* 16:729-733, 1989
- van er Tempel, H, Tulleken JE, van Rifswijk, et al, Effects of fish oil supplementation in rheumatoid arthritis, *Ann Rheum Dis*, 49:76-80, 1990
- Blok WL, Katan MB, Meer JWM, Modulation of inflammation and cytokine production by dietary (n-3) fatty acids, *J Nutr* 126:1515-33, 1996
- Clandinin MT, Jumpsen J, Relationship between fatty acid acretion, membrane composition and biological functions, *J Ped* 125; 5:S25-S32, 1994

## Aircast references:
- Peterson KS, Knees a sore spot for aging boomers, *USA Today*, Apr 17, 1997, 4D
- Stuessi E, et al, Biomechanical study of stabilization effect of Aircast ankle brace, *Int Series on Biomech* 6A: 159-164, 1987
- Coffman J, et al, A comparison of ankle taping and the Aircast sport stirrup on athletic performance, *Ath Train* 24:123, Sum 1989
- Gross M, et al, Comparison of Swede-O-Universal Ankle Support and Aircast Sport-Stirrup orthoses and ankle tape in restricting eversion-inversion before and after exercise, *J Orth Sport Phys Ther* 13:11-19, Jan 1991

## Chiropractic references:
- Meade TW, Dyer S, Browne W, Frank AO, Randomised comparison of chiropractic and hospital outpatient management for low back pain: results from extended follow up, *Brit Med J*, 311:349-351, 1995

## Infection references:
- DiFabio A, *Rheumatoid Diseases Cured At Last*, Franklin TN, 1982 Rheumatoid Disease Foundation, Rt 4, Box 137, Franklin TN 37064. Ask for the 1997 update, entitled only ARTHRITIS.
- The Arthritis Trust of America, 5106 Old Harding Rd, Franklin TN 37064-9400, phone 615-646-1030, has a huge and fascinating book list, including *Cell Wall Deficient Forms: Stealth Pathogens* (Mattman LH), *How To Deal With Back Pain & Rheumatoid Joint Pain* (Batmanghelidj F), *Oxygen Healing Therapies* (Altman N), *Hydrogen Peroxide Therapy* (Farr CH), *Root Canal Coverup* (Meinig G), etc. I suggest you start with DeFabio's 1997 update of his original book, merely called *Arthritis.*

- O'Dell JR, Treatment of rheumatoid arthritis with minocycline or placebo, *Arthritis & Rheumatism*, 40; 5:842-848, 1997
- Siegel LB, Gall EP, Viral infection as a cause of arthritis, *Amer Fam Phys*, 54; 6:2009-2015, Nov, 1, 1996
- Rook GAW, et al: A reapprisal of the evidence that rheumatoid arthritis and several other idiopathic diseases are slow bacterial infections, *Ann Rheum Dis* 52:S30-8; 1993
- Williams MH, Brostoff J, Roitt IM, Possible role of Mycoplasma fermentens in pathogenesis of rheumatoid arthritis, *Lancet* 2:277-80, 1970
- Van Barr HMJ, et al, Tetracyclines are potent scavengers of the superoxide radical, *Br J Dermatol* 117:131-4, 1987
- Greenwald RA, Goulb LM, Lavietes Be, et al, Tetracyclines inhibit human synovial collagenase in vivo and in vitro, *J Rheumatol* 14:28-32, 1987
- Golub LM, et al: Tetracyclines inhibit connective tissue breakdown: new therapeutic implications for an old family of drugs, *Crit Rev Oral Med Pathol* 2:297-322, 1991
- Hakkarainen K, et al, Mycoplasmas and arthritis, *Ann Rheumat Dis*, 51:1170-1172, 1992
- Rook GAW, et al, A reappraisal of the evidence that rheumatoid arthritis and several other idiopathic diseases are slow bacterial infections, *Ann Rheumat Dis*, 52:S30-S38, 1993
- Gaby AR, Alternative treatments for rheumatoid arthritis, *Alternative Medicine Review*, 4; 6:392-402, Dec 1999
- Jansson E, Makisara P, Vainio K, et al, An 8-Year study on mycoplasma in rheumatoid arthritis, *Ann Rheumat Dis*, 30:506-508, 1971
- Jansson E, Makisara P, Tuuri S, Mycoplasma antibodies in rheumatoid arthritis, *Scand J Rheuamtol* 4:1654-168, 1975
- Stuckey M, Quinn Pa, Gelfand EW, Identification of T-strain mycoplasma in a patient with polyarthritis, *Lancet* 2:917-920, 1978
- Cassell GH, Cole BD, Mycoplasmas as agents of human disease, *N Engl J Med*, 304:80-89, Jan 8, 1981
- Sewell KE, Furrie E, Trentham DE: The therapeutic effect of minocycline in experimental arthritis. Mechanism of action, *J Rheumatol* 33(Suppl): S106, 1991
- Kloppenburg M, Breedveld FC, Miltenburg AMM, et al, Antibiotics as disease modifiers in arthritis, *Clin Exper Rheumatol* 11 (suppl 8):S113-5, 1993
- Langevitz P, et al, Treatment of resistant rheumatoid arthritis with minocycline: An open study, *J Rheumatol* 19:1502-4, 1992
- Clark HW, et al, Detection of Mycoplasma antigens in immune complexes from rheumatoid arthritis synovial fluids, *Ann Allergy* 60:394-8, May 1988
- Clark HW, The potential role of mycoplasmas as auto-antigens and immune complexes in chronic vascular pathogenesis, *Am J Primatol* 24:235-243, 1991
- Greenwald RA, Goulb LM, Lavietes B, et al, Tetracyclines inhibit human synovial collagenase in vivo and in vitro, *J Rheumatol* 14:28-32, 1987

408

- Golub LM, et al, Tetracyclines inhibit connective tissue breakdown: new therapeutic implications for an old family of drugs, *Crit Rev Oral Med Pathol* 2:297-322, 1991

- Tilley BC, Alarcon GS, Heyse SP, et al, Minocycline in rheumatoid arthritis: a 48-week, double-blind, placebo-controlled trial, *Ann Intern Med*, 1995; 122:81-89

- Ingman T, Sorsa T, Suomalainen K, et al, Tetracycline inhibition and the cellular source of collagenase in gingival crevicular fluid in different periodontal diseases. A review article, J *Periodontol* 64; 2:82-88, 1993

- Thong YH, Ferrante A, Effect of tetracycline treatment of immunological responses in mice, *Clin Exp Immunol* 39:728-732, 1980

- Editorial: Antibiotics as biological response modifiers, *Lancet* 337:400-401, 1991

- Nicolson GL, Chronic infections as a common etiology for many patients with Chronic Fatigue Syndrome, Fibromyalgia Syndrome and Gulf War Illnesses, *Intern J Med.*, 1: 42-46, 1998

- Nicolson GL, Nicolson NL, Nasralla M, Mycoplasmal infections and Chronic Fatigue Illness (Gulf War Illness) associated with deployment to Operation Desert Storm, *Intern J Med*, 1: 80-92, 1998

- Nicolson GL, New treatments for chronic infections found in Fibromyalgia syndrome, Chronic Fatigue Syndrome, and Gulf War Illnesses, *Intern J Med*, 1: 118-122, 1998

- Nicolson GL, Considerations when undergoing treatment for chronic infections found in Chronic Fatigue Syndrome, Fibromyalgia Syndrome and Gulf War Illnesses. (Part 1). Antibiotics recommended when indicated for treatment of Gulf War Illness/CFIDS/FMS (Part 2). *Intern J Med*, 1: 115-117, 123-128, 1998

- Nasralla M, Haier J, Nicolson GL, Polymerase chain reaction-hybridization for detection of mycoplasmal infections in blood of Chronic Fatigue Syndrome and Fibromyalgia Syndrome patients, *CFIDS Chronicle* in press, 1998

- Nicolson GL, Nasralla M, Hier J, Nicolson NL, Diagnosis and treatment of chronic mycoplasmal infections in Fibromyalgia Syndrome and Chronic Fatigue Syndrome: relationship to Gulf War Illness, *Biomed Therapy* in press, 1998

- Van Barr HMJ, et al, Tetracyclines are potent scavengers of the superoxide radical, *Br J Dermatol* 117:131-134, 1987

- Le CH, Morales A, Trentham DE, Minocycline in early diffuse scleroderma, *Lancet*, 352:1755-1756, Nov 28, 1998

- Breedveld FC, Trentham DE, Suppression of collagen and adjuvant arthritis by a tetracycline, *Arthritis Rheum* 31 (Suppl) R3, 1988

- Sewell KE, Furrie E, Trentham DE, The therapeutic effect of minocycline in experimental arthritis. Mechanism of action, *J Rheumatol* 33(SUPPL): S106, 1991

- Skinner M, Cathcart ES, Mills JA, et al, Tetracycline in the treatment of rheumatoid arthritis, *Arthritis Rheum* 14:727-732, 1971

- Kloppenburg M, Breedveld FC, Miltenburg AMM, et al, Antibiotics as disease modifiers in arthritis, *Clin Exp Rheumatol* 11 (suppl 8): S113-S115, 1993

- Langevitz P, et al, Treatment of resistant rheumatoid arthritis with minocycline; An open study, *J Rheumatol* 19:1502-1504, 1992
- Tilley B, et al, Minocycline in rheumatoid arthritis: A 48 week double-blind placebo controlled trial, *Ann Intern Med*, 122:81, 1995
- Clark HW, et al, Detection of mycoplasma antigens in immune complexes from rheumatoid arthritis synovial fluids, *Ann Allergy* 60:394-398, May 1988
- Holoshitz J, Koning F, Coligan JE, et al, Isolation of CD4-CD8- mycobacteria-reactive T lymphocyte clones from rheumatoid arthritis synovial fluid, *Nature* 339:226-229, 1989
- Granfors K, Jalkanen S, Toivanen A, et al, Yersinia antigens in synovial-fluid cells from patients with reactive arthritis, *N Engl J Med*, 320:216-221, 1989
- Urtasun RC, Rabin HR, Parington J, Human pharmacokinetics and toxicity of high-dose metronidazole administered orally and intravenously, *Surgery*, 145-148, Jan 1983
- Wyburn-Mason R, *The Causation of Rheumatoid Disease and Many Human Cancers, A New Concept In Medicine*, The Rheumatoid Disease Foundation, Franklin TN, 1983
- Notkins AL, Koprowski H, How the immune response to a virus can cause disease, *Sci Amer*, 228:22-31, 1973
- Rappaport EM, Rosien AX, Rosenblum LA, Arthritis due to intestinal amebiasis, *Ann Intern Med*, 34:1224-1232, 1951

**Magnet references:**
- Philpott WH, *Magnetic Resonance Bio-OxidativeTherapy for Rheumatoid Degenerative Diseases*, 17171 SE 29th St, Choctaw OK 73020, ph. 405-390-1444, fax 405-390-2968
- Philpott WH, *Biomagnetic Handbook*, The Arthritis Trust of America, Franklin TN (or ibid)
- Holcomb RR, Parker RA, Harrison MS, Biomagnetics in the treatment of human pain — past, present, future, *Environmental Medicine*, 8; 2:24-30, 1991
- Newman MS, *Introductory and Research Articles About Bio-Magnetic Therapeutic Modalities*, JB Graphics Publ., Burley WA 98322, 1996
- Becker RO, *Cross Currents: The Perils of Electropollution: The Promise of Electromedicine*, Jeremy Tarcher Inc. Los Angeles, 1990
- Becker RO, *The Body Electric: Electromagnetism and the Foundation of Life*, William Marrow & Co, NY 1986
- Becker RE, Marino A, *Electromagnetism and Life*, State University of New York Press, Albany NY 1982
- Foley-Nolan D, Barry C, Roden D, et al, Pulsed high frequency (27 mhz) electromagnetic therapy for persistent neck pain: a double-blind, placebo-controlled study of 20 patients, *Orthopedics* 13; 4:445-51, April 1990
- Binder A, Parr B, Fitton-Jackson S, et al, Pulsed electromagnetic field therapy of persistent rotator cuff tendonitis, *Lancet*, 695-8, Mar 31, 1984

• Tata DB, Vanhouten NF, Triton, TR, et al, Non-invasive, permanent magnetic field modality induces lethal effects on several rodent and human cancers, *Proc Amer Assoc Cancer Res* 35:386, Mar 1994

• Raylman RL, Clavo C, Wahl RL, Exposure to strong static magnetic field slows the growth of human cancer cells, in vitro, *Bioelectromagnetics* 17:358-63, 1996

• Harper DW, Wright EF, Magnets as analgesics, *Lancet* 47, July 2, 1977

• Weinberger a, Nyska A, Giler S, Treatment of experimental inflammatory synovitis with continuous magnetic field, *Israel J Med Sci*, 32; 12:1197-1201, 1966

• Hallet M, Cohen LG, Magnetism: a new method for stimulaton of nerve and brain, *J Amer Med Assoc* 4:538-41, July 28, 1989

• Sandyk R, The influence of pineal gland on migraine and cluster headaches and effects of treatment with picotesla magnetic fields, *Internat J Neurosci* 67:145-71, 1992

## Yoga references:
• Carrico Mara, and the editors of Yoga Journal, *Yoga Journal's Yoga Basics*, Berkeley CA, 1-800-436-9642. A good start with instructive photographs.

• Schatz MP, Back Care Basics, *A Doctor's Gentle Yoga Program For Back and Neck Pain Relief*, Rodmell Press, 2550 Shattuck Ave, Ste 18, Berkeley CA 94704, ph 510-841-3223

• Pierce MD, Pierce MG, *Yoga For Your Life*, Rudra Press, POB 13390, Portland OR 97213, 1996

• Tobias M, Sullivan TP, *Complete Stretching*, Alfred A. Knopf, NY, 1992

• Dworkis S, *Extension*, Poseidon Press, Rockefeller Center, 1230 Avenue of the Americans, NY, NY 10020, 1994

• Jain SC, Effect of yoga training on exercise tolerance in adolescents with childhood asthma, *J Asthma*, 28:437-432, 1991

• Jain S, A study of response pattern of non-insulin dependent diabetes to yoga therapy, *Diabet Res Clin Pract*, 19:69-74, 1991

• Rodriguez AA, Therapeutic exercise and chronic neck and back pain, *Arch Phys Med Rehab*, 73:870-875, 1992

## Hyperbaric references:
• Perlmutter D, *BrainRecovery.com*, The Perlmutter Health Center, Naples FL, 2000, 941-649-7400 or brainrecovery.com

• Neubauer RA, Walker M, *Hyperbaric Oxygen Therapy*, Avery Publ Group, Garden City Park, NY,, 1998, 1-800-548-5757

## Fibromyalgia references:
• St. Amand P, Marelle CC, *What Your Doctor May Not Tell You About Fibromyalgia*, Warner Books, 1999, NY

## Anti-depression references:

• Puttinit PS, Carusol, Primary fibromyalgia syndrome and 5-hydroxy-L-tryptophan: a 90 day open study, *J Int Med Res* 20:182-189, 1992
• Rogers SA, *Depression Cured At Last!*, Prestige Publishing, 1998, Syracuse NY, 1-800-846-6687 or prestigepublishing.com
• Sahley BJ, Birkner, KM, *Heal With Amino Acids*, Pain & Stress Publications, San Antonio TX 78229, 1-800-669-2256 or painstresscenter.com

## Arthritis references:

• Rea WJ, *Chemical Sensitivity, Vol 1-4*, CRC Press, Boca Raton, 1992-98
• Rudge SR, Effect of menstrual cyclicity on disease activity in rheumatoid arthritis, *Int Med* 6; 1:111-119, 1985
• Hirat F, del Carmine R, Steinberg AD, et al, Presence of autoantibody for phospholipase inhibitory protein, lipomodulin, in patients with rheumatic diseases, *Proc Natl Acad Sci USA*, 78; 5:3190-3194, 1981
• Ressel OJ, Disc regeneration: reversibility is possible in spinal osteoarthritis, *ICA Internat Rev Chiroprac*, 39-60, Mar/Apr 1989

## Connecting:

• Order from Sacred Melody Bookstore, 3535 James St., Syracuse NY, 13206, 315-437-1095, Gillham, W, *What God Wishes Christians Knew About Christianity* (Harvest House Publ, Eugene, Oregon 97402), and Stedman, R, *Adventuring Through the Bible*, 1-800-653-8333
• Faid RW, *A Scientific Approach To Christianity*, 1990, New Leaf Press, PO Box 311, Green Forest, AR 72638
• Faid RW, *The Scientific Approach To Biblical Mysteries*, guideposts.com

## Chapter 8

• Tassman G, Zafran J, Zayon G, Evaluation of a plant proteolytic enzyme for the control of inflammation and pain, *J Dent Med* 9:73-77, 1964
• Chandra D, Gupta S, Anti-inflammatory and anti-arthritic activity of volatile oil of Curcuma long (Haldi), *Indian J Med Res*, 60:138-142, 1971
• Arora R, Basu N, et al, Anti-inflammatory studies on Curcuma long (tumeric), *Indian J Med Res* 59:1289-1295, 1971
• Srimal R, Dhawan B, Pharmacology of diferuloyl methane (curcumin), a non-steroidal anti-inflammatory agent, *J Pharm Pharmac* 25:447-4452, 1973
• Ghatak N, Basu N, Sodium curcuminate as an effective anti-inflammatory agent, *Ind J Exp Biol* 10:235-236, 1972

## Cesium references:

• Brewer AK, The high pH therapy for cancer; tests on mice and humans *Pharmacology, Biochemistry & Behavior*, 21; suppl. 1:1-5, 1984

- Keith Brewer International Science Library, 325 N Central Ave, Richland WI 53581, phone 608-647-6513, has collated all the research about cesium and its ability to turn around cancer cells.
- Sartori HE, Cesium therapy in cancer patients, *Pharmacology, Biochemistry & Behavior*, 21; suppl. 1:11-13, 1984
- Neulieb R, Effects of oral intake of cesium chloride: a single case report, *Pharmacology, Biochemistry & Behavior*, 21; suppl 1:15-16, 1984
- Tufte MJ, Tufte FW, The response of colon carcinoma in mice to cesium, zinc, and vitamin A, *Pharmacology, Biochemistry & Behavior* 21 suppl 1:25-26, 1984
- Cukierman S, Yellen G, Miller C, The K+ channel of sarcoplasmic reticulum. A new look at Cs+ block, *Biophys J*, 48:477-484, 1985
- Messiha FS, Lithium, rubidium and cesium: cerebral pharmacokinetics and alcohol interactions, *Pharmacology, Biochemistry & Behavior*, 21; suppl.1:87-92, 1984
- Sartori HE, Nutrients and cancer: an introduction to cesium therapy, *Pharmacology, Biochemistry & Behavior*, 21; suppl. 1:7-10, 1984

**Angina references:**
- Hodis HN, Mack WJ, Azen SP, et al, Serial coronary angiographic evidence that antioxidant vitamin intake reduces progression of coronary artery atherosclerosis, *J Amer Med Assoc*, 273; 23:1849-1854, 1996
- Willett WC, Stampfer MJ, Hennekens CH, et al, Intake of trans fatty acids and risk of coronary heart disease among women, *Lancet* 341:581-585, Mar 6, 1993
- Ornish D, Brown SE, Gould KL, et al, Can lifestyle changes reverse coronary heart disease?, *Lancet* 336:129-133, 1990
- Whitman GJR, Nibori K, Momeni R, et al, The mechanisms of coenzyme Q10 as therapy for myocardial ischemia reperfusion injury, *Mol Aspects Med* 18 suppl (S195-S203) 1997
- Sinatra ST, Refractory congestive failure successfully managed with high dose coenzyme Q10 administration, *Mol Aspects Med*, 18 suppl (S299-S305), 1997
- Anderson TW, et al, Ischemic heart disease, water hardness and myocardial magnesium, *Cand Med Assoc J*, 113:199-203, 1975
- Chipperfield B, Chipperfield JR, Heart muscle magnesium, potassium and zinc concentrations after sudden death from heart disease, *Lancet* II: 293-296, 1973
- Morton BC, et al, Magnesium therapy in acute myocardial infarction — a double-blind study, *Magnesium* 3:346-352, 1984
- Brodsky MA, Magnesium, myocardial infarction and arrhythmias, *J Amer Coll Nutr*, 11; 5:607 (ABSTR 36), 1992
- Cherchi A, et al, Propionyl carnitine in stable angina, *Cardiovasc Drugs Ther* 4:481-486, 1990
- Judy WV, et al, Myocardial preservation by therapy with coenzyme 10 during heart surgery, *Clin Invest* 71:S155-S 161, 1993
- Mortensen SA, Perspectives on therapy of cardiovascular diseases with coenzyme Q10 (ubiquinone), *Clin Invest*, 71:S116-S123, 1993

- Willis RA, Folkers K, et al, Tamagawa H, Lovastatin decreases coenzyme Q levels in humans, *Proc Natl Acad Sci*, 87:8928-8930, 1990
- Folkers KS, Vadhanavikit S, Mortensen SA, Biochemical rationale and myocardial tissue data on the effective therapy of cardiomyopathy with coenzyme Q10, *Proc Natl Acad Sci*, 82; 3:901-904, 1985
- Folkers K, Heart failure is a dominant deficiency of coenzyme Q10 and challenges for future clinical research on CoQ10, *Clin Investig* 71; s51-s54, 1993
- Karlsson J, Semb B, Muscle ubiquinone and plasma antioxidants in effort angina, *J Nutr Environ Med* 6:255-266, 1996
- Baggio e, Gandini R, Carmosino G, et al, Italian multicenter study on the safety and efficacy of coenzyme Q10 as adjunctive therapy in heart failure (interim analysis), *Clin Investig* 71:s145-s149, 1993
- Jameson S, Statistical data support prediction of death within 6 months on low levels of coenzyme Q10 and other entities, *Clin Investig* 1:s145-s149: 137-139, 1993
- Morisco C, Trimarco B, Condorelli M, Effect of coenzyme Q10 therapy in patients with congestive heart failure: a long-term multicenter randomized study, *Clin Investig* 71:s145-s149: 134-136, 1993
- Hanaki Y, Sugiyama S, et al, Coenzyme Q10 and coronary artery disease, *Clin Investig* 71:s145-s149: 112-115, 1993
- Conte a, Palmieri L, Bertelli A, Protection of adenylate pool and energy charge by L-carnitine and coenzyme Q during energy depletion in rat heart slices, *Int J Tiss Reac* XII (3): 187-191, 1990
- Thomsen JH, Shug AL, et al, Improved pacing tolerance of the ischemic human myocardium after administration of carnitine, *Amer J Cardiol* 43:300-306, Feb 1979
- Azum j, Sawamura A, Awata N, Hasgawa H, Kishimoto S, et al, Double-blind randomized crossover trial of taurine in congestive heart failure, *Curr Therap Res*, 1983

## Silverlon references:
- Chu CS, McManus AT, Matylevich NP, Mason AD, Pruitt BA, Enhanced survival of autoepidermal-allodermal composite grafts in allosensitive animals by use of silver nylon dressing and direct current, *J Trauma* 273:39-42.1996
- Becker RO, Spadaro JA, Treatment of othropedic infections with electrically generated silver ions, *J Bone Jt Surg*, 60-A: 871, 1978
- Webster DA, Spadaro JA, Kramer S, Becker RO, Silver anode treatment of chronic osteomyelitits, *Clin Orthop* 1961,105, 1981
- Chu CS, McManus AT, Pruitt BA, et al, Therapeutic effects of silver nylon dressing with weak direct current on Pseudomonas aeruginosa infected burn wounds, *J Trauma* 28:1488, 1988

## Gulf War references:
- See all of Dr. Garth Nicolson's references on Gulf War in "Sterilize Yourself" section, plus *Chemical Sensitivity, Tired or Toxic?*, and *Depression Cured at Last!* (1-

800-846-6687). Also see Dr William J. Rea's 4-volume book, *Chemical Sensitivity* (1-800-428-2343).

## Diabetic references:
- Nagamatsu M, et al, Alpha lipoic acid improves nerve blood flow, reduces oxidative stress, and improves distal nerve conduction in experimental diabetic neuropathy, *Diabetes Care*, 18; 8: 1160-1167, Aug 1995
- Sen CK, Roy S, Han D, Packer L, Regulation of cellular thiols in human lymphocytes by a-lipoic acid, *Free Rad Biol Med* 22; 7: 1241-1257, 1997
- Wagh SS, Natraj W, Meron KKG, Mode of action of lipoic acid in diabetes, *J Biososci*, 11: 59-74, 1987
- Onofrj M, Fulgente T, et al, L-acetylcarnitine as a new therapeutic approach for peripheral neuropathies with pain, *Int J Clin Pharm Res*, 1995; 15: 9-15
- Quatraro A, Roa P, et al, Acetyl-l-carnitine for symptomatic diabetic neuropathy, *Diabetalogia*, 1995; 38: 123

## Theologic:
- *The Holy Bible.* For a very enjoyable interpretation, I heartily recommend:
- Stedman RC, *Adventuring Through the Bible. A Comprehensive Guide to the Entire Bible,* Discovery House Publishers, Box 3566, Grand Rapids MI 49501, 1997 (1-800-653-8333)
- *The New Living Bible,* 1-800-950-2092 or 1-612-333-0725
- *The Comparative Study Bible. A Parallel Bible presenting the New International Version, New American Standard Bible, Amplified Bible and King James Version,* Zondervan Publishing House, 1984, Grand Rapids MI 49506
- Gillham, Bill, *What God Wishes Every Christian Knew About Christianity,* 1998, Harvest House Publ., Eugene OR 97402
- Faid RW, *A Scientific Approach To Christianity,* 1990, New Leaf Press, PO Box 311, Green Forest, AR 72638
- Faid RW, *The Scientific Approach To Biblical Mysteries,* guideposts.com